# English-Italian Medical Dictionary and Phrasebook

## Italian-English

first edition 2013

ISBN is 1493639129
EAN-13 is 978-1493639120

by A.H.Zemback

© All rights reserved

# Contents

| | | |
|---|---|---|
| Introduction/demographics | | 4 |
| History and physical: | Chief complaint | 5 |
| | Common complaints | 6 |
| | Past Medical & Surgical History | 8 |
| | Family/social history | 9 |
| | Allergies/medications | 9 |
| | Review of systems (ROS) | |
| |     Lymph, bone, blood, endocrine | 10 |
| |     HEENT | 11 |
| |     Respiratory/cardiac | 12 |
| |     GI/GU | 13 |
| |     Women's health | 15 |
| |     Peripartum/neonatal | 17 |
| |     Neurologic/psychiatric | 18 |
| | Physical exam | 19 |
| | Joint exams | 27 |
| | Counseling | 31 |
| | Dates, numbers, time | 33 |
| | Body parts | 36 |
| English-Italian: | abasia→coronoid | 38 |
| | corpulence→Hansen's disease | 70 |
| | haploid→myelopathy | 98 |
| | myocardial→salpingography | 125 |
| | salpingostomy→zymogen | 151 |
| Italian-English: | a caso→colinergico | 175 |
| | colinesterasi→fulminante | 201 |
| | fumare→mucocele | 228 |
| | mucoide→risonanza | 255 |
| | risultato→zucchero | 283 |
| Postscript | | 311 |

| Introduction/ demographics | English | Italian |
|---|---|---|
| | How are you? | Como sta? |
| | Good morning, good afternoon, good evening | Buon giomo, buon pomeriggio, buon sera. |
| | My name is ... | Mi chiamo... |
| | What is your name? | Come si chiama? |
| | Please write your name. | Potrebbe scrivere il suo nome. |
| | Do you speak English? | Parla inglese? |
| | Say that one more time, please. | Potrebbe ripetere per favore? |
| | Can you speak slowly, please? | Potrebbe parlare lentamente? |
| | Come with me. | Venga con me. |
| | Sit down, please. | Si accomodi, per favore. |
| | What is your address? | Dove abita? |
| | What is your telephone number? | Qual è il tuo numero di telefono? |
| | Can you give us the name and telephone number or address of someone to be contacted? | Potrebbe darce il nome, il numero di telefone o l'indirizzo di una persona da contattare? |
| | Are you married? | È sposato? |
| | What is your age? | Quanti anni ha? |

| Chief complaint | English | Italian |
|---|---|---|
| | What is your health concern today? | Che cos'è che non va? |
| | When did this problem start? | Da quanto tempo ha questi dolori? |
| | How long have you been feeling ill? | Da quanto tempo si sente? |
| | Have you had an accident? | Ha avuto degli incidente? |
| | What medicine have you taken? | Che medicina ha preso? |
| | Do you feel pain now? | Ha dolori? |
| | Is the pain severe? | Il dolore è intenso? |
| | Is your pain burning? | Il dolore è bruciante? |
| | Is your pain stabbing, cramping? | Il dolore è come una pugnalata, a crampi? |
| | Is the pain constant...? | Si tratta di un dolore costante? |
| | or does it come and go? | O va e viene? |
| | Does the pain radiate? Where does it radiate to? | Il dolore si irradia? Dove? |
| | Touch the spot where it hurts with one finger. | Indichi con un dito il punto esatto dov'è il dolore. |
| | What makes it better? | Che cosa le fa meglio? |
| | What makes it worse? | Che cosa le fa peggio? |
| | When do you get the pain... | Quando le vengono i dolori... |
| | at night, before meals, after meals? | di notte, dopo mangiato? |
| | Have you been in the hospital before? (for female) | É mai stato ricoverato in questo oespedale? (É mai stata ricoverata in questo oespedale?) |
| | What were you treated for? (for female) | Per quale motivo e'stato ricoverato? (Per quale motivo e'stata ricoverata? ) |

| Common complaints | English | Italian |
|---|---|---|
| | My lower back hurts. | Ho male alla schiena. |
| | My neck is stiff. | I mio collo è rigido. |
| | I have a sore throat. | Ho mal di gola. |
| | I have a fever. | Ho febbre. |
| | I have night sweats. | Sudo la notte. |
| | I am coughing a lot. | Ho molta tosse. |
| | It hurts when I swallow. | Mi fa male inghiottire. |
| | I have an earache. | Ho mal d'orecchi. |
| | I have poor vision. | Ho disturbi visivi. |
| | I have a toothache. | Mi fa male il dente. |
| | My tooth is loose. | Il dente si muove. |
| | My dentures are loose and my gums hurt. | La dentiera si muove e mi fa male alle gengive. |
| | My filling fell out. | Un'otturazione si è tolta. |
| | My gums bleed when I brush my teeth. | Le gengive mi sanguinano quando mi lavo i denti. |
| | I have shoulder pain. | Ho un mal di spalla. |
| | I have elbw pain. | Ho un mal di gomito. |
| | I have wrist pain. | Ho un mal di polso. |
| | I havc kncc pain. | Ho un mal di ginocchio. |
| | I have ankle pain. | Ho un mal di caviglia. |
| | I am dizzy. | Mi gira la testa. |
| | I am very nervous. | Sono molto nervoso. |
| | I can't sleep. | Soffro di disturbi di insonnia. |
| | I am tired. | Sono stanco. |
| | I have chest pain. | Ho male al petto. |
| | My heart beats very fast. | Ho palpitazioni di cuore. |
| | I have a headache. | Ho mal di testa. |
| | I have trouble breathing. | Ho l'affanno. |
| | I am short of breath at night. | Ho l'affanno di notte. |
| | I am short of breath with exertion. | Ho l'affanno con movimenti. |
| | I have to sleep sitting up. | Devo dormire seduto. |
| | I have blackouts. | Vedo macchie nere. |
| | I am coughing a lot. | Ho molta tosse. |
| | It hurts when I cough. | Mi fa male tossire. |
| | I have missed my periods. | Mi sono scomparse le regole. |
| | I think I am pregnant. | Penso che sono incinta. |
| | I have morning sickness. | Vomito la mattina. |
| | I am pregnant. | Sono incinta. |
| | I have pain during my menstrual period. | Ho dolore durante il mio periodo mestruale. |

| Common complaints | English | Italian |
|---|---|---|
| | I have a vaginal infection. | Ho un'infezioine vaginale. |
| | I am on a birth control pill. | I sono il controllo delle nascite. |
| | I have not had my period for... months. | Non ho avuto il mio periodo da allora... |
| | I have a stomach ache. | Ho un mal di stomaco. |
| | I cannot eat. | Non posso mangiare. |
| | I have heartburn. | Ho bruciori allo stomaco. |
| | I am nauseated. | Ho nausea. |
| | I feel like vomiting. | Sto per vomitare. |
| | I have indigestion. | Soffro di disturbi di digestione. |
| | I have no appetite. | Non ho appetito. |
| | I have diarrhea | Ho diarrea. |
| | I am constipated. | Ho stitichezza. |
| | I have blood in my stool. | Le mie feci congengono sangue. |
| | My stools are light colored. | Le mie feci sono chiare. |
| | I get up at night to urinate. | Mi alzo la notte per orinare. |
| | My urine is cloudy. | La mia orina è torbida. |
| | I have bloody urine. | La mia orina è con sangue. |
| | I have pain with urination. | Quando orino ho die dolori. |
| | I feel sick. | Sto molto male. |
| | I feel weak. | Mi sento debole. |
| | I have sprained my... | Ho preso una storta al... |
| | I have pain in this joint. | Ho un dolore in questa giuntura. |
| | I think I broke my arm. | Mi son rotto il mio braccio. |
| | I think I broke my leg. | Mi son rotto il mia gamba. |
| | I have a rash. | Ho dell'orticaria. |
| | I have a boil. | Ho un foruncolo. |
| | I have a burn. | Ho un bruciatura. |
| | I have a wound. | Ho un ferita. |
| | I am injured. (for female) | Sono ferito. (Sono ferita) |
| | I am limping. | Sto zoppicando. |
| | He hurt his head. | Ha ferito la sua testa. |
| | He is unconscious. | È svenuto. |
| | He is bleeding a lot. | Sta sanguinando molto. |
| | He has a broken bone. | Egli ha un osso rotto. |
| | My baby nurses well. | Il mio bambino succhia bene. |
| | My baby suckles poorly. | Il mio bambino succhia poco. |
| | I don't have enough (breast) milk. | Non c'è sufficientemente latte nel seno. |
| | My nipples are cracked. | I miei capezzoli sono screpolati. |
| | I need a breast pump. | Ho bisogno di una pompa aspira latte. |

| Past Medical and Surgical History | English | Italian |
|---|---|---|
| | Are you being treated for any chronic health problem? | Avete una storia di qualsiasi problema di salute cronico? |
| | Do you have a history of: | Ha una storia di... |
| | asthma | asma |
| | epilepsy | epilessia |
| | hypertension | pressione sanguigna alta |
| | thyroid disease | malattia tiroide |
| | diabetes | diabete |
| | hepatitis | epatite |
| | cancer | cancro |
| | heart problems | problemi cardiaci |
| | pneumonia | polmonite |
| | malaria | malaria |
| | whooping cough | tosse convulsiva |
| | typhoid fever | tifo |
| | tuberculosis | tubercolosi |
| | HIV/AIDS | virus dell'immunodeficienza unama/ sindrome da immunodeficienza acquista |
| | What date did you start the ARV? (this is an HIV medicine) | Quando ha iniziato la terapia con ARV? ('e un farmaco per l'infezione da HIV) |
| | What was the date and value of the last CD4? (a test to measure how bad the HIV infection is) | Quando ha eseguito l'ultimo dosaggio dei CD4? Che valore ha? (e' un test che misura la severita' dell'infezione da HIV) |
| | Do you have a vaccination record? | Ha una tessera delle vaccinazioni? |
| | Have you have pneumonia or meningitis? | Hanna avuto la polmonite o la meningite? |
| | Have you had surgery in the past? | Ha mai avuto operazioni? |
| | What surgery was done? | Quale intervento chirurgico è stato fatto? |
| | What year was the surgery done? | In che anno è stato fatto l'intervento chirurgico? |

| Family/social history | English | Italian |
|---|---|---|
| | Is your mother living? | Sua madre è viva? |
| | Is your father living? | Suo padre è vivo? |
| | Do you know what he died from? | Mi sa dire la causa della morte di suo padre? |
| | Do your brothers/sisters have health problems? | Vostri fratelli o sorelle hanno problemi di salute? |
| | Do you have any children? | Ha figli? |
| | Do you drink alcohol? | Beve? |
| | How many drinks per day? | Quanto al giorno? |
| | Do you drink alcohol every day? | Bevi alcol ogni giorno? (c'è un termine local per "alcool"?) |
| | Do you smoke cigarettes? | Fuma? |
| | How many cigarettes per day? | Quante sigarette al giorno? |
| | What kind of work do you do? | Che lavoro fa? |

| Medications/ allergies | English | Italian |
|---|---|---|
| | I am allergic to... | Sono allergico alla... |
| | Have you had reactions to medications? | È allergico a qualche cosa? |
| | Which medications? | Sono allergico alla... |
| | Do you take (modern) medication at home? | Attualmente sta prendendo medicine? |
| | Have you taken traditional medication? | Prende altre meicine o rimedi naturali? |
| | Are you taking Bactrim? | Stai prendendo Bactrim? |
| | I want to see the medication bottle. | Voglio vedere il flacone del farmaco. |
| | What is the name of the medication? | Come si chiama la medicazione? |

| Review of systems: lymph, bone, blood | English | Italian |
|---|---|---|
| | Do you have skin problems? | Avete problemi di pelle? |
| | Do you have a rash? | Ha mai notato sfogo? |
| | Do you have any blisters or sores? | Ha mai notato ulcerazioni del pelle? |
| | Do you have any problems with dry skin? | Ha mai notato la pelle secca? |
| | Have you had lice? | Ha avuto pidocchi? |
| | Have you been bitten by ticks? | E'stato punto dalle zecche? |
| | Have you seen any rats in your home? | Ha visto ratti nella sua caserma? |
| | Were you bitten by a dog or another animal? | E'stato morso da un cane o da qualche altro animale? |
| | Do you have lymph node enlargement or pain? | Avete l'ingrandimento linfonodale o dolore? |
| | Do you have bone pain? | Avete dolore osseo? |
| | Do you have joint pain? | Hai dolori articolari? |
| | Do you have joint swelling? | Avete gonfiore delle articolazioni? |
| | Do you have pain in the back or the neck? | Avete dolore al collo o mal di schiena? |
| | Have you ever had a blood transfusion? | Ha mai avuto trasfusioni di sangue? |
| | Do you have bleeding problems? | Avete problemi di sanguinamento? |
| | Do you urinate frequently? | Urina spesso? |
| | Are you very thirsty? | Ha molta sete? |
| | Have you lost weight? | Ha subito diminuzione di peso? |
| | Is the ankle pain so severe you cannot walk on it? | Hai dolore alla caviglia così grave che non può camminare? |
| | Does your knee give way or lock up? | Il suo ginocchio cede o si blocca? |
| | Do you feel pain when you move your shoulder? | Ti senti dolore quando si sposta la tua spalla? |
| | Have you had any broken bones? | Avete avuto qualche osso rotte? |

| Review of systems: HEENT | English | Italian |
|---|---|---|
| | Have you suffered from a head trauma in the past? | Hai avuto un trauma cranico in passato? |
| | Do you have dizziness? | Ha mai sofferto di giramento di testa? |
| | Have you blacked-out? | Ha avuto perdita di coscienza? |
| | Can you see well? | Ci vede bene? |
| | Do you have double vision? | Ha mai veduto doppio? |
| | Do you have spots in front of your eyes? | Ha mai veduto macchie davanti agli occhi? |
| | Do you have blurred vision? | La sua vista è offuscata? |
| | Do you have pain in bright light? | Avverte dolore agli occhi quando e' esposto alla luce intensa? |
| | Can you hear well? | Ci sente bene? |
| | Have you noticed any hearing loss? | Ha notato una diminuzione dell'udito? |
| | Which ear is effected? | In quale orecchio? |
| | Do you have pain in your ears? | Ha mai avuto dolore all'orecchio? |
| | Do you have drainage from your ears? | Ha ami avuto secrezioni dall'orecchio? |
| | Do you have hearing loss in only one ear? | Ha perdita di udito in un solo orecchio? |
| | Do you have nosebleeds? | Ha mai avuto sangue dal naso? |
| | Do you have bleeding gums? | Ha mai avuto sangue dalle gengive? |
| | Do you have ulcers in your mouth? | Ha mai avuto ulcere nella bocca? |
| | Do you have a toothache? | Avete un mal di denti? |
| | Do you have a broken tooth? | Avete un dent rotto? |
| | Do you have lumps or swelling in your mouth? | Avete grumi o gonfiore in bocca? |
| | Do you have hoarseness (a change in your voice)? | Ha mai avuto raucedine? |
| | Do you have a sore throat? | Avete un mal di gola? |
| | Do you have neck stiffness? | Avete rigidità del collo? |

| Review of systems: respiratory/cardiac | English | Italian |
| --- | --- | --- |
| | Are you short of breath? | Ha difficoltà a respirare? |
| | Do you have difficulty breathing when you lay down? | Ha mai avuto difficoltà nel respirare quando è sdraiato? |
| | Do you have pain when you take a deep breath? | Ha dolore quando si respira profondamente? |
| | Do you have wheezing? | Ha mai avuto respiro fischiante? |
| | Do you have a cough? | Ha tosse? |
| | How long have you had the cough? | Quanto tempo è stato tosse? |
| | Do you cough up phlegm? | Ha tosse con catarro? |
| | Do you have a lot of sputum? | Produci un sacco di espettorato? |
| | Do you have bloody sputum? | Ha mai avuto sputo di sangue? |
| | What color is your sputum. | Di che colore è il tuo sputo? |
| | Have you had tuberculosis? | Avete avuto tubercolosi? |
| | Do you have chest pain? | Ha mai avuto dolore al petto? |
| | Do you have palpitations? | Ha mai avuto palpitazione di cuore? |
| | Do you have leg edema? | Ha mai avuto gonfiore delle caviglie? |
| | Do you have weakness? | Ti senti debole? |

| Review of systems: GI/GU | English | Italian |
| --- | --- | --- |
| | Do you have abdominal pain? | Avete dolori addominali? Hai dolore nella pancia? |
| | Do you have abdominal pain after you eat? | Ha dolore addominale dopo aver mangiato? |
| | When did this problem start? | Quando ha iniziato a questo problema? |
| | Has it been weeks, months, years? | E'stato settimane, mesi o anni? |
| | Are you in pain now? | Sente dolore adesso? |
| | Touch the spot where you have pain with one finger. | Indichi con un dito il punto esatto dov'è il dolore. |
| | Does it hurt all the time? | Le fa male di continuo? |
| | Does the pain come and go? | Il dolore va e viene? |
| | Is the pain better than yesterday? | Il dolore è meglio di ieri? |
| | Do you have fever? | Ha avuto febbre? |
| | Do you have chills? | Ha preso freddo? |
| | Do you have night sweats? | Ha mai avuto sudori di notte? |
| | Do you have a good appetite? | Ha buon appetito? |
| | Have you vomited? | Ha vomito? |
| | What did the vomit look like? | Com' era il vomito? |
| | Have you vomited blood? | Ha vomitato sangue? |
| | Do you have nausea? | Ha sofferto di nausea? |
| | Did you have a bowel movement today? | Ha avuto movimenti intestinali oggi? |
| | When was your last stool? | Quando ha evacuato l'ultima volta? |
| | Are you constipated? | Ha mai avuto stitichezza? |
| | Can you pass gas? | Fa aria dall'intestino? |
| | Do you have diarrhea? | Ha diarrea? |
| | How frequently? | Quante volte? |
| | What did the stools look like? | Come sono le feci? |
| | Is the stool black or bloody? | Le sue feci sono mai state nerastre, sanguinolente? |
| | What color is your stool? | Di che colore sono le sue feci? |
| | Do you have anal itching? | Avete prurito anale? |
| | Do you have pain with swallowing? | Ha mai avuto dolore nell'inghiottire? |
| | Do you have difficulty swallowing? | Ha mai avuto difficoltà nell'inghiottire? |

| Review of systems: GI/GU | English | Italian |
|---|---|---|
| | Do you have a burning pain in your stomach? | Ha bruciore alla stomaco? |
| | Have you seen worms in your stools? | Ha mai visto vermi nelle feci? |
| | Have you had a gastroscopy? | Avete avuto una gastroscopia? |
| | Do you have pain when you urinate? | Prova dolori orinando? |
| | Do you have penile discharge? | Ha mai sofferto di secrezioni dagli organi genitali? |
| | Do you have a sore on your penis? | Ha mai sofferto di ulcere o piaghe delgi pene? |
| | What does your urine look like? | Di che colore sono le urine? |
| | Is your urine cloudy? | L'urina è torbida? |
| | Do you have sharp pains in your back where the last rib meets the spine? | Ha mai avuto dolore alla parte bassa della schiena? |
| | Do you have an aching pain under your scrotum? | Avete un dolore facente male sotto tuo scroto? |
| | Do you have difficulty staring to urinate? | Ha ami osservato nell'urinare difficoltà quando comincia ad urinare? |
| | Do you have dribbling after you finish? | Ha mai sgocciolamento quando crede di aver finito? |
| | How often do you urinate at night? | Urinare spesso di notte? |
| | Do you have the urge to urinate after just urinating and are you only urinating small amounts? | Voi avete il bisogno di urinare dopo urinare solo e sei solo urinare piccole quantità? |
| | Is the urine stream slow? | Il flusso urinario è lento? |
| | Do you leak urine when you cough or sneeze? | Ha mai avuto perdite di urina quando tossisce o starnutisce? |
| | Do you have blood in the urine? | Ha mai avuto urine con sangue? |
| | Have you every passed a kidney stone? | Ha mai avuto calcoli renale? |
| | Do you have incontinence? | Lei è mai capiato di non poter trattenere le urine? |
| | Have you have a positive test for syphilis? | Ha mai avuto un esame del sangue con risultato positivo sifilide? |

| Review of systems: Women's Health | English | Italian |
|---|---|---|
| | Have you noticed any breast lumps? | Ha mai notato nodoli nel suo seno? |
| | Do you have nipple discharge? | Ha secrezione da capezzolo? |
| | Do you have swelling around or below your nipples? | Ha gonfiore intorno o sotto i capezzoli? |
| | Have you reached change of life? | Ha raggiunto la menopausa? |
| | Are you pregnant? | È incinta? |
| | How many months pregnant are you? | Di quanti mesi? |
| | Could you possibly be pregnant? | Potrebbe esseere gravida? |
| | We will do a pregnancy test. | Dovrà essere sottomessa ad un esame di gestazione. |
| | Are your periods regular? | Ha mestruazioni regolan? |
| | Are your periods painful? | Ha mai avuto dolori durante i periodi mestruali? |
| | Is the flow heavy? | La mestruazione è abbondante? |
| | When did your last period start? | Quando ha avuto l'ultima volta le mestruazioni? |
| | How many days do your periods last? | Quanti giorni durano? |
| | Do you bleed between periods? | Ha perdite di sangue all'infuori della mestruazione? |
| | Do you take birth control pills? | Prende anticoncezionali orali? |
| | Do you have pain during intercourse? | Ha dolori durante i rapporti sessuali? |
| | Do you have vaginal itching? | Avete prurito vaginale? |
| | Do you have vaginal pain? | Avete dolore vaginale? |
| | Do you have unusual discharge from the vagina; a lot or a little? | Avete insolite secrezioni dalla vagina; molto o pocco? |
| | How many times have you been pregnant? | Quante volte sei stata incinta? |
| | How many children do you have? | Ha bambini, quanti? |

| Review of systems: Women's Health | English | Italian |
|---|---|---|
| | Were your deliveries normal? | I parti sono stati normali? |
| | Have you had any miscarriages? | Ha avuto aborti? |
| | Did you have problems in your previous pregnancies? | Hai avuto problemi durante le precedenti gravidanze? |
| | Did you have any severe bleeding after any of your deliveries? | Hai mai avuto gravi emorragie dopo uno dei suoi parti precedenti? |
| | Do you know your blood type? | Conosci il tuo gruppo sanguigno? |
| | During your pregnancy did you have any bleeding or swelling of the ankles? | Durante la vostra gravidanza le caviglie si gonfiano o hai avuto sanguinamento vaginale? |
| | Are you in labor? | É in travaglio? |
| | When did your contractions start? | Quando hanno avuto inizio le contrazioni? |
| | Are the contractions regular or irregular? | Sono le contrazioni regolari o irregolari? |
| | How many minutes between contractions? | Quanti minuti tra le contrazioni? |
| | Did your water break? | Le acque si sono rotte? |
| | Is this your first baby? | Questo è il tuo primo bambino? |
| | Do you feel the baby move? | Ti senti muovere il bambino? |

| Review of systems: neonatal and peripartum | English | Italian |
|---|---|---|
| | How old is your baby? | Che età ha il bambino? |
| | What was your baby's birth weight? | Qual è stato il peso di nascita del vostro bambino? |
| | How are you feeding the baby, with breast or bottle? | Come nutre il bambino, con latte materno/latte? |
| | Is the baby nursing well? | Il bambino e'allattato in modo adeguato? |
| | Has the baby had a convulsion? | I bambino ha una convulsione (attacco)? |
| | What color was the amniotic fluid? | Di che colore era il liquido amniotico? |
| | Were you ill before the delivery? | Eri malato prima che il bambino é nato? |
| | What is the baby's temperature. | Qual è la temperatura del bambino? |
| | We need to warm the baby up. | Bisogna riscaldare il bambino. |
| | We need to put the baby under the bili-light to warm him/her. | Abbiamo bisogno di mettere il bambino sotto una lampada speciale per tenerlo caldo. |
| | We need to give the baby oxygen. | Dobbiamo dare l'ossigneo del bambino. |
| | Does the child cry often? | Piange molto il bambino? |
| | Is the child gaining weight? | Cresce di peso il bambino? |
| | Does the child have a good appetite? | Ha appetito il bambino? |
| | What kinds of pain does the child complain of? | Che dolori ha il bambino? |
| | Is the child drinking ok? | Il bambino è bere bene? |
| | Is the child eating ok? | Il bambino sta mangiando bene? |
| | Have you seen worms in the vomit or stool? | Ha visto vermi nel vomito o nelle feci? |

| Review of systems: neuro & psychiatric | English | Italian |
|---|---|---|
| | Do you have facial weakness? | Avete debolezza facciale? |
| | Do you have facial numbness? | Avete intorpidemento facciale? |
| | Do you have leg weakness? | Avete debolezza gamba? |
| | Do you have leg numbness? | Avete intorpidemento gamba? |
| | Do you have arm weakness? | Avete debolezza del braccio? |
| | Do you have arm numbness? | Avete intorpidemento braccio? |
| | Were you unconscious? | Ha mai perduto la coscienza? |
| | Have you had any convulsions? | Ha mai sofferto di convulsioni? |
| | Do you have tremors? | Ha mai osservato tremori? |
| | Do you have headaches? | Ha mai sofferto di mal di testa? |
| | Have you had vision loss in one eye? | Hanno avuto perdita di visione in un occhio solo? |
| | Do you have problems with your balance? | Avete problemi con il vostro equilibrio? |
| | Do you have problems walking? | Avete difficoltà piedi? |
| | Do you have pain that travels from your buttock down the back of your leg? | Ha dolore che parte dalla natica e scende lungo la parte posteriore della gamba? |
| | Do you have memory problems? | Ha mai sofferto perdita della memoria? |
| | Do you have anxiety? | È nervoso o stanco? |
| | Do you have depression? | Lei soffre di depressione? |
| | How is your mood? | Come sta il tuo umore? |
| | Do you hear voices? | Ha mai sofferto di sensazione di voci nella testa? |
| | Do you sleep well? | Dorme bene? |

| Physical exam | English | Italian |
|---|---|---|
| | Appearance, height | apparenza, all'altezza |
| | pulse, blood pressure respiratory rate temperature weight (pounds/kilograms) | polso, pressione sanguigna, frequenza respiratorio, temperatura, peso (libbra/kilogrammo) |
| | skin | pelle |
| HEENT | visual acuity "Cover your right eye. Read the letters on the wall. Now, cover your left eye." | acutezza visiva "Copra l'occhio destro. Legga le lettere sulla parete. Ora, copra l'occhio sinsitro." |
| | conjunctivae, sclerae | congiuntiva, sclera |
| | pupils "I am going to shine a light into your eyes." | pupilla "Io vado a brillare di una luce negli occhi." |
| | optic disc | disca ottica |
| | ear canal, tympanic membrane "I am going to look into your ears." | condotto auricolare, membrana timpanica "Vado a guardare nelle orecchie." |
| | AC> BC bilaterally? Rinne. "Cover this ear with your hand. Tell me when you cannot feel the vibration." Move the tuning fork off the mastoid process and next to but not touching the ear. "Tell me when the sound stops." | conduzione aira > conduzione ossea, Rinne. "Coprire questo orecchio con la mano. Dimmi quando non può sentire le vibrazioni." (Spostare il Diaspason fuori il processo mastoideo e tenerlo accanto a, ma non toccare l'orecchio.) "Dimmi quando si ferma il suono." |
| | Weber "Is the sound the same in both ears? (with a tuning fork that is vibrating, resting on top of the patient's head) | Weber "Il suono è lo stesso in entrambe le orecchie? (con un diapason che vibra sulla testa del paziente a riposo.) |
| | nasal mucosa "I am going to look into your nose." | mucosa nasale "Ho intenzione di gaurdare nel tuo naso." |
| | nasal septum | setto nasale |
| | turbinates | turbina |
| | soft palate | palato molle |
| | sinuses | chiuso |
| | teeth | dente |
| | mouth, gums, teeth, uvula, Stenson's and Wharton's ducts "Open your mouth, please." | bocca, gengiva, dente, ugula, condotto di Wharton, condotto di Stenson, "Apra la bocca." |

| Physical exam | English | Italian |
|---|---|---|
| | "Stick out your tongue please." | "Mi mostri la lingua, per favore." |
| | "Say ahh!" | "Dica 'a' "! |
| Pulmonary | Auscultation, "Breathe in deeply." | "Respiri profondament." |
| | percussion | percussioni |
| | "Lie down on your back, please." | "Si distenda, per favore." |
| | "Lie on your left side." | "Si giri sul fianco sinistro." |
| | "Lie on your right side." | "Si giri sul fianco destro." |
| | tenderness "Does it hurt here?" | "Le fa male qui, se premo." |
| | cva tenderness | tenerezza angolo costovertebrale |
| Cardiac | heart rate, rhythm "Breathe normally." | frequenza cardiaca, ritmo "Respiri normalmente." |
| | heart murmur? | soffio cardiaco? |
| | carotid "Hold your breath." | carotide "Trattenga il respiro." |
| | jugular venous pressure | pressione venosa glugular |
| Breast | nipple discharge? | secrezione capezzolo |
| | breast tenderness? | dolenzia mammella |
| | breast exam | esame del seno |
| Peripheral vascular | carotid, radial, aortic pulsation "Hold your breath." | pulsazione carotide, radiale, aortico "Trattenga il respiro." |
| | femoral, dorsalis pedis and posterior tibial pulsation | pulsazione femorale, dorsales pedis, tibiale posteriore |
| | leg edema? | edema arto inferiore |
| Abdomen | "Lie down please." | "Si distenda, per favore." |
| | "Show me where it hurts." | "Mi indichi dove ha dolore." |
| | "Does it hurt when I touch here?" | "Le fa male qui, se premo?" |
| | umbilicus | ombelico |
| | inguinal hernia? | ernia inguinale? |
| | palpation | palpazione |
| | auscultation | ascoltazione |
| | fluid wave, superficial abdominal veins? | onda fluida, vena addominale superficiale ? |
| Ob/gyn | Uterine height (cm) | altezza uterino |
| | fetal heart tones | battito cardiaco fetale |
| | urinalysis | analisi delle urine |
| | presentation: | presentazione |
| |   brow presentation | presentazione frontale |
| |   breech presentation | presentazione podalica |
| |   transverse presentation | presentazione transvero |
| | speculum exam | esame del spèculo |
| | vaginal exam | esame del vaginale |
| | gestational age | età gestazionale |
| | amniotic fluid | liquido amniotico |

| Physical exam | English | Italian |
|---|---|---|
| Perinatal | Apgar, 1 minute | Punteggio di Apgar |
| | Breathing effort: If the infant is not breathing-score is 0. If the respirations are slow or irregular-score is 1. If the infant cries well-score is 2. | Atività respiratoria: assente = 0, debole o irregolare = 1, vigorosa con pianto = 2. |
| | Heart rate evaluated by stethescope. If there is no heartbeat-score is 0. If the heart rate is less than 100 beats per minute-score is 1. If the heart rate is over 100 beats per minute-score is 2. | Atività cardiaca: assente = 0, < 100/minuto = 1, > 100/minuto = 2. |
| | Muscle tone. If the muscles are loose and floppy-score is 0. If there is some tone-score is 1. If there is active motion-score is 2. | Tono muscolare: assente (atonia) = 0, flessione assennata = 1, normale atteggiamento inflessione delle estremità = 2. |
| | Grimace response or reflex irritability in response to a mild pinch. If there is no reaction-score is 0. If there is grimacing-score is 1. If there is grimacing and a cough, sneeze, or vigorous cry-score is 2. | Eccitabilità dei riflessi: (risposta al catetere nasofaringeo). Assente = 0, scarsa = 1, stamuto, pianto vivace, tosse o stemuto= 2. |
| | Skin color: If the color is pale blue-score is 0. If the body is pink and the extremities blue-score 1. If the entire body is pink-score is 2. | Colore della pelle: cianotico o pallido = 0, tronco roseo, estremità cianotiche = 1, completamente roseo = 2. |
| | Apgar at 5minutes | Apgar 5 minuti |
| | Fontanelle | fontanella |
| GU/rectal | circumcision? | circoncisione? |
| | genital herpes? | herpes genitale? |
| | testicular exam | esame testicolare |
| | hemorrhoids,nodules, prostate on rectal exam | emorroide, nodulo, esamo prostata |
| | "I want to check your rectum for hemorrhoids. This might be uncomfortable. Bend over please." | "Voglio esaminaare per vedere se hai le emorroidi. Questo potrebbe essere scomodo. Chinarsi, per favore." |
| | guaiac:positive or negative | guajaco: positivo o negativo |
| Neurologic | "Sit up please." | "Si metta in posizione eretta, per favore." |
| Cranial nerves | N1 Olfactory: coffee, peppermint? "Close your eyes and tell me what you smell." | N1 nervo olfattorio: caffè, menta piperita? "Chiuda gli occhi e mi dica che odore sente? (metti del caffe' e poi della menta piperita vicino il loro naso) |

| Physical exam | English | Italian |
|---|---|---|
| | N2 Optic: Snellen chart confrontation. "Read the letters on this chart. Follow my finger with your eyes, without moving your head." | N2 nervo ottico, tavola ottometrica di Snellen "Leggere le lettere su questo grafico. Segua il mio dito con gli occhi, senza muovere la testa." |
| | N3,4,6 Oculomotor, Trochlear, Abducens. EOM's "Follow my finger." | N3,4,6 nervo oculomotore, trocleare, abducente. "Segua il mio dito." |
| | N5 Trigeminal "Clench your jaw." "Move your jaw back and forth." | N5 nervo trigemino "Stringere la mascella. Spostare avanti e indietro la mascella." |
| | Ophthalmic branch: forehead, Maxillary branch: cheek, Mandibular branch: chin, "Do you feel this?" | Ramo oftalmico: fronte, ramo mascellare: quancia, ramo mandibola: mento. "E' in grado di sentire quando la tocco qui?" |
| | N7 Facial: "Raise your eyebrows." | N7 nervo facciale: "Sollevare le sopracciglia." |
| | "Close your eyes tightly, smile big." | "Chiudere bene gli occhi. Sorriso largamente." |
| | N8 Acoustic: whisper, Rinne "Can you hear me talking? Try to repeat what I say." | N8 nervo acustico "Mi sente quando parlo? Cerchi di ripetere quello che dico." |
| | "Tell me when you can't feel the vibration." | "Dimmi quando non può sentire questa vibrazione." |
| | N9 Glossopharyngeal: swallow (hoarsenss?) "Swallow please." | N9 nervo glossofaringeo "Inghiotta, please." |
| | N10 Vagus: swallow, soft palate, gag reflex "Open your mouth widely. Stick out your tongue please. Now, close it." | N10, nervo vago: palato molle, reflesso faringeo. "Apra bene. Per piacere, mostri la lingua. Li chiuda" |
| | N11 Spinal accessory nerve: "Turn your head to the right, now to the left. Shrug your shoulders." | N11 nervo spinale accessorio "Volti la testa a destra contro la mia mano. Ora, a sinistra. Scrollare le spalle." |
| | N12 Hypoglossal: tongue midline | N12 nervo hypoglossal. È la linea mediana di lingua? |
| Coma score | Glasgow coma score | Scala di Glasgow |
| | Opens eyes to: spontaneous (4), to speech (3), to pain (2), none (1) | Apertura occhi: 4) spontanea, 3) allo stimolo verbale, 2) allo stimolo doloroso, 1) nessuna |
| | Best motor: "Hold up two fingers" obeys commands (6), localizes (5), withdraws (4), abnormal flexion (3), abnormal extension (2), none (1) | Risposta motoria: 6) obbedisce ai comandi, 5) localizzazione dello stimolo doloroso, 4) flessione/ ritrazione allo stimolo doloroso, 3) anormale flessione allo stimolo doloroso, 2) extensione allo stimolo doloroso, 1) nessuna risposta |

| Physical exam | English | Italian |
|---|---|---|
| | Best verbal: oriented (5), confused (4), inappropriate (3), garbled (2), none (1) | Risposta verbale: 5) paziente orientato, conversazione appropriata, 4) confusione, frasi sconnesse , 3) parla e pronuncia parole, ma incoerenti, 2) suoni incomprensibili, 1) nessun suono emesso |
| Motor | Motor function | Funzione motoria |
| | biceps brachii, elbow flexion | biceps, flessione del gomito |
| | "Pull your arm up, like this." | "Tirare il braccio verso l'alto, come questo." |
| | wrist extensors | estensori del polso |
| | "Bend your wrist up, like this." | "Piegare il polso, come questo." |
| | triceps brachii, elbow extension | tricipite, estensione del gomito |
| | "Straighten your arm out, like this." | "Raddrizzare il braccio, come questo." |
| | finger flexors, distal phalanx middle finger | flessori del dito, falange distale, dito medio |
| | "bend the tip of this finger" | "Piegare la punta di questo dito." |
| | finger abduction, little finger | abduzione di dito, dito mignolo |
| | "hold the small finger tightly. (Don't let me squeeze your fingers together.)" | Chiuda saldamente il mignolo. (Apra le sue dita e non lasci che le stringa.)" |
| | iliopsoas, hip flexors | psoas, flessione articulazione coxo-femorale |
| | "Move this knee to your chest, now the other knee." | "Spostare questo ginocchio verso il petto. Ora, l'altro ginocchio." |
| | quadriceps, knee extensors | quadricipite femorale, estensori del ginocchio |
| | "Straighten your leg out, like this." | "Raddrizzare la gamba, come questo." |
| | tibialis anterior, ankle dorsiflexors | muscolo tibiale anteriore, dorsiflessori di caviglia |
| | "Pull your foot up, like this." | "Tirare il piede, come questo." |
| | extensor hallucis longus, long toe extension | longus di hallucis dell'estensore, estensione alluce |
| | "Raise your toe up, like this." | "Sollevare questo dito del piede." |
| | gastrocnemius, ankle plantar flexors | gastrocnemio, caviglia flessione plantare |
| | "Push your foot down, like this." | "Spingere il piede verso il basso, come questo." |
| Sensory | Sensation "say 'yes' if you can feel this" | "E' in grado di sentire quando la tocco qui?" |

| Physical exam | English | Italian |
|---|---|---|
| | "Is the sensation dull or sharp? Say sharp or dull." | "E in grado di sentire se quest'oggetto è smussato o tagliente? Dire tagliente o smussato." |
| | C-4 (top of acromioclavicular joint) | C4 (cima acromioclavicolare) |
| | C-5 (lateral side of antecubital fossa) | C4 (funzione laterale dell fossa antecubital) |
| | C-6 (thumb) | C6 (pollice) |
| | C-7 (middle finger) | C7 (dito medio) |
| | C-8 (little finger) | C8 (dito mignolo) |
| | T-4 (nipple line) | T4 (linea mammillare) |
| | T-10 (umbilicus) | T10 (ombelico) |
| | L-2 (mid-anterior thigh) | L2 (metà anteriore della coscia) |
| | L-3 (medial femoral condyle) | L3 (condilo femorale mediale) |
| | L-4 (medial malleolus) | L4 (malleolo mediale) |
| | L-5 (dorsum of the foot, at third MTP joint) | L5 (dorsum del piede, terzo metatarso falangea guinto) |
| | S-1 (Lateral heel) | S1 (tallone laterale) |
| | S-2 (popliteal fossa of the knee, in the midline) | S2 (popliteal fossa, piano mediano) |
| | S-3 (ischial tuberosity) | S3 (tuberosità ischiatica) |
| | S4-5 (perianal area) | S4-5 (regione perianale) |
| Reflexes | Reflexes; "I am going to tap you here with this reflex hammer." | Riflessi "La tocchero' qui con questo martelletto per i riflessi." |
| | triceps right and left | tricipiti, destra e sinistra |
| | biceps, right and left | biciptale, destra e sinistra |
| | brachioradial, right and left | brachio-radiale, destra e sinistra |
| | patella, right and left | rotuleo, destra e sinistra |
| | ankle, right and left | achilleo, destra e sinistra |
| | babinski, right and left (great toe extension= positive) | Babinski, destra e sinistra (estensione alluce = positivo) |
| Cerebellar function | Tandem walk | piedi tandem |
| | "Walk like this, one foot in front of other." (Or, say walk like this and demonstrate.) | "Camminare come questo." |
| | heel walk, toe walk, | tallone camminando, punta di piedi camminando |
| | "Walk on your heels, now on toes." | "Cammini sui talloni. Ora, cammini sulle punte dei suoi piedi." |
| | romberg "Stand up, hold your arms out, close your eyes." | Segno di Romberg "Si alzi, per favore. Tenga le braccia in questo modo. Chiudi gli occhi." |
| | rapid alternating movement (2nd finger, thumb) "Do this, fast". | "Fare questo movimento, rapidamente." |

| Physical exam | English | Italian |
|---|---|---|
| | heel-shin "Close your eyes. Move your right heel from your left knee to the ankle. Now, move your left heel from your right knee down to the ankle." ( Open your eyes, let me demonstrate.) | calcagno-cresta tibiale: "Chiudi gli occhi. Sposti il tallone destro dal ginocchio sinistro alla caviglia sinistra. Ora sposti il suo tallone sinistro dal suo ginocchio destro alla caviglia destra." (Apri gli occhi, e lasci che le dimostri come fare.) |
| | finger nose finger "Touch my finger with your finger then touch your nose." | dito-naso-dito "Toccare il mio dito con il dito, quindi toccare il naso." |
| | stereognosis (key, pencil, cup) "Close your eyes; what is this in your hand?" | stereognosia (chiave, matita, tazza) "Chiudi gli occhi. Che cosa le ho messo in mano." |
| | graphesthesia (draw #3 in hand) "Close your eyes, what is the number written in your hand?" | grafestesia (Disegnare il numero 3 in mano.) "Chiudi gli occhi. Qual è il numero scritto in mano?" |
| | point localization: "Close your eyes, tell me what part of your body is being touched." | posizione del punto "Chiudi gli occhi. Dimmi quale parte del tuo corpo sto toccando." |
| | two point discrimination: "Do you feel one or two points of contact?" | discriminazione di due punti: "Ti senti un punto di contatto o due?" |
| Memory assessment | SLUMS Examination | |
| | Saint Louis University Mental Status Examination | Esame dello stato mentale di St. Louis University |
| | What day of the week is it? (1) | Quale giorno della settimana è? |
| | What is the year? (1) | Che anno è? |
| | What state are we in? (1) | In quale stato siamo? |
| | Please remember these five objects. I will ask you what they are later. Apple Pen Tie House Car | Per favore si ricorda questi cinque oggetti. Le chiedero' di indicarmi quali sono piu' tardi. Mela, penna, cravatta, casa, auto. |
| | You have $100 and you go to the store and buy a dozen apples for $3 and a tricycle for $20. How much did you spend? (1)   How much do you have left?  (2) | Le hai  100 euro e va al negozio a comprare una dozzina di mele per 3 euro e un triciclo per 20 euro. Quanto spende in tutto? (1) Quanti soldi le sono rimasti? (2) |
| | Please name as many animals as you can in one minute. (0) 0-4 animals, (1) 5-9 animals, (2) 10-14 animals, (3) 15+ animals | Per favore, dica il maggior numero di nome di animali che può in un minuto. (0) 0-4 (zero- quattro) animali, (1) 5-9 (cinque-nove) animali, (2) 10-14 (dicei-quattordici) animali, (3) 15+ (piu' di quindici) animali |

| Physical exam | English | Italian |
|---|---|---|
| | What were the five objects I asked you to remember? Apple Pen Tie House Car. One point for each correct answer. | Quali erano i cinque oggetti che le ho chiesto di ricordare? mela, penna, cravatta, casa, auto. Un punto per ogni risposta corretta. |
| | I am going to give you a series of numbers and I would like you to give them to me backwards. For example, if I say 42, you say 24. (0) 87, (1) 649, (2) 8537 | Le leggerò una serie di numeri e vorrei che li ripetesse in ordine inverso. Ad esempio, se dico 42, dica 24. (0) 87 {otto sette}, (1) 649 {sei quattro nove}, (2) 8537 {otto cinque tre sette} |
| | This is a clock face. Please put in the hour markers and the time at ten minutes to eleven o'clock. (2) Hour markers correct? (2) Time correct? | Questo è il quadrante di un orologio. Per favore metta le lancette delle ore e dei minuti a dieci minuti alle 11. (2) Le lancette delle ore sono corrette? (2) Il tempo è corretto?. |
| | Place an X in the triangle. □△◇, (1) Which of the figures is the largest? (1) | Mettere una X nel triangolo. □△◇ (1) Quale delle figure è la più grande? (1) |
| | I am going to read you a story. Please listen carefully because afterwards, I'm going to ask you some questions about it. Maria was a very successful cook. She made a lot of money on the stock market. She then met Giovanni, a devastatingly handsome man. She married him and had three children. They lived in Rome. She then stopped work and stayed at home to bring up her children. When they were teenagers, she went back to work. She and Giovanni lived happily ever after. | Le leggero' una storia. Per favore ascolti attentamente perché dopo, le faro' alcune domande. Maria era una cuoca di successo. Ha fatto un sacco di soldi. Poi ha incontrato Giovanni un uomo irresistibilmente bello. Lei lo sposò ed ebbe tre figli. Loro vivevano a Roma. Successivamente lei smise di lavorare e rimase a casa per crescere i suoi figli. Quando i figli diventarono adolescenti, lei tornò a lavoro. Lei e Giovannia vissero felici e contenti. |
| | What was the female's name? (2) | Come si chiamava la femmina? (2) |
| | What work did she do? (2) | Che lavoro ha fatto? (2) |
| | When did she go back to work? (2) | Quando e'tornata al lavoro? (2) |
| | What nation did she live in? (2) | In quale nazione viveva? |
| | Add total score, with high school education: 27-30 normal, 21-26 mild cognitive disorder, 1-20 dementia. Without high school education: 25-30 normal, 20-24 mild cognitive disorder, 1-19 dementia. | Aggiungere il punteggio totale, con scuola secondaria di secondo grado 27-30 normale, 21-26 disturbo cognitivo lieve, 1-20 demenza. Senza scuola secondaria di secondo grado: 25-30 normale, 20-24 disturbo cognitive lieve, 1-19 demenza |

| Joint exam | English | Italian |
|---|---|---|
| | Shoulder test for impingement. Apley scratch test: Use your right hand to touch the left scapula by reaching over the left clavicle. Next, use your right hand to touch the right scapula. Thirdly, move your right thumb to the middle of your back between the scapulae. "Move your arm like I do" | Test di Apley; Test per la sindrome da conflitto della cuffia dei rotatario. "Muovi il braccio come faccio io." |
| | Shoulder test for impingement.Neers test: Place one hand on the patient's scapula, grasp their forearm with your other hand (their thumb should be facing down). Slowly forward flex the arm. "I am going to put my hand on your shoulder blade and move your arm." | Test di Neers. "Mettero' la mia mano sulla sua spalla e le muovero' il braccio." |
| | Supraspinatus isometric test: the patient holds their arm at 20 degrees abduction and the examiner attempts adduction. "Hold your arm like this and try to raise it." | Tenga il braccio in questo modo e cerchi di alzarlo." |
| | Supraspinatus function. Painful arc sign: "I am going to raise your arm, let me know when you have pain." | Segno dell' arco dolorso "Le sollevero'il braccio: mi faccia sapere quando sente dolore." |
| | Supraspinatus function. Drop arm test: raise the arm to 180 degrees abduction then instruct the patient: "Slowly lower your arm to your side". If the arm falls quickly the test is positive. | Test di caduta del braccio: "Abbassi lentamente il braccio lungo il fainco." Se il braccio cade rapidamente il test e'positivo. |
| | Supraspinatus function. Jobe's or empty can test: hold the arm straight at the elbow at 90 degrees abduction, 30 degrees forward flexion and internally rotate the shoulder. Hand the patient a cup and instruct: "Turn this cup upside down." Pain during this motion is a positive sign. | Funzione del sovraspinato. Test di Jobe o della lattina vuota. "Capovolga questa tazza. Il movimento le provica dolore?" |
| | External rotation test for infraspinatus impingement. Have the patient abduct the shoulders 30 degrees, flex at the elbow 90 degrees. Hold the outside of the forearm and direct them to "Push outward." | Test per i rotatori esterni del braccio " Spinga il braccio verso l'esterno" |
| | Subscapularis;Push off test: have the patient put their arm behind their back with the palm facing outward and push against the examiner's hand. "Move your hand like this and push against my hand." | Test della spinta esterna. "Muova la mano in questo modo e la spinga contro la mia." |

| Joint exam | English | Italian |
|---|---|---|
| | Tinel test for ulnar nerve entrapment: tap over the ulnar groove and ask "Do you have pain or numbness. If so, where?" (Pain and numbess at 4th, 5th fingers indicates a positive test.) | Test di Tinel per l'intrappolamento del nervo ulnare: toccare il solco ulnare e chiedere "ha dolore o intorpidimento. Se sì, dove? "(Dolore e intorpidimento al 4°, 5° dito indica un test positivo.) |
| | Phalen maneuver for carpal tunnel syndrome: hold the wrist in forced flexion. Pain is a positive indication. "Where do you have pain when I do this?" | Manovra di Phalen. "Dove sente dolore quando premo il polso in questo modo?" |
| | Finkelstein test for de Quervain's tenosynovitis. Have the patient cover the thumb with their fingers of the same hand. Deviate the wrist towards the ulna. Pain is indicative of tenosynovitis. "Hold your hand like this. Does this hurt?" | Test di Finkelstein per tenosinovite di de Quervain. "Tenga la mano in questo modo. Le fa male?" |
| | Scaphoid compression test. The thumb is held and pushed toward the scaphoid. Pain indicates a possible scaphoid fracture. "Tell me if you feel pain." | Test di compressione dello scafoide. "Mi dica se sente dolore." |
| | Hip assessment. Perform internal and external rotation of the hip and ask, "Does this hurt?" | Esame dell'anca. "Questa fa le male?" |
| | Patrick test for hip or sacroiliac pathology: examiner flexes, abducts, externally rotates and extends the leg so that the ankle of that leg is on top of the opposite knee. "I am going to move your leg, does this hurt?" | Test di Patrick. "Le mouvero'la gamba: mi dica se sente dolore." |
| | Piriformis test Patient is in lateral decubitus position with hip flexed at 60 degrees and knee at full extension. Examiner places a hand on the patient's shoulder and exerts mild pressure on the flexed leg at the knee. A positive test is noted by radicular pain caused by impingement of the sciatic nerve by the tight piriformis muscle. "Lay on your side." | Test di Piriforme. "Si metta su un fianco e me dica se sente dolore." |
| | Ely's test to assess rectus femoris flexibility. Patient lays prone with legs fully extended. Examiner passively flexes the knee to full ROM. If the ipsilateral hip rises it is suggestive of a tight rectus femoris muscle. "Lay on your abdomen." | Test di Ely."Si metta in posizione prona." |
| | Fulcrum test Patient is seated on a table with legs dangling. Examiner places their forearm under the thigh for use as a fulcrum. Pressure is applied with the other hand over the knee and up the femur. Pain elicited may indicate a stress fracture. "Sit on the edge of the bed." | Test di l'instabilita': "Si sieda sul bordo del letto." |

| Joint exam | English | Italian |
|---|---|---|
| | Straight leg raise "Lay down, I am going to lift your leg, let me know where you feel pain."; | Test di sollevamento della gamba tesa. "Si distenda, per favore. Le sollevero' la gamba; mi dica dove sente dolore." |
| | Sensation of anterolateral thigh to assess for meralgia paresthetica; "I am going to touch you with this cotton ball, let me know when you feel it." | Meralgia parestesica. "Ho intenzione di toccarle con questa palla di cotone; mi dica quando lo sente." |
| | Knee collateral ligament assessment. valgus stress for medial instability. "Lay down. I am going to check your knee." Place one hand on lateral thigh while the other hand is used to apply outward pressure on the calf. | exame del legamento collaterale del ginocchio per instabilità mediale. "Si distenda, per favore. Ho intenzione di esaminare il ginocchio." |
| | Knee collateral ligament assessment. varus stress for lateral instability "Lay down. I am going to check your knee." Place one hand on the medial thigh while the other hand is used to apply inward pressure on the calf. | exame del legamento collaterale del ginocchio per instabilità laterale. "Si distenda, per favore. Ho intenzione di esaminare il ginocchio." |
| | Lachman's test for anterior cruciate ligament injury (ACL) "Lay down, bend your knee." Place the knee at 30 degrees flexion, stabilize the the femur with one hand while pulling the proximal tibia anteriorly. Laxity indicates ACL injury. | Test di Lachman. "Si distenda, piegare il ginocchio." |
| | Pivot shift test for ACL injury. "Lay down." With the knee in full extension the examiner rotates the tibia and applies valgus stress then flexes the knee. If acl injury is present a "clunk" sound will be heard. | Test per lesione del legamento crociato anteriore. "Si distenda." |
| | Anterior drawer for ACL injury. "Lay down and bend your knee." to 90 degrees. The examiner hold the proximal tibia with both hands, sits on the patient's foot and pulls the tibia anteriorly to look for laxity. | Test per lesione del legamento crociato anteriore. "Si distenda, piegi il ginocchio." |
| | Posterior drawer test for posterior cruciate ligament injury (PCL) Patient is supine with the hips flexed at 45 degrees and knees at 90 degrees, Examiner sits on the patient's feet, grasps the tibia with both hands and applies backward pressure. Laxity is a sign of a torn posterior cruciate ligament. "Lay on your back and bend your knee." | Test per lesione del legamento crociato posteriore. "Si distenda, piegi il ginocchio. Ho intenzione di stare in piedi e applicare una pressione verso la tibia." |
| | Thessaly test: for knee meniscal injury"Stand up. Bend your knee and then turn it like this." Patient should hold the examiner's hand, stand on one leg with the knee flexed at 20 degrees. THe pt then internally and externaly rotates their knees. Pain or locking is a positive test. | Test di Thessaly. "Alzarsi, piegi il ginocchio e poi trasformi come questo." |

| Joint exam | English | Italian |
|---|---|---|
| | Apley test for knee meniscal injury "Lay on your abdomen." With patient prone bend the knee to 90 degrees and apply downward pressure while internally and externally rotating the foot. Pain indicates a positive test. | Test di Apley. "Giaccia sul suo addome. Mi dica se si sente dolore." |
| | Ottawa knee rules X ray indicated if any of following are present: 1. age over 55 "What is your age?" 2. Tenderness of patella: "Do you have pain here?" 3. Tenderness of fibular head: "Do you have pain here." Inability to flex the knee to 90 degrees: "4. Bend your knee as much as possible." 5. Inability to transfer weight to each leg. "Stand on your right leg only, now on your left leg only." | Regole del ginocchio di Ottawa. La radiografia è indicata se i seguenti sono presenti: 1) oltre 55 anni di età. "Quanti anni ha?" 2) tenerezza rotuleo. "Ha dolore qui?" 3) tenerezza testa fibular "Ha dolore qui?" 4) Incapacità di flettere il ginocchio a 90 gradi. "Piegi il ginocchio quanto più possibile." 5) Incapacità di trasferire il peso di ciascuna gamba. "Stia sulla sua gamba destra solo. Ora stia sulla gamba sinistra solo." |
| | Ottawa ankle rules, part 1. An ankle x ray is indicated if there is inability to bear weight in the ER or there is tenderness at the posterior edge or tip of the medial or lateral malleolus (distal 6cm). "Can you walk? Do you have pain when I touch here?" | Regole della caviglia di Ottawa. 1) Una radiografia della caviglia è indicata se egli non può sopportare il peso al pronto soccorso o se c'è la tenerezza a margine posteriore o la punta del malleolo mediale o laterale (distale 6 centimetri). "Si può camminare? Ha dolore quando le tocco qui?" |
| | Ottawa ankle rules, part 2. A foot x ray is indicated if there is inability to bear weight in the ER or there is tenderness at the base of the 5th metatarsal or over the navicular bone. "Can you walk? Do you have pain when I touch here?" | Regole della caviglia di Ottawa. 2) Una radiografia del piede è indicata se egli non può sopportare il peso al pronto soccorso o se c'è la tenerezza alla base del quinto osso metatarsale o sopra l'osso navicolare. "Si può camminare? Ha dolore quando le tocco qui?" |
| | Thompson test for achilles tendon rupture. The patient lays prone with their feet hanging over the end of the bed. The calf muscles are squeezed and if the Achilles tendon is ruptured there is no plantar flexion of the foot."Lay on your abdomen." | Test di Thompson per rottura del tendine d'Achille. "Giaccia sul suo ventre. Ho intenzione di spremere il muscolo del polpaccio." |

| Counseling | English | Italian |
|---|---|---|
| **Pulmonary** | You need to go for an x ray. | Ha bisogno di una radiografia. |
| | I have the result of your sputum. | Ho il risultato del suo esame sull'espettrato. |
| | You have... | Soffre di... |
| | tuberculosis | tubercolosi |
| | pneumonia | polmonite |
| | Your lungs are... | I suoi polmoni sono... |
| | one is infected, the other is healthy. | un polmone è infetto, l'altro è sano. |
| | You must stop smoking. | Deve smettere di fumare. |
| **Infectious disease** | You are sick with malaria. | Lei ha un malaria. |
| | You have typhoid fever. | Lei ha un tifo. |
| | You have intestinal worms. | Lei ha un teniasi. |
| | Your illness can be healed. | La malattia può essere guarita. |
| **Gastroenterology** | There is an ulcer in your stomach. | Ha un'ulcera nello stomaco. |
| | You need to quit drinking beer completely. | Deve smettere completamente di bere birra. |
| | You have a tumor in your stomach. | Ha un tumore allo stomaco. |
| **Surgery** | You need to have an operation today. | Deve subire un intervento chirurgico. |
| | When have you last eaten? | Che cosa ha mangiato o bevuto? |
| | You need to have this wound sewed up (sutured). | Dovrei darle dei punti. |
| | You need a cast on your leg. | Dovremo ingessarle la gamba. |
| | You need to stay in the hospital. | Dovrebbe rimanere in ospedale. |
| **Pharmacy** | I will give you medication. | Le dò una ricetta. |
| | You take this medicine once (two, three, four)times per day. | Prenda questa medicina una volta (due, tre, quattro volte) al giorno. |
| | Do not stop this medication! | Non smettere di prendere questo medicina! |
| | Take this medication only if you want to. | Prenda questa medicina solo se vuole. |
| | Take this medication before eating. | Prenda questa medicina prima i pasti. |
| | Take this medication with food. | Prenda questa medicina con il cibo. |
| | Take this medication on an empty stomach. | Prenda questa medicina a digiuno. |
| | Take this medication after meals. | Prenda questa medicina dopo i pasti. |

| Counseling | English | Italian |
|---|---|---|
| | Take this medication in the morning. | Prenda questa medicina la mattina. |
| | Take this medication at night. | Prenda questa medicina alla sera. |
| | Take this medication in case of pain. | Prenda questa medicina se si ha dolore. |
| **Maternity/Ob** | Congratulations, you are pregnant! | Congratulazioni, lei è incinta! |
| | The baby is due on this date... | Il parto avverrà prevedibilmente verso il... |
| | The nurse is on her way. | L'infermiera sta arrivando. |
| | She will help with the delivery. | Lei aiuterà con il parto. |
| | You had a boy. You had a girl. | Ha un bimbo. Ha una bimba. |
| | You had twins. | Ha due gemelli. |
| | You will need a cesarean section. | Avrà bisogno di un taglio cesareo. |
| **Procedures** | "I need to take a blood sample." | "Desidero farle un prelievo di sangue." |
| | "Please give me a urine sample in this cup." | "La prego, mi faccia avere un campione d'orina in questa bottiglia." |
| | "Please give me a stool specimen in this container." | "La prego, mi faccia avere un campione di feci in questa barrattolo." |
| | "Please give me a sputum sample in this cup." | "La prego, mi faccia avere un campione d'espettorato in questa tazza." |
| | "I need to put this tube in your nose." | "É necessario inserire questo sondino nel naso." |
| | "I need to start an IV." | " É necessario inziare un'infusione endovenosa." |
| | I need to give you a shot 1) in the arm, 2) in the leg | Le devo fair un'iniezione 1) nel braccio 2) in gamba. |
| **Orthopedics** | You have a broken leg. | Ha una frattura alla gamba. |
| | You have a broken arm. | Ha una frattura al braccio. |
| | You have tendinitis. | Ha una tendinite. |
| | You have fluid in your joint. | Hai liquido nel tuo giuntura. |
| | We have to put a cast on your arm/leg. | Le dobbiamo ingessare il/la braccio/gamba. |
| **General** | What you have is not serious. | Quello che ha non è grave. |
| | Your condition is grave. | La sua condizione è grave. |
| | Please come back if you have more problems. | Non esiti a tornare se dovesse avere altri problemi. |
| | Please return in one week. | Venga in una settimana. |

| Date/time, numbers | English | Italian |
|---|---|---|
| | January | gennaio |
| | February | febbraio |
| | March | marzo |
| | April | aprile |
| | May | maggio |
| | June | glugno |
| | July | luglio |
| | August | agosto |
| | September | settembre |
| | October | ottobre |
| | November | novembre |
| | December | dicembre |
| | Sunday | domenica |
| | Monday | lunedì |
| | Tuesday | martedì |
| | Wednesday | mercoledì |
| | Thursday | giovedì |
| | Friday | venerdì |
| | Saturday | sabato |
| | 0 (zero) | zero |
| | 1 one | uno |
| | 2 two | due |
| | 3 three | tre |
| | 4 four | quattro |
| | 5 five | cinque |
| | 6 six | sei |
| | 7 seven | sette |
| | 8 eight | otto |
| | 9 nine | nove |
| | 10 ten | dieci |
| | 11 eleven | undici |
| | 12 twelve | dodici |
| | 13 thirteen | tredici |
| | 14 fourteen | quattordici |
| | 15 fifteen | quindici |
| | 16 sixteen | sedici |
| | 17 seventeen | diciassette |
| | 18 eighteen | diciotto |
| | 19 nineteen | diciannove |
| | 20 twenty | venti |
| | 21 twenty-one | ventuno |
| | 30 thirty | trenta |

| Date/time, numbers | English | Italian |
|---|---|---|
| | 31 thirty-one | trentuno |
| | 40 forty | quaranta |
| | 50 fifty | cinquanta |
| | 60 sixty | sessanta |
| | 70 seventy | settanta |
| | 71 seventy-one | settantuno |
| | 72 seventy-two | settantadue |
| | 73 seventy-three | settantatre |
| | 74 seventy-four | settantatre |
| | 75 seventy-five | settantaquattro |
| | 76 seventy-six | settantasei |
| | 77 seventy-seven | settantasette |
| | 78 seventy-eight | settantotto |
| | 79 seventy-nine | settantanove |
| | 80 eighty | ottanta |
| | 81 eighty-one | ottantuno |
| | 82 eighty-two | ottantadue |
| | 90 ninety | novanta |
| | 91 ninety-one | novantuno |
| | 92 ninety-two | novantadue |
| | 100 one hundred | cento |
| | 200 two hundred | duecento |
| | 300 three hundred | trecento |
| | 400 four hundred | quattrocento |
| | 500 five hundred | cinquecento |
| | 600 six hundred | seicento |
| | 700 seven hundred | settecento |
| | 800 eight hundred | ottocento |
| | 900 nine hundred | novecento |
| | 1000 one thousand | mille |
| | 1500 one thousand five hundred | milleinquecento |
| | 2000 two thousand | duemila |
| | 2500 two thousand five hundred | duemila e cenquecento |
| | 5000 five thousand | cinquemila |
| | When is the meeting? | Quando è l'incontro? |
| | At what time? | A che ora? |
| | At 8p.m. (this evening) | A 20 (questa sera). |
| | At noon. | A mezzogiorno. |
| | It is 9 a.m. | Si tratta di nove del mattino. |
| | It is 2:30 p.m. | Si tratta di 2:30 del pomeriggio. |
| | today | oggi |
| | tomorrow | domani |
| | yesterday | ieri |
| | soon | presto |

| Date/time, numbers | English | Italian |
|---|---|---|
| | right now | adesso |
| | now | ora |
| | morning | mattino |
| | afternoon | pomeriggio |
| | evening | sera |
| | night | notte |
| | last week | la settimana scorsa |
| | this week | questa settimana |
| | next week | la settimana prossima |
| | last year | anno scorso |
| | this year | quest'anno |
| | next year | anno prossimo |
| | one week | una settimana |
| | two weeks | due settimane |
| | one month | un mese |
| | two months | due mesi |
| | three months | tre mesi |
| | four months | quattro mesi |
| | five months | cinque mesi |

| Body parts | English | Italian |
|---|---|---|
| | head | testa |
| | hair | pelo |
| | forehead | fronte |
| | face | faccia |
| | eye (eyes) | occhio (occhi) |
| | pupil | pupilla |
| | eyebrow | sopracciglia |
| | eyelash | ciglio |
| | eyelid | palpebra |
| | nose | naso |
| | ear (ears) | orecchio (orecchi) |
| | tongue | lingua |
| | tooth (teeth) | dente (denti) |
| | cheek | guancia |
| | lips | labbra |
| | tonsils | tonsille |
| | throat | gola |
| | mouth | bocca |
| | chin | mento |
| | mandible | mandibola |
| | neck (anterior) | collo |
| | adam's apple | pomo d'Adamo |
| | clavicle | clavicola |
| | shoulder | spalla |
| | axilla | ascella |
| | humerus | omero |
| | arms | braccia |
| | upper arm | braccio |
| | elbow | gomito |
| | lower arm | avambraccio |
| | wrist | polso |
| | hand (hands) | mano (mani) |
| | thumb | pollice |
| | finger (fingers) | dito (dita) della mano |
| | 5th finger | mignolo |
| | 4th finger | anulare |
| | 3rd finger | dito medio |
| | 2nd finger | dito indice |
| | knuckle | nocca |
| | fingernail | unghia |
| | lower back | spina dorsale |
| | scapula | scapola |
| | chest | petto; torace |

| Body parts | English | Italian |
|---|---|---|
| | heart | cuore |
| | lung | polmone |
| | breast (breasts) | seno |
| | nipple | capezzolo |
| | abdomen | addome |
| | liver | fegato |
| | stomach | stomaco |
| | gallbladder | cistifellea |
| | intestines, small | intestino tenue |
| | colon | intestino crasso |
| | rectum | retto |
| | spleen | milza |
| | kidney | rene |
| | ureter/urethra | uretere/uretra |
| | pancreas | pancreas |
| | urinary bladder | vescica |
| | umbilicus | ombelico |
| | umbilical cord | cordone ombelicale |
| | buttocks | natiche |
| | vagina | vagina |
| | clitoris | clitoride |
| | uterus | utero |
| | anus | ano |
| | penis | pene |
| | scrotum/testicle | scroto/testicolo |
| | pelvis | bacino |
| | femur/thigh | coscia |
| | leg | gamba |
| | knee | ginocchio |
| | patella | rotula |
| | lower leg | gamba |
| | shin | stinco |
| | calf | polpaccio |
| | ankle | caviglia |
| | achilles' tendon | tendine d'Achille |
| | heel | tallone |
| | foot (feet) | piede (piedi) |
| | big toe | alluce |
| | toe (toes) | dito (dita) del piede |
| | toenail | unghia dei piedi |

| English | Italian |
|---|---|
| **abasia** *Inability to walk due to impaired coordination.* | abasia |
| **abdomen** *The portion of the body bordered by the diaphragm and the pelvis.* | addome |
| **abdomen, lower** | basso addome |
| **abdominal girth** *Waist circumference.* | circonferenza addominale |
| **abdominal reflexes** *Elicited by stroking the abdomen lightly from mid-axillary line to umbilicus. A normal response is contraction of the umbilicus toward the stimulated side.* | addominale riflesso |
| **abdominocentesis** *Puncturing of the abdominal wall for drainage purposes.* | addominocentesi |
| **abducens nerve** *A motor nerve (6th cranial nerve) that controls the lateral rectus muscle of the eye.)* | nervo abducente |
| **abducent** *Abducting or to separate.* | abducente |
| **abductor pollicis brevis** *Abducts the thumb.* | abduttore pollicis brevi |
| **abductor pollicis longus** *Abducts and flexes the thumb.* | abduttore pollicis lungo |
| **aberrant** *Different than normal.* | anomalo |
| **ablation** *Surgical removal or amputation.* | ablazione |
| **abnormal** | anormale |
| **ABO system** *The system using human blood antigens to determine blood type.* | sistema ABO |
| **abortion** *Premature expulsion of the fetus from the uterus.* | aborto |
| **above** | oltre |
| **abrupt** *Suddenly or hastily.* | improvviso |
| **abruptio placentae** *The premature detachment of a normally implanted placenta resulting in maternal decompensation.* | abruptio placentae |
| **abscess** *A localized collection of pus.* | ascesso |
| **absence of** | mancanza |
| **absolute** | totale |
| **absorption (intestinal absorption)** | assorbimento |
| **abuse (sexual abuse)** | abusi |
| **acalculia** *The inability to perform mathematical calculations.* | acalcolia |
| **acanthoma** *An adult cornifying squamous carcinoma.* | acantoma |
| **acanthosis** *Hypertrophy of the prickle cell layer of the skin.* | acantosi |
| **acanthosis nigricans** *A skin disorder characterized by dark, thick, velvety skin in the body folds and creases.* | acantosi nigricans |
| **acapnia** *A condition of lower than normal carbon dioxide level in the blood.* | acapnia |
| **acariasis** *Mite infestation.* | acariasi |
| **acaricide** *A treatment for mite infestation.* | acaricide |
| **acarus** *A mite.* | acaro |
| **acatalasia** *A condition characterized by the congenital absence of the enzyme catalase.* | acatalasia |
| **acathisia** *The inability to sit quietly or to have motor restlessness.* | acatisia |
| **accelerate** *(To accelerate the healing process).* | accelerare |
| **access** *Means of entry.* | accesso |
| **accessory** *Complimentary or concomitant.* | accessorio |

| English | Italian |
|---|---|
| **accessory nerve (XI)** *Supplies motor innervation to the sternocleidomastoid and trapezius.* | nervo accessorio |
| **accident** | accidente |
| **acclimatization** *The process of becoming adapted to a new environment.* | ambientamento |
| **accommodation** *A term used to describe the ability of the eye to adjust to various distances.* | accomodazione |
| **accomplish, to** *Achieve.* | compiere |
| **according to** | secondo |
| **accretion** *The expected growth of tissue from the intake of nutrients.* | concrescenza |
| **acephalous** *A absence of a head.* | acefalo |
| **acetabular** *Referring to the acetabulum.* | concavità |
| **acetabulum** *The cup-shaped cavity with which the head of the femur articulates.* | acetabulo |
| **acetaminophen** *Mild analgesic drug used for pain relief.* | acetaminofene |
| **acetonemia** *The presence of acetone in the blood.* | acetonemia |
| **acetonuria** *The presence of acetone in the urine.* | acetonuria |
| **acetylcholine** *A reversible acetic acid ester of choline.* | acetilcolina |
| **acetylsalicylic acid** *The chemical name for common aspirin.* | acido acetilsalicilico |
| **achalasia** *Inability to relax the smooth muscle fibers of the gastrointestinal tract. In the case of esophageal achalasia one has dilatation and hypertrophy of the esophagus.* | acalasia |
| **achieve, to** *To complete something one was striving for.* | conseguire |
| **Achilles tendon reflex** *The normal response to tapping the achilles tendon with a reflex hammer is the plantar flexion of the foot.* | riflesso achilleo |
| **achilliodynia** *Pain around the calcaneal tendon.* | achillodinia |
| **achillobursitis** *Inflammation around the calcaneal tendon.* | borsite achille |
| **achlorhydria** *The absence of hydrochloric acid in gastric secretions.* | acloridria |
| **acholia** *The lack of bile.* | acolia |
| **achondroplasia** *A congenital inadequacy of enchondral bone formation resulting in a type of dwarfism.* | acondroplasia |
| **achromatic spindle** *The threads between the poles of the spindle in karyokinesis.* | fusiforme acromatico |
| **achromatopsia** *Inability to differentiate yellow, blue, red or their intermediates.* | acromatopsia |
| **achylia** *The absence of chyle.* | achilia |
| **acid phosphatase** *A phosphate derived chemical that is optimally active in an acidic environment.* | fosfatasi acida |
| **acid** *Substance with a pH less than 7.* | acida |
| **acid-base balance** *The equilibrium of the electrolytes in the body.* | bilancio acido-base |
| **acidemia** *A lower than normal pH in the blood.* | acidemia |
| **acidity** *Referring to an acid state.* | acidità |
| **acinous gland** *The exocrine part of the pancreas.* | ghiandola acinoso |
| **acinus** *A very small grape shaped portion of an acinous gland.* | acino |
| **acne** *Inflamed or infected sebaceous glands.* | acne |
| **acne rosacea** *A chronic disease characterized by the presence of flushing of the skin of the nose, forehead and cheeks.* | acne congestiva |
| **acne vulgaris** *Chronic acne occurring on the face, chest and back of youth.* | acne volgare |
| **acorea** *The absence of the pupil of the eye.* | acorea |
| **acoustic crest** *A prominence on ampulla of the semicircular ducts.* | cresta acustico |
| **acoustic neuroma** *A nonmalignant tumor that can cause deafness, tinnitus and vertigo.* | neurinoma dell'acustico |

| English | Italian |
|---|---|
| **acoustic** *Referring to the auditory system.* | acustico |
| **Acquired Immunodeficiency Syndrome (AIDS)** *Presence of an AIDS defining illness or having a CD4 of less than 200/mm3.* | Sindrome da immunodeficienza acquisita |
| **acrocephaly** *A condition characterized by a pointed head.* | acrocefalia |
| **acrocyanosis, Raynaud's disease** *A benign condition in which the feet and hands are cyanotic, cold and sweating.* | acrocianosi |
| **acrodermatitis** *Inflammation of the skin of the hands and/or feet.* | acrodermatite |
| **acrodynia** *An infantile condition exhibited by swollen bluish-red extremities and later polyarthritis..* | acrodinia |
| **acromegaly** *Hyperplasia of the nose, jaw, fingers and toes.* | acromegalia |
| **acromioclavicular joint** *Referring to the junction of the acromion and clavicle.* | articolazione acromioclavicolare |
| **acromion** *The flattened process extending laterally from the spine of the scapula which forms the most prominent point of the shoulder.* | acromion |
| **acrophobia** *The morbid fear of heights.* | acrofobia |
| **acrotic** *Referring to great weakness or absence of a pulse.* | acrotico |
| **actin** *A protein in the muscle that, along with myosin, facilitates muscle contraction and relaxation.* | actina |
| **actinic dermatosis** *A skin disease caused by exposure to radiation from the sun, ultraviolet waves or gamma radiation.* | actinic dermatitis |
| **actinomycosis** *A chronic bacterial infection that effects the face and neck and is caused by Actinomyces israelii. In rare cases it can cause a pulmonary infection.* | actinomicosi |
| **actinon** *A radioactive element, radon-219; short lived isotope of radon.* | attinon |
| **action potential** *The alteration in electrical potential associated with the movement along a nerve cell.* | potenziale d'azione |
| **activity** | attività |
| **actomyosin** *Myosin and actin complex present in muscles.* | actinomicina |
| **acuity** *1. Relating to accuracy of hearing, as in hearing acuity. 2. Severity of illness as in, "What is the patient's acuity?"* | acutezza |
| **acupuncture** *Traditionally an aspect of Chinese medicine involving insertion of needles into the skin.* | agopuntura |
| **acute** *Abrupt onset.* | acuto |
| **adactylia** *A congenital condition exhibited by the absence of toes and fingers.* | adattilo |
| **Adam's apple** *A prominence on the anterior neck caused by the thyroid cartilage of the larynx.* | pomo d'Adamo |
| **Adams-Stokes Syndrome** *Characterized by bradycardia, syncope and convulsions.* | malattia di Adams-Stokes |
| **add, to** *To count.* | aggiungere |
| **addiction** *An abnormal dependency.* | tossicodipendenza |
| **Addison's disease** *A disease of the adrenal gland exhibited by anemia, hypotension and a bronze tone to the skin.* | morbo di Addison |
| **adduction** *To bring toward the midline.* | adduzione |
| **adductor** *A muscle that brings a part to the midline.* | adduttore |
| **adenectomy** *The removal of a gland.* | adenectomia |
| **adenitis** *The inflammation of a gland.* | adenite |
| **adenocanthoma** *Malignant tumor comprised of glandular tissue.* | adenoacatoma |
| **adenocarcinoma** *Cancer from glandular tissue.* | adenocarcinoma |
| **adenofibroma** *Connective tissue with glands that form a tumor.* | adenofibroma |
| **adenohypophysis** *The anterior portion of the pituitary gland.* | adenoipofisi |
| **adenoid** *Referring to a gland.* | adenoide |
| **adenoidectomy** *Removal of the adenoids.* | adenoidectomia |

| English | Italian |
|---|---|
| **adenoiditis** *Inflammation of the adenoids.* | adenoidite |
| **adenoids** *Pharyngeal tonsils.* | adenoidi |
| **adenolymphoma** *A salivary gland tumor, also called Warthin's tumor.* | adenolinfoma |
| **adenomyoma** *A tumor characterized by the overgrowth of endometrial and uterine muscle tissue.* | adenomioma |
| **adenomyosis** *A condition characterized by the overgrowth of endometrial and uterine muscle tissue.* | adenomiosi |
| **adenopathy** *Generally referring to a condition of the lymphatic glands.* | adenopatia |
| **adenosine triphosphate (ATP)** *A chemical that represents the energy reserve of the muscle.* | adenosindifosfato |
| **adenosine diphosphate** *A product of hydrolysis of ATP.* | adenosindifosfato |
| **adenosine monophosphate** *A nucleotide, it is produced when ATP is converted to ADP.* | adenosinmonofosfato |
| **adenovirus** *A type of a virus that can cause upper respiratory tract infections.* | adenovirus |
| **adequate** *Sufficient.* | sufficiente |
| **adherence** *To stick to something figuratively or literally.* | fedeltà |
| **adhesion** *The abnormal adherence of tissue exposed to inflammation or after surgery.* | aderenza |
| **adhesive capsulitis** *Also known as frozen shoulder.* | tenosinovite scapolo-omerale cronica |
| **adhesive tape** *Tape used to secure dressings or intravenous lines to the body.* | nastro adesivo |
| **adiadochokinesia** *The inability to perform rapid alternating movements.* | adiadococinesia |
| **Adie's pupil** *Characterized by a weak light reaction and a strong but slow near response.* | pupilla di Adie |
| **adipose** *Referring to fat. (adipose tissue)* | adiposo |
| **adipsia** *Absence of thirst which can be caused by SIADH, hydrocephalus or injury/tumor to/of the hypothalamus.* | adipsie |
| **aditus** *The entrance to an organ or part.* | adito |
| **adjust, to** *To modify a plan.* | adattarsi |
| **adjustment** *A modification of a plan.* | modifica |
| **adjuvant** *Term used to describe the medical treatment after initial therapy, as in adjuvant radiation therapy after initial chemotherapy.* | adiuvante |
| **admission (to hospital)** | andare (all'ospedale) |
| **adnexa** *The appendages, for example, of the uterus are the ovaries, fallopian tubes and the ligaments of the uterus.* | annesso |
| **adolescence** | adolescenza |
| **adrenal** *Referring to being near the kidney.* | soprarenale |
| **adrenal cortex** *The outer layer of the adrenal gland.* | corteccia surrenale |
| **adrenal gland** *A gland located on the superior aspect of both kidneys.* | surrene |
| **adrenal medulla** *The innermost part of the adrenal gland.* | midollare del surrene |
| **adrenalectomy** *Excision of the adrenal gland.* | surrenectomia |
| **adrenaline (epinephrine)** *A hormone secreted by the adrenal glands and a synthetic medication used for treatment of allergic reactions and cardiac arrest.* | adrenalina |
| **adrenergic** *That which is activated or transmitted by epinephrine.* | adrenalinico |
| **adrenocorticotrophic hormone (ACTH)** *A hormone that influences the cortex of the adrenal glands.* | ormone adrenocorticotropo |
| **Adson maneuver** *A test used to screen for thoracic outlet syndrome.* | manovra di Adson |
| **advanced stage** *A late period of a disease.* | stadio tardo |
| **adventitia** *Outermost.* | avventizio |

| English | Italian |
|---|---|
| **adverse effect** *In reference to medication use, it is an undesirable consequence of the drug.* | effetto indesiderato |
| **advise, to** *To give counsel.* | consigliare |
| **aerobe** *An organism that grows in the presence of oxygen.* | aeroba |
| **aerodontalgia** *The dental pain that occurs with low atmospheric pressure, like during airflight.* | aerodontalgia |
| **aerophagy or aerophagia** *A condition associated with hysteria in which one swallow repeatedly swallows air and then belches.* | aerofagia |
| **afebrile** *Absence of fever.* | afebbrile |
| **affect** *The expression of emotions or feelings.* | affetto |
| **affected** | affettato |
| **affective disorders** *Manic-depressive psychosis.* | psicosi affettivo |
| **afferent loop syndrome** *The obstruction of the duodenum or jejunum after gastrojejunostomy, resulting in duodenal distension.* | sindrome dell'ansa afferente |
| **afferent** *Moving toward the center.* | afferente |
| **affinity** *To have a natural liking for.* | affinità |
| **afibrinogenemia** *Marked deficiency of fibrinogen in the blood.* | afibrinogenemia |
| **aflatoxin** *A toxin produced by Aspergillus flavus.* | aflatossina |
| **after-load** *Referring to the amount of pressure the heart needs to pump against. If one has left heart failure it is beneficial to reduce after-load.* | post-carico |
| **after-pains** *The pain experienced after childbirth caused by uterine contractions.* | dolore del secondamento |
| **after-taste** *The sensation of a prolonged savor following eating/drinking.* | retrogusto |
| **afterbirth** *The tissue expelled after the birth of a child that includes the placenta and allied membranes.* | placenta (espulsa dopo il parto) |
| **agar** *Media used for bacterial cultures.* | agar |
| **age** *Length of life.* | età |
| **agenesis** *The absence of an organ. (cerebellar agenesis)* | agenesia |
| **agglutination** *The process of adherence of a mass.* | agglutinazione |
| **aggression** *Violent or hostile behavior.* | aggressione |
| **aging** *Becoming older.* | invecchiamento |
| **agitation** *A state of extreme emotional disturbance.* | agitazione |
| **aglutition** *The inability to swallow.* | afagia |
| **agnathia** *Congenital abnormality characterized by the absence of the mandible.* | agnazia |
| **agnosia** *A condition exhibited by the loss of sensory stimuli.* | agnosia |
| **agonist** *A synthetic compound that activates cells normally activated by natural chemicals.* | agonista |
| **agony** *Anguish or torment.* | agnoscia |
| **agoraphobia** *The fear of being in a large open space.* | agorafobia |
| **agranulocytosis** *A condition characterized by leukopenia and neutropenia.* | agranulocitosi |
| **agraphia** *The inability to express one's thoughts in writing.* | agrafia |
| **agreement** *Accordance in opinion or feeling.* | accordo |
| **ague** *A term used to describe recurrent fever and shivering typically associated with malaria.* | febbre malarica |
| **Aicardi syndrome** *A rare genetic anomaly in which the corpus callosum is absent or insufficient. It is characterized by seizures, microphthalmos, coloboma and developmental delays.* | sindrome di Aicardi |
| **AIDS** *Acquired Immunodeficiency Syndrome* | aids |
| **air** | aria |
| **air embolism** *The blockage of an artery or vein by an air bubble.* | embolia gassosa |

| English | Italian |
|---|---|
| **air flow** *The rate of air movement.* | ventilazione |
| **air hunger** *The sensation of shortness of breath.* | respiro di Kussmaul |
| **akathisia** *A condition exhibited by motor restlessness and inability to sit quietly.* | acatisia |
| **akinesia** *An absence of movement or sparsity of movement.* | acinesia |
| **akinesthesia** *Lack of perception of movement.* | acinestesia |
| **albinism** *Congenital absence of pigment in the eyes, skin and hair.* | albinismo |
| **albino** *A person who lacks pigment in the eyes, skin and hair.* | albino |
| **albumin** *A protein that is soluble in water and coagulates if heated.* | albumina |
| **albuminuria** *The presence of albumin in the urine.* | albuminuria |
| **alcohol** *Ethanol or ethyl alcohol.* | alcol |
| **alcoholic** *A person with alcohol dependence.* | alcolizzato |
| **alcoholism** *An addiction to alcohol.* | alcolismo |
| **aldehyde** *A substance derived by oxidizing and containing a CHO group from alcohol.* | aldeidico |
| **aldosterone** *A steroid secreted by the adrenal cortex that regulates electrolytes.* | aldosterone |
| **aldosteronism** *A condition characterized by the excessive secretion of aldosterone.* | aldosteronismo |
| **alert** *Being in a watchful, ready state.* | vigile |
| **alexia** *Inability to read due to a central brain lesion.* | alessia |
| **algae** *Nonflowering plants containing chlorophyll but without stems, roots, or leaves.* | alghe |
| **algid** *cold* | algida |
| **algophilia** *Sexual perversion; getting pleasure in giving or receiving pain.* | algofobia |
| **algorithm** *Any procedure designed to solve a problem in a step-by-step or mechanical fashion.* | algoritmo |
| **alimentary** *Referring to the gastrointestinal tract.* | alimentare |
| **alkali** *A class of compounds that form soluble carbonates.* | alcali |
| **alkaline** *Referring to something with properties of an alkali.* | alcalino |
| **alkalinuria** *The urine in an alkaline state.* | alcalinuria |
| **alkaloid** *Plant derived nitrogenous organic compound.* | alcaloide |
| **alkalosis** *A condition in which the pH is increased.* | alcalosis |
| **alkaptonuria** *A condition exhibited by the urine turning dark upon standing because of the presence of alkapton bodies in it.* | alcaptonuria |
| **allantois** *A posterior portion of the hind-gut of an embryo.* | allantoide |
| **allele** *A type of a gene; in humans there are two alleles per chromosome pair.* | allele |
| **allergen** *Compound that causes an allergic reaction.* | allergene |
| **allergy** *An immune response by the body to a compound it is hypersensitive to.* | allergia |
| **alleviate, to** | alleviare |
| **allograft** *A tissue transplant of from someone of the same species but different genotype.* | eterotrapianto |
| **allopathy** *Treatment of disease with minute amounts of natural substances.* | allopatia |
| **alopecia** *The absence of hair in areas where it normally exists.* | alopecia |
| **alpha wave** *Electroencephalographic waves with a frequency of 8-13 per second.* | onda Alfa |
| **alpha-fetoprotein** *A glycoprotein that has a high serum level in hepatocellular and nonseminomatous germ cell tumors.* | alfa-fetoproteina |
| **alteration** *The process of change or modification.* | modifica |

| English | Italian |
|---|---|
| **altitude sickness** *A general term used for an illness that occurs at high altitude.* | malattia di altitudine |
| **alveolar** *Referring to the alveolus.* | alveolare |
| **alveolus** *A small sac like structure commonly used for the pulmonary alveolus.* | alveolo |
| **Alzheimer's disease** *A dementia of unknown cause or pathogenesis.* | malattia di Alzheimer |
| **amalgam** *An alloy that includes mercury as one ingredient.* | amalgama |
| **amalgamate,to** *To make an amalgam by dissolving a metal in mercury.* | amalgamare |
| **amastia** *A development condition exhibited by the absence of breasts.* | amastia |
| **amaurosis** *Blindness that occurs without an ocular lesion but may include the optic nerve.* | amaurosi |
| **amaurosis fugax** *This transient monocular blindness is considered a sign of an impending stroke.* | amaurosi fugax |
| **amaurotic pupil** *A pupil that will not respond to light when directly exposed but will respond when the other eye is exposed to light.* | pupilla amaurotico |
| **ambidextrous** *Ability to use both hands equal ability.* | ambidestro |
| **ambisexual** *Referring to both sexes.* | ambisessuale |
| **amblyopia** *Decreased vision without an ocular lesion.* | ambliopia |
| **ambulation** *Relating to walking.* | passeggio |
| **ambulatory electrocardiographic monitoring** *A continuous recording of the electrocardiogram used to detect occult dysrhythmias.* | monitoraggio ambulatoriale electrocardiografico |
| **ameba** *A one-celled protozoan.* | ameba |
| **amebiasis** *A condition in which one is infected with amebae, mostly commonly Entamoeba histolytica.* | amebiasi |
| **amebic liver abscess** *A pus filled fluid collection within the liver caused by amoebe.* | ascesso epatico amebico |
| **amebicide** *A compound used to treat amebiasis.* | amebicida |
| **amelia** *A congenital anomaly exhibited by the absence of limbs.* | amelia |
| **ameliorate** *To make something better or to improve.* | migliorare |
| **amenorrhea** *The absence of menses.* | amenorrea |
| **amentia** *The absence of mental ability.* | amenza |
| **ametria** *Obsolete term for congenital uterine agenesis.* | ametra |
| **ametropia** *Abnormal refractive ability of the eyes resulting in hypermetropia, myopia or astigmatism.* | ametropia |
| **amino acid** *A compound containing a carboxyl and an amino group.* | amminoacido |
| **ammonia** *A colorless alkaline gas.* | ammoniaca |
| **amnesia** *The inability to remember past events.* | amnesia |
| **amnesia, antegrade** *The inability to remember events which occurred after the insult that caused the condition.* | amnesia anterograda |
| **amnesic stroke** *Cerebral infarct exhibited by loss of memory.* | ictus amnesico |
| **amniocentesis** *Transabdominal aspiration of amniotic fluid.* | amniocentesi |
| **amniography** *X-ray of the gravid uterus after insertion of opaque dye.* | amniografia |
| **amnion** *The membrane lining the placenta which produces the amniotic fluid.* | amnio |
| **amniotic fluid** *The fluid surrounding the fetus.* | liquido amniotico |
| **amorphus** *A fetus with no heart and no definitive shape.* | amorfo |
| **amount** *The total or the aggregate.* | quantità |
| **ampulla** *The dilated end of a duct.* | ampolla |
| **ampulla chyli** *Also called cisterna chyli; it is a dilated area of the thoracic duct that collects lymph from several areas.* | ampolla chyli |
| **amputation** *Typically referring to the surgical removal of a limb.* | amputazione |
| **amygdala** *Any almond shaped structure such as the tonsil* | mandorla |

| English | Italian |
|---|---|
| **amylase** *An enzyme involved in the hydrolysis of starch.* | amilase |
| **amyloidosis** *The accumulation of amyloid in body tissues.* | amiloidosi |
| **amyotonia** *A condition associated with the lack of muscle tone.* | amiotonia |
| **amyotrophic lateral sclerosis** *A progressive neurodegenerative disorder.* | sclerosi laterale amiotrofica |
| **amyotrophy** *Atrophy of muscle tissue.* | amiotrofia |
| **anabolism** *The formation of molecules in organisms from simpler molecules.* | anabolismo |
| **anacrotic** *Referring to a prominent bulge on the ascending portion of a pulse recording.* | anacroto |
| **anaerobe** *An organism that lives in the absence of oxygen.* | anaerobico |
| **anal** *Near or referring to the anus.* | anale |
| **anal fistula** *An opening in the skin that tracts to the anal canal thus causing some fecal material to leak from the opening in the skin.* | fistola anale |
| **analeptic** *A medication used as a stimulant to the central nervous system.* | analettico |
| **analgesia** *The absence of pain.* | analgesia |
| **analgesic** *A medication used to remove pain.* | analgesico |
| **analogous** *To resemble or be similar to.* | analogo |
| **anaphase** *A stage in mitosis following metaphase.* | anafase |
| **anaphoresis** *Reduced activity of the sweat glands.* | anforesi |
| **anaphylaxis** *An exaggerated response to a foreign substance.* | anafilassi |
| **anaplasia** *The loss of normal differentiation of tumor cells.* | anaplasia |
| **anastomosis** *Surgical formation of a connection between two previously separate parts.* | anastomosi |
| **anatomical chart** *A pictorial diagram of part of the anatomy.* | diagramma anatomico |
| **anatomical dead space** *The area between the mouth and pulmonary alveoli.* | spazio morto anatomico |
| **anatomical** *Referring to the anatomy.* | anatomico |
| **anatomical snuff-box** *The area on the back of the hand near the base of the thumb that is between the extensor pollicis longus and extensor pollicis brevis.* | tabacchiera anatomica |
| **anatomy** *The study of body structure.* | anatomia |
| **ancylostomiasis** *A type of nematode parasite, also called hookworm.* | anchilostomiasi |
| **androgen** *A compound that produces masculinizing characteristics.* | androgeno |
| **androgynous** *Referring to a female pseudohermaphroditism (a genetic female with masculine characteristics).* | androgino |
| **android pelvis** *A pelvis shaped like a man's.* | pelvi maschile |
| **androsterone** *A hormone excreted in the urine of men and women.* | androsterone |
| **anemia** *Lower than normal red blood cell count.* | anemia |
| **anencephaly** *The congenital absence of the cranial vault and cerebral hemispheres.* | anencefalia |
| **aneroid** *The absence of liquid.* | aneroide |
| **anesthesia** *Loss of sensation.* | anestesia |
| **anesthetic** *A chemical that produces anesthesia.* | anestetico |
| **anesthetist** *A person who administers anesthesia.* | anestetista |
| **aneurysm** *A condition exhibited by the dilatation of the walls of an artery or vein to form a blood-filled sac.* | aneurisma |
| **angiectasia** *Dilation of a blood or lymph vessel.* | telangiectasia |
| **angina pectoris** *Exercise induced myocardial ischemia.* | angina pectoris |
| **angioedema** *Also called angioneurotic edema, it is caused by a histamine reaction. It can produce welts in mild cases but in severe cases can cause swelling of the lips and tongue.* | angioedema; edema angioneurotico |

| English | Italian |
|---|---|
| **angiogram** *Radiologic imaging of blood vessels.* | angiogramma |
| **angiography** *Roentgenographic imaging of blood vessels.* | angiografia |
| **angioma** *A tumor comprised of blood or lymph vessels.* | angioma |
| **angioneurotic** *Caused by a neurosis affecting the blood vessels, like vasospasm.* | angioneurotico |
| **angioneurotic edema** *A condition exhibited by sudden edema of skin and mucous membranes.* | edema angioneurotico |
| **angioplasty** *Surgical alteration of blood vessels.* | angioplastica |
| **angiosarcoma** *A sarcoma comprised of blood vessels.* | angiosarcoma |
| **angiospasm** *A spasm of a blood vessel.* | angiospasmo |
| **angiotensin** *A blood protein that increases aldosterone secretion.* | angiotensina |
| **angiotensin converting enzyme inhibitors (ACEI)** *A class of medicines that prevent conversion of angiotensin I to angiotensin II, a potent vasoconstrictor.* | inibitore dell'enzima convertitore dell'angiotensina |
| **angitis or angiitis** *The inflammation of a lymph or blood vessel.* | angioite |
| **anguish** *Significant mental or physical pain.* | angoscia |
| **anhidrosis** *A condition exhibited by reduced quantity of sweat.* | anidrosi |
| **anhidrotic** *Something the reduces the quantity of sweat.* | anidrotico |
| **anhydrous** *Lacking water.* | anidro |
| **aniseikonia** *A condition in which the ocular image of an object is viewed differently by each eye.* | aniseiconia |
| **anisocoria** *Pupillary diameter inequality.* | anisocoria |
| **anisocytosis** *Variation in size of erythrocytes.* | anisocitosi |
| **anisomelia** *Unequal size of arms or legs.* | anisomelia |
| **anisometropia** *Refractive power inequality between the two eyes.* | anisometropia |
| **ankle** *The area of the ankle joint.* | caviglia |
| **ankle clonus** *An abnormal response exhibited by alternating plantar- and dorsiflexion noted after the examiner rapidly dorsiflexes the foot.* | clono del piede |
| **ankle edema or dependent edema** *Extracellular fluid volume noted by swelling or pitting.* | edema caviglia |
| **ankle joint** *The articulation of the tibia/fibula and talus.* | articolazioine tibioastragalica |
| **ankle support** *A mechanical device or banding to support the ankle.* | sostegno caviglia |
| **ankle swelling** *Enlargement of the ankle region with or without pitting.* | gonfiore caviglia |
| **ankyloglossia** *Limitation of tongue motion because of a short frenulum.* | anchiloglossia |
| **ankylosing spondylitis** *A type of arthritis found in the spine that is exhibited by bony fusion.* | spondilite anchilosante |
| **ankylosis** *Abnormal immobility of a joint.* | anchilosi |
| **annular** *Referring to a ring.* | anulare |
| **anomia** *Inability to name or recognize familiar objects.* | afasia anomica |
| **anonychia** *Congenital absence of fingernails or toenails.* | anonichia |
| **anoperineal** *Referring to the anus and perineum.* | ano-perianale |
| **anorchous** *The absence of testicles.* | anorchidismo |
| **anorectal** *Referring to the anus and rectum.* | anorettale |
| **anorexia nervosa** *A mental disorder characterized by the desire to avoid eating and to lose weight.* | nervosa anoressia |
| **anorexia** *The loss of appetite.* | anoressia |
| **anorrectal abscess** *A localized collection of pus in the anorrectal region.* | accesso anorettale |
| **anosmia** *Lack of the sense of smell.* | afasia anosmica |
| **anovulatory** *Lack of ovulation.* | anovulazione |
| **anovulatory cycle** *A menstrual cycle in which no ovum is released.* | ciclo anovulare |
| **anoxemia** *Reduction in blood oxygen concentration.* | anossiemia |

| English | Italian |
|---|---|
| **anoxia** *Reduced oxygen levels in body tissues.* | anossia |
| **antacid** *A medication, usually with a calcium or magnesium base that binds with acid in the stomach.* | antiacido |
| **antagonist** *A muscle or agent that acts in counteract to effects of another muscle or agent.* | antagonista |
| **antiemetic** *A medication used to control nausea.* | antiemetico |
| **antemortem** *Refers to: before death.* | prima della morte |
| **antenatal** *Refers to events before birth.* | antepartum |
| **anterior root** *A motor nerve root that is in the anterior part of the spinal cord between the anterior and lateral funiculi.* | fascio anteriore |
| **anterior** *Toward the front.* | anteriore |
| **anterograde** *Moving forward.* | anterogrado |
| **anteroinferior** *Toward the front and lower part.* | anteroinferiore |
| **anterolateral** *Toward the front and away from the midline.* | anterolaterale |
| **anteromedian** *Toward the front and toward the midline.* | anteromediana |
| **anteroposterior** *From front to the back. (An AP x-ray has the beam directed from the front to the back.)* | anteroposteriore |
| **anterosuperior** *Toward the front and the upper part.* | anterosuperiore |
| **anteversion** *The forward leaning of an organ.* | antiversione |
| **anthelmintic** *An agent used to destroy worms.* | antelmintico; vermifugo |
| **anthracosis** *Pneumoconiosis caused by coal dust.* | pneumoconiosi |
| **anthrax** *An infectious disease caused by Bacillus anthracis; there are cutaneous, inhalation and gastrointestinal syndromes.* | antrace |
| **anti-inflammatory** *Medication used to reduce inflammation.* | antiinfiammatorio |
| **antibiotic** *A medication that inhibits or kills microorganisms.* | antibiotico |
| **antibody** *A protein that combines with and counteracts foreign substances.* | anticorpo |
| **anticholinergic** *Parasympathetic blocker.* | anticolinergico |
| **anticholinesterase** *Cholinesterase blocker.* | anticolinesterasi |
| **anticoagulant** *Medication used to inhibit coagulation.* | anticoagulante |
| **anticodon** *A series of three nucleotides that form a unit of genetic code for transfer RNA.* | anticodon |
| **anticonvulsant** *Medication used to treat seizures.* | anticonvulsivante |
| **antidepressant** *Medication used to treat depression.* | antidepressivo |
| **antidiuretic hormone** *Vasopressin.* | ormone antidiuretico |
| **antidote** *A medication that neutralizes a toxin.* | antidoto |
| **antigen** *A foreign substance, like bacteria, that induces an immune response.* | antigene |
| **antiglobulin test (Coombs' test)** *Test used to detect erythroblastosis fetalis.* | test di Coomb |
| **antihemophilic factor** *Also called factor VIII. A deficiency of the factor causes hemophilia.* | fattore antiemofilico |
| **antihistamine** *Medication used to treat conditions exhibited by a histamine response* | antiistamina |
| **antilymphocyte** *A serum globulin that has antibodies to lymphocytes.* | antilinfocito |
| **antilymphocyte globulin** *The gamma globulin portion of antilymphocyte serum.* | globulina antilinfocito |
| **antimalarial** *Medication used to treat malaria.* | antimalariale |
| **antimetabolite** *A substance that impedes metabolism.* | antimetabolita |
| **antimigraine** *Medication used to treat headaches.* | antiemicrania |
| **antimitotic** *Impeding mitosis.* | antimitotico |
| **antimycotic** *Inhibition of fungal growth.* | antimicotico |

| English | Italian |
|---|---|
| **antinuclear factor** *Also called antinucleic antibody (ANA); it is found in conditions such as lupus and rheumatoid arthritis.* | fattore antinucleare |
| **antiperistaltic** *An agent that impedes normal peristalsis.* | antiperistaltico |
| **antipruritic** *Medication used to treat pruritus.* | antiprurito |
| **antipyretic** *Medication used to treat fever.* | antipiretico |
| **antiseptic** *A substance that inhibits microorganism growth.* | antisettico |
| **antiserum** *A substance that contains antibodies to specific antigens.* | antisiero |
| **antispasmodic** *Medication used to treat muscle spasm.* | antispastico |
| **antithrombin** *A substance that inhibits thrombin, thus decreasing the body's ability to coagulate.* | antitrombina |
| **antithyroid** *A substance inhibiting the effect of the thyroid.* | antitiroide |
| **antitoxin** *A substance that inhibits the effect of a toxin.* | antitossina |
| **antitussive** *Medication used to diminish a cough.* | antitosse |
| **antivenin** *An antitoxin formulated for various types of snake bites.* | antiveleno |
| **antrotomy** *To cut open the antrum.* | antrotomia |
| **antrum** *Referring to a cavity or chamber.* | antro |
| **anuria** *The lack of urine excretion.* | anuria |
| **anus** *The body opening distal to the rectum.* | ano |
| **anxiety** *Nervousness or unease.* | ansia |
| **anxiety neurosis** *Abnormal presence of anxiety.* | neurosi d'ansia |
| **anxious** *Experiencing nervousness or unease.* | ansioso |
| **aorta** *The large artery originating at the left ventricle and going to the pelvis where it bifurcates.* | aorta |
| **aortic insufficiency** *A dysfunction of the aortic valve allowing backflow of blood into the heart.* | insufficienza aortico |
| **aortic** *Referring to the aorta.* | aortico |
| **aortic stenosis** *Narrowing of the aortic orifice.* | stenosi valvolare aortica |
| **aortic valve** *The valve situated between the left ventricle and the aorta.* | valvola aortica |
| **apart** *Separated by a distance.* | in disparte |
| **apathy** *Lack of interest in one's environment or indifference.* | apatia |
| **aperistalsis** *Lack of intestinal peristalsis.* | mancanza di peristalsi |
| **aperture** *An opening or hole, as in the hole the light passes through in a camera.* | apertura |
| **apex** *The highest point of something.* | apice |
| **apex of heart** *Normally found 8cm to the left of the midsternal line in the 5th intercostal space.* | apice cardiaco |
| **Apgar score** *A scoring system for newborns that utilizes heart rate, respiratory effort, muscle tone, responsiveness and skin color.* | Punteggio di Apgar |
| **aphagia** *The lack of eating.* | afagia |
| **aphakia** *The congenital absence of the lens of the eye.* | afachia |
| **aphasia** *Diminished ability to communicate via speech or writing.* | afasia |
| **aphid** *A minute insect that feeds on plants.* | afide |
| **aphonia** *The loss of voice.* | afonia |
| **aphthous stomatitis** *Grouped small lesions that occur on the tongue or in the mouth.* | stomatite aftosa |
| **apicectomy** *Removal of the apex of the petrous portion of the temporal bone.* | apicectomia |
| **aplastic anemia** *Bone marrow failure causing a decrease in all types of blood cells.* | anemia aplastica |
| **apnea** *Absence of respiration.* | apnea |
| **apocrine gland** *A gland that releases some of its cytoplasm in secretions; an example is axillary sweat glands.* | ghiandola sudoripara |

| English | Italian |
|---|---|
| **aponeurosis** *A tendinous expansion that connects with muscle to move a part.* | aponeurosi |
| **apophysis** *Generally a bony outgrowth that forms a process or tubercle.* | apofisi |
| **apoplexy** *Extravasation of blood within an organ. For example, neonatal apoplexy is consistent with intracranial hemorrhage.* | apoplexy |
| **appearance** *The way someone looks or presents.* | aspetto |
| **appendectomy** *Surgical excision of the appendix.* | appendicectomia |
| **appendicitis** *Inflammation of the appendix.* | appendicite |
| **appendix** *An appendage of the cecum.* | appendice |
| **apperception** *The ability to interpret sensory impressions.* | appercezione |
| **application** *The forms one fills out to obtain a grant.* | modulo di domanda |
| **applicator** *A device used to apply a topical medication.* | applicatore |
| **appointment** *A previously scheduled time to see a person.* | appuntamento |
| **apprehensive** *A fear that something unpleasant will happen.* | apprensivo |
| **approval** *Accepting something as satisfactory.* | approvazione |
| **approximate** *Nearly but not totally accurate.* | approssimativo |
| **approximate, to** *To bring together, as in wound margins.* | approssimarsi |
| **approximately** *Nearly but not completely.* | approssimativamente |
| **apraxia** *The inability to carry out intentional movements when paralysis is not present.* | aprassia |
| **apt** *Suitable in the circumstances.* | appropriato |
| **aptitude** *A natural talent for something.* | attitudine |
| **aptyalism** *Diminished or absence of saliva.* | aptialismo |
| **acquaint, to** *To make someone familiar with something.* | conoscere |
| **aqueous humor** *The fluid between the cornea and lens, anterior to the globe.* | umore acqueo |
| **aqueous** *Use of water as a solvent or medium.* | acqueo |
| **arachnodactyly** *A condition exhibited by abnormally long and slender fingers.* | aracnodattilia |
| **arachnoid** *Refers to that which resembles a spider web.* | aracnoide |
| **arbovirus** *Virus that is transmitted by arthropods; responsible for diseases such as Yellow fever and dengue fever.* | arbovirus |
| **arcuate nucleus** *Small masses of gray matter found on the medulla oblongata.* | nucleo arcuato |
| **arcus** *Narrow opaque band.* | arco |
| **areola** *The pigmented skin surrounding a nipple.* | areola |
| **argininosuccinicaciduria** *Presence of arginosuccinic acid in the urine; associated with mental retardation.* | argininosuccinicadiduria |
| **argue, to** *To debate or reason. (quarrel)* | sostenere |
| **Argyll Robertson symptom** *Presence of small pupils that do not react to light but will constrict when the person focuses on a near object.* | segno di Argyll-Robertson |
| **argyria** *The greyish discoloration of the skin and conjunctiva.* | argiria |
| **arm** *One of two upper extremities.* | braccio |
| **armpit** *A common term for axilla.* | ascella |
| **around** *On every side of.* | intorno |
| **arousal reaction** *The change in brain wave patterns upon awakening.* | reazione di risveglio |
| **arrhenoblastoma** *An ovarian tumor that results in masculine secondary sex characteristics.* | arrenoblastoma |
| **arrhythmia** *An abnormal heart rhythm.* | aritmia |
| **arterial blood gas** *Measurement of the arterial concentration of carbon dioxide and oxygen.* | gas ematici arterioso |
| **arterial** *Referring to an artery.* | arterioso |

| English | Italian |
|---|---|
| **arteriectomy** *Surgical excision of an artery.* | arteriectomia |
| **arteriography** *Roentgenography of an artery after infusion of contrast media.* | arteriografia |
| **arterioplasty** *Surgical repair of an artery.* | arterioplastica |
| **arteriosclerosis** *Hardening and thickening of arterial walls.* | arteriosclerosi |
| **arteriotomy** *Creation of an opening in an artery.* | arteriotomia |
| **arteriovenous malformation** *A sac like structure created by the abnormal communication of an adjacent artery and vein.* | malformazione arterovenoso |
| **arteritis** *Inflammation of an artery.* | arterite |
| **artery** *Vessel that carries oxygenated blood from the heart to the periphery.* | arteria |
| **arthralgia** *Joint pain.* | artralgia |
| **arthritis** *Joint inflammation.* | artrite |
| **arthrodesis** *Surgical fusion of a joint.* | artrodesi |
| **arthrodynia** *Joint pain.* | artralgia |
| **arthrography** *Joint roentgenography.* | artrografia |
| **arthroplasty** *Plastic surgery involving a joint.* | artroplastica |
| **arthroscopy** *Viewing of the inside of a joint with a specially designed scope.* | artroscopia |
| **arthrotomy** *Surgical opening of a joint.* | artrotomia |
| **articular** *Referring to a joint.* | articolare |
| **artifact** *An aberration from the normal.* | artefatto |
| **artificial** *Not natural produced.* | artificiale |
| **arytenoid** *Referring to the cartilage in the posterior larynx.* | cartilagine aritenoide |
| **asbestos** *A heat resistant silicate material.* | amianto |
| **asbestosis** *Lung disease caused by the inhalation of asbestos.* | asbestosi |
| **ascaricide** *Agent that destroys ascaris.* | trattamento per ascariasi |
| **ascaris** *A nematode from genus intestinal lumbricoid parasite, also called round worm.* | ascaris lumbricoides |
| **ascending colon** *The portion of the colon between the cecum and the right colic flexure.* | colon ascendente |
| **ascertain, to** *Synonym of "to determine".* | appurare |
| **ascites** *Serous fluid in the abdominal cavity.* | ascite |
| **ascorbic acid** *Commonly known as vitamin C; a deficiency of this vitamin causes scurvy.* | acido ascorbico |
| **asepsis** *Lack of infection.* | asepsi |
| **aseptic** *Being free of septic matter.* | asettico |
| **asexual** *Without sex or sex organs.* | asessuale |
| **asleep** *To be in a dormant or inactive state.* | addormentato |
| **Asperger's syndrome** *A condition characterized by disturbed social interaction; if was named after the Austrian scientist who first described it.* | sindrome di Asperger |
| **aspermia** *Absence of sperm.* | aspermatismo |
| **asphyxia** *A condition exhibited by a lack of oxygen and subsequent loss of consciousness or death.* | asfissia |
| **aspiration biopsy** *Removal of fluid from a cavity for pathologic analysis.* | biopsia per aspirazione |
| **aspiration pneumonia** *Taking air or matter into the lungs.* | polmonite aspirazione |
| **aspirator** *A device used to remove fluid from a cavity.* | aspiratore |
| **aspirin** *Common name for acetylsalicylic acid.* | aspirina |
| **assay** *A procedure for measuring the activity of a biological sample.* | saggio; prova |
| **assessment** *An medical evaluation.* | valutazione medica |
| **assistance** *The act of helping.* | assistenza |

| English | Italian |
|---|---|
| **assisted ventilation** *The act of helping one breathe through artificial means.* | ventilazione meccanica assistita |
| **asteatosis** *A condition exhibited by diminished sebaceous secretion.* | asteatosi |
| **astereognosis** *Lack of ability to recognize objects by touching them.* | astereognosi |
| **asterixis** *Commonly known as a flapping tremor, it is characterized by involuntary jerking movements of the hands and is seen commonly in hepatic encephalopathy.* | asterissi |
| **asthenia** *Diminished strength and energy.* | astenia |
| **asthenopia** *Visual fatigue accompanied by ocular pain.* | astenopia |
| **astragalus** *Synonym of talus.* | astragalo |
| **astringent** *An agent causing contraction of the skin.* | astringente |
| **astrocytoma** *A tumor comprised of astrocytes.* | astrocitoma |
| **astroglia** *The neurologic tissue which is composed of astrocytes.* | macroglia |
| **asymmetry** *Lack of symmetry.* | asimmetria |
| **asymptomatic** *The absence of symptoms.* | asintomatico |
| **asynclitism** *Oblique presentation of the head during delivery.* | asinclitismo |
| **at random** *Occurring by chance alone.* | a caso |
| **atavism** *The inheritance of characteristics from remote rather than immediate ancestors.* | atavismo |
| **ataxia** *Lack of muscular coordination.* | atassia |
| **atelectasis** *Incomplete expansion or collapse of a lung.* | atelectasia |
| **atherogenic** *Something that causes atheromatous lesions in arterial walls.* | aterogenico |
| **atheroma** *Degenerative arteriosclerosis.* | ateroma |
| **athetosis** *An involuntary symptom exhibited by continuous slow, writhing movements, mostly in the hands.* | atetosi |
| **athlete's foot** *Common term for tinea pedis.* | piede d'atleta |
| **atlas** *The first cervical vertebra.* | atlante |
| **atomizer** *A device for propelling a fine mist.* | atomizzatore |
| **atony** *Absence of normal muscle tone.* | atonia |
| **atresia** *Closure of a body orifice as in atresia ani in which there is a congenital imperforate anus.* | atresia |
| **atrial flutter** *Sawtooth waves on an electrocardiogram with atrial rate of 250-330 per minute.* | flutter atriale |
| **atrial natriuretic factor** *A chemical secreted by the right atrium that promotes sodium excretion in the urine.* | fattore natriuretico atriale |
| **atrial** *Referring to the atrium.* | atriale |
| **atrial septal defect** *An abnormal communication between the atria of the heart.* | difetto del setto atriale |
| **atrio-ventricular block** *An interruption of the electrical conduction at the atrio-ventricular node.* | blocco atrioventricolare |
| **atrioventricular bundle** *Also called bundle of His.* | fascio di His |
| **atrioventricular** *Referring to the atrium and ventricle.* | atrioventricolare |
| **atrium** *Referring to a chamber used as an entrance, as in the entrance to the heart.* | atrio |
| **atrophic** *Referring to atrophy.* | atrofico |
| **atrophy** *A diminution in the size of a part.* | atrofia |
| **atropine** *A parasympathetic agent derived from Atropa belladonna.* | atropina |
| **attack** *A fit or paroxysm.* | parossismo |
| **atypical** *Not usual.* | atipico |
| **audiogram** *The recording of a one's hearing in decibels.* | audiogramma |
| **audiologist** *A specialist in the field of hearing.* | audiologo |
| **audiometer** *A device used to measure hearing.* | audiometro |

| English | Italian |
|---|---|
| **auditory** *Referring to hearing.* | acustico |
| **auditory agnosia** *Caused by a temporal lobe lesion, it is characterized by inability to recognize sounds as words.* | agnosia acustico |
| **aural** *Referring to the ear.* | dell'orecchio |
| **auricle** *The external portion of the ear.* | auricola |
| **auricular** *Referring to the auricle.* | auricolare |
| **auriculotemporal** *The area of the ear and temple.* | auricolotemporale |
| **auscultation** *The act of listening to sounds emanating from the body.* | auscultazione |
| **autism** *A mental condition exhibited by difficulty in forming relationships, communicating and uses abstract thought.* | autismo |
| **autistic** *Referring to autism.* | autistico |
| **autoantibody** *An antibody that acts against the organism's own tissue.* | autoanticorpo |
| **autoantigen** *A normal tissue constituent that prompts a cell-mediated response.* | autoantigene |
| **autoclave** *A device used for sterilization with the use of steam under pressure.* | autoclave |
| **autogenous** *Self-generated.* | autogeno |
| **autograft** *Grafting tissue from one part of person to another part of the same person.* | innesto autogeno |
| **autohypnosis** *Self-hypnosis.* | autoipnosi |
| **autoimmunization** *The body's ability to promote an immune response without external resources.* | autoimmunizzazione |
| **autolysis** *A state of self destruction of cells within a body.* | autolisi |
| **autonomic nervous system** *Responsible for regulation of cardiac muscle, smooth muscle and glandular activity.* | sistema nervoso autonomo |
| **autopsy** *Examination of a body post-mortem in an attempt to determine cause of death.* | autopsia |
| **autosomal** *Referring to an autosome.* | autosomico |
| **autotransfusion** *The reinfusion of one's own blood.* | autotransfusione |
| **availability** *A person or thing that is available.* | disponibilità |
| **available** *Attainable, obtainable.* | disponibile |
| **avascular** *An area with no blood supply.* | non vascolare |
| **avascular necrosis** *Bone death caused by poor blood supply.* | necrosi avascolare |
| **avian flu** *A viral disease found in birds and fowl that can be transmitted to humans; it is exhibited by respiratory and gastrointestinal symptoms but can lead to encephalitis.* | influenza aviaria |
| **avian** *Referring to birds.* | aviaria |
| **avitaminosis** *A state of vitamin deficiency.* | avitaminosi |
| **avoidable** *That which can be stopped or inhibited.* | evitabile |
| **awakening** *The state of being conscious.* | risveglio |
| **away from** *Separated from.* | iontano da |
| **axilla** *The hollow beneath the arm.* | ascella |
| **axillary** *Referring to the axilla.* | ascellare |
| **axis** *The second cervical vertebra.* | seconda vertebra cervicale |
| **axon** *The structure along which nerve impulses are transmitted from the cell body to other cells.* | assone |
| **azo itch** *A pruritus noted in people who use azo dyes.* | prurito azo |
| **azoospermia** *The absence of spermatozoa in the semen.* | azoospermia |
| **Azorean disease** *A form of hereditary ataxia found in peoples of Azorean descent. Also called Machado-Joseph disease or Portuguese-Azorean disease.* | malattia delle Azzorre |
| **azotemia** *Prerenal disease.* | azotemia |

| English | Italian |
|---|---|
| **azoturia** *An excess of urea in the urine.* | azoturia |
| **Babinski's sign** *A reflex that occurs when the plantar surface of the foot is stimulated. The great toe turns upward- normal in infancy but when it turns upward in an adult it means there is central nervous system injury.* | segno di Babinski |
| **baby** *A newborn.* | neonato |
| **baby-scale** *A device used to weigh an infant.* | bilance neonati |
| **bacillary** *Referring to bacilli.* | bacillare |
| **bacillus** *A rod-shaped bacterium.* | bacillo |
| **back pain** *Discomfort on the dorsal surface of the torso.* | dorsalgia |
| **bacteremia** *The presence of bacteria in the blood.* | batteriemia |
| **bacteria** *Plural for any organism of the order Eubacteriales.* | batterio |
| **bacterial** *Referring to bacteria.* | batterico |
| **bactericidal** *An agent that destroys bacteria.* | battericida |
| **bacteriostatic** *An agent that impedes bacterial growth.* | batteriostatico |
| **bacteriuria** *The presence of bacteria in the urine.* | batteriuria |
| **bagassosis** *A pulmonary disorder contracted from inhalation of the waste of sugar cane (bagasse dust).* | bagassosi |
| **Bainbridge reflex** *Increase in heart rate due to increased pressure in the right atrium.* | riflesso Bainbridge |
| **Baker cyst** *A synovial fluid collection in the popliteal fossa.* | cisti poplitea |
| **balanitis** *Inflammation of the glans of the penis.* | balanite |
| **ballottement** *Presence of movement of a floating object by palpation.* | ballottamento |
| **balm** *A topical medical preparation.* | balsamo |
| **bandage** *A strip of gauze used to immobilize or support.* | banda |
| **banding** *The process of encircling with a thin piece of material.* | bendaggio |
| **barber's itch** *Ringworm that is transmitted by contaminated shaving equipment.* | tinea barbae |
| **barium enema** *Administration of barium into the rectum followed by roentgenography to check for rectal or colon abnormalities.* | clisma baritato |
| **Barretts's esophagus** *A condition characterized by varying degrees of esophageal injury from gastric acid.* | esofago di Barrett |
| **Bartholin's cyst or abscess** *This is a purulent fluid collection in the Bartholin cysts which are located in the perivaginal area.* | cisti Bartholin |
| **Bartter's syndrome** *An autosomal recessive renal disorder with a defect in chloride reabsorption and secondary hyperaldosteronism.* | sindrome di Bartter |
| **basal ganglia** *Structures adjacent to the thalamus that are involved with coordination of movement.* | gangli basale |
| **basal** *Referring to the base.* | basale |
| **basilar** *Referring to the base or lower segment.* | basilare |
| **basilic vein** *A vein in the hand that joins the brachial veins to form the axillary vein.* | vena basilica |
| **basin** *A small bowl used for washing.* | bacino |
| **basophil** *A polymorphonuclear granulocyte.* | basofilo |
| **bear, to** *To endure or resist.* | supportare |
| **bear, to** *To give birth to a child.* | dare alla luce |
| **bearing down** *As in during labor.* | espulsivo |
| **beat** *As in heart beat.* | battito |
| **Bechterew-Mendel reflex** *Plantar flexion of the toes when the examiner percusses the dorsum of the foot; seen with pyramidal lesion.* | riflesso Bechterew-Mendel |
| **bed** *A mattress resting on a frame.* | letto |
| **bed rest** *A medical order requiring one to stay in bed.* | sostegno per ammalati allettati |

| English | Italian |
|---|---|
| **bedbug Cimex lectularius**. *A small insect that is parasitic and hides in clothing or bedding.* | Cimex lectularius; cimice |
| **bedpan** *A metal or plastic vestibule one sits on while in bed to defecate.* | padella da letto |
| **bedridden** *Term used to indicate one is so ill they cannot get out of bed.* | allettato |
| **bee sting** *A piercing from a bee.* | puntura di api |
| **beforehand** *In advance or previously.* | prematuro |
| **behavior disorder** *An abnormal mental state.* | malattia mentale |
| **Behçet syndrome** *Characterized by recurrent oral and genital ulcers, uveitis, iridocyclitis and frequently arthritis.* | sindrome di Behcet |
| **Bell's palsy** *Unilateral facial paralysis related to dysfunction of the seventh cranial nerve.* | paralisi di Bell |
| **below** *Under.* | sotto |
| **belt** *A strap used to hold clothing up.* | cintura |
| **benign** *Not harmful.* | benigno |
| **bereavement** *The sorrow one feels with the loss of a loved one.* | lutto |
| **berylliosis** *A lung exhibited by granulomas and caused by inhalation of beryllium.* | berilliosi |
| **best** *Optimal or ideal.* | migliore |
| **betablocker** *A substance that inhibits adrenergic stimulation. It is used to reduce pulse, blood pressure and to treat angina.* | beta-bloccante |
| **beyond** *On the farther side.* | oltre |
| **bezoar** *A concretion composed of either hair, vegetable/fruit fibers or hair and vegetable/fruit fibers that is found in the stomach.* | bezoar |
| **Bezold-Jarisch reflex** *A reflex in the vagus, originating in the heart, resulting in sinus bradycardia, hypotension and peripheral vasodilation.* | riflesso Bezold-Jarisch |
| **biased** *Prejudiced.* | fare inclinare |
| **biceps** *A muscle with two heads usually referring to the biceps brachii which is used for forearm flexion.* | muscolo bicipite |
| **biceps reflex** *The biceps brachii tendon is hit with a reflex hammer and results in flexion of the forearm as a normal response. This assesses the C5-C6 region.* | riflesso bicipite |
| **bicuspid** *Having two points as in bicuspid valve or a premolar tooth.* | bicuspide |
| **bifid** *Presence of two branches.* | bifido |
| **bifurcate ligament** *A ligament on the dorsum of the foot that includes the calcaneonavicular and calcaneocuboid ligaments.* | legamento biforcuto |
| **bifurcate** *When one branch divides into two branches.* | biforcuto |
| **bilateral** *Referring to both sides.* | bilaterale |
| **bile** *An alkaline fluid secreted by the liver to aid digestion.* | bile |
| **bile ducts** *The structures that are conduits for passage of bile from the liver and gallbladder to the duodenum.* | dotti biliari |
| **bile pigments** *The golden brown or green-yellow color associated with bile.* | pigmenti biliari |
| **bile salts** *Normally occurring salts of bile acids.* | salato biliari |
| **Bilharzia** *Historical name of a genus of flukes or nematodes now known as Schistosoma.* | schistosoma |
| **biliary** *Referring to bile, bile ducts or gallbladder.* | biliare |
| **bilious** *Something that contains bile.* | bilioso |
| **bilirubin** *A pigment found in bile that is responsible for the yellow color seen in patients with elevated serum levels of bilirubin.* | bilirubina |
| **biliuria** *The presence of bile in the urine.* | biliuria |
| **biliverdin** *A green pigment formed by oxidation of bilirubin.* | biliverdina |
| **bill** *A financial statement that indicates how much one owes.* | conto |

| English | Italian |
|---|---|
| **Bill maneuver** *During childbirth, use of forceps at midpelvis to help extract the head.* | manovra di Bill |
| **bimanual** *Use of two hands, as in bimanual pelvic examination in which the right hand touches the cervix uteri and the left hand presses above the mons pubis.* | bimanuale |
| **binaural** *Referring to both ears.* | biauricolare |
| **binocular** *Referring to both eyes.* | binoculare |
| **binovular** *Derived from two different ova.* | biovulare |
| **bioassay** *A laboratory test determination as compared to normal.* | saggio biologico |
| **bioavailability** *The portion of a drug that is able to be utilized by the body after it is introduced to the body.* | biodisponibilità |
| **biochemistry** *The study of chemistry and physiochemical processes in living organisms.* | biochimica |
| **biology** *The study of living organisms.* | biologia |
| **biopsy** *The removal and examination of bodily tissues or fluids.* | biopsia |
| **biotin** *A vitamin involved in the synthesis of fatty acids and glucose.* | biotina |
| **birth** *The process of bearing offspring from the uterus.* | nascita |
| **birth control** *Any method of limiting contraception.* | contraccezione; controllo delle nascite |
| **birth defect** *A congenital anomaly.* | difetto congenito |
| **birth rate** *The number of live births per 1000 of a given population per year.* | tasso di natalità |
| **bistoury; scalpel** *A surgical knife.* | bisturi |
| **bitemporal hemianopsia** *A visual defect seen commonly in pituitary tumors in which the visual defect is in the temporal portion of each eye.* | emianopsia bitemporale |
| **bitter (taste)** *Having a harsh, unpleasant taste.* | amaro |
| **black** *Referring to the color, as in the color of coal.* | nero |
| **black fly** *From the family Simuliidae, a gnat that can cause disease in humans; also called buffalo fly.* | mosca nera |
| **black stools** *Common term for melena.* | feci nere |
| **blackout** *Common term for loss of consciousness.* | lipotimia momentanea da brusca |
| **blackwater fever** *A term used to describe the fever associated with malaria when the urine is reddish-black.* | febbre dell'ematuria |
| **bladder, urinary** *Vestibule for urine prior to being expelled via the urethra.* | vescica urinaria |
| **blast injury** *Trauma from a wave of air pressure.* | lesione da scoppio |
| **blastomycosis** *Infection caused by organisms of genus Blastomyces.* | blastomicosi |
| **bleach** *A solution that includes sodium hypochlorite.* | candeggina |
| **bleeding** *Loss of blood.* | emorragia |
| **bleeding time** *The time of bleeding after a controlled standardized puncture of the earlobe.* | tempo di emorragia |
| **blemish** *A small mark on one's skin.* | macchia |
| **blennorrhea** *Discharge from the mucous membranes, usually referring to gonorrhea.* | blenorragia |
| **blepharitis** *Inflammation of the eyelids.* | blefarite |
| **blepharospasm** *A spasm of the orbicularis oculi muscle that causes closure of the eyelid.* | blefarospasmo |
| **blind** *Absence of sight.* | cieco |
| **blind loop syndrome** *A condition in which there is a non-functional section of the bowel that is thought to be responsible for malabsorption and Vitamin B12 deficiency.* | sindrome dell'ansa cieca |
| **blind spot** *An area of insensitivity to light located at the point of entry of the optic nerve on the retina.* | punto cieco |

| English | Italian |
|---|---|
| **blindness** *Absence of visual perception.* | cecità |
| **blinking** *To open and close the eyelid rapidly.* | ammiccamento |
| **blister** *Common term for bulla.* | vescicola; bolla |
| **bloated** *Sensation of having an abnormally large amount of air in the viscera.* | rigonfio |
| **Boerhaave Syndrome** *Rupture of the esophagus from vigorous vomiting, with resultant mediastinitis.* | sindrome di Boerhaave |
| **blood** *Plasma containing erythrocytes, leukocytes and platelets.* | sangue |
| **blood alcohol level** *A quantitative measurement of the amount of alcohol in the blood.* | livello di alcol nel sangue |
| **blood bank** *An area where blood products are stored for later use.* | emobanca |
| **blood brain barrier** *A matrix of capillaries that move blood between the blood and brain, as well as, limiting some substances from passing.* | barriera ematoencefalica |
| **blood cells** *A common term that does not differentiate between erythrocyte or leukocyte.* | cellule ematiche |
| **blood clot** *A mass of coagulated blood.* | coagulo sanguigno |
| **blood grouping** *Testing blood to determine which type should be used for transfusion.* | gruppo sanguigno |
| **blood pressure** *Written as the measurement in mmHg at the time of systole of the left ventricle over the time of diastole.* | tensione arteriale |
| **blood sedimentation rate (ESR)** *The settling time of erythrocytes in a prepared sample. This is a measure of the abnormal concentration of substances that are associated with pathological states.* | velocità di eritrosedimentazione |
| **blood stream** *Common term or the arterial or venous systems.* | corrente sanguigna |
| **blood tubing** *(used for infusion of blood)* | tubo per trasfusione di sangue |
| **blood type** *Determined and listed in the ABO system.* | gruppo sanguigno |
| **blood volume** *The amount of blood cells/plasma in the circulatory system.* | volume ematico |
| **blue** *A color between green and violet.* | blu |
| **blue diaper syndrome** *A disorder of tryptophan absorption. Excess tryptophan is metabolized to indicans in the bowel, excreted in the urine and oxidized in the diaper to indigo, thus the blue diaper.* | sindrome del pannolino blu |
| **blunt** *Having a flat or rounded end.* | ottuso |
| **blurred vision** *Low visual acuity.* | vista offuscata |
| **blurt out, to** *To speak without considering the repercussions.* | spifferare |
| **blush, to** *To have an increased volume of blood flow to one's face causing a red tint to the skin.* | arrossare |
| **body surface area** *Dubois formula is: (weight in kilograms)to the 0.425th power x (height in centimeters) to the 0.725th power x 0.007184.* | superficie corporea |
| **body weight** *Relative mass as measured in kilograms or pounds.* | peso corporeo |
| **bolus** *A fluid bolus is a phrase used for rapid infusion of fluid.* | bolo |
| **bone** *Skeletal tissue formed by osteoblasts.* | osso |
| **bone graft** *The transfer of bone to aid in the healing of a complex fracture.* | trapianto osseo |
| **bone marrow** *The soft material filling the cavity of bones.* | midollo osseo |
| **bone marrow puncture** *The aspiration of marrow to look for pressure of disease.* | biopsia del midollo osseo |
| **bone scan** *Bone imaging using technetium 99m (99mTc) diphosphate.* | scintigrafia osseo |
| **bonesetter** *A person who sets bones without being a physician.* | assesta-ossa |
| **border** *Margin.* | bordo, margine |
| **born, to be** *Being present as a result of birth.* | di essere nato |
| **bottle** *A container used for the storage of liquids.* | flacone |

| English | Italian |
|---|---|
| **bougienage** *Passage of a bougie through a body orifice with the goal of increasing the diameter of the orifice.* | cateterismo a scopo dilatante |
| **brace, to** *Application of a splint.* | immobilizzare (con ferula un osso fratturato) |
| **brace** *A splint.* | apparecchio ortopedico |
| **brachial artery** *A continuation of the axillary artery and branches into the radial and ulnar among others.* | arteria brachiale |
| **brachial plexus** *A cluster of nerves coming off the last four cervical and first thoracic spinal nerves form the nerve supply the the chest and arms.* | plesso brachiale |
| **brachial plexus neuropathy** *Characterized by acute arm or shoulder pain followed by focal muscle weakness.* | neuropatia del plesso brachiale |
| **brachial** *Referring to the arm.* | brachiale |
| **brachium cerebelli** *Synonym of pedunculus cerebellaris superior (upper portion the cerebellum).* | peduncolo crebellare superiore |
| **Bracht maneuver** *Delivery of a fetus in a breech position.* | manovra di Bracht |
| **brachycephaly** *The presence of a short broad skull.* | brachicefalia |
| **bradycardia** *Lower than normal cardiac rate measured in beats per minute.* | bradicardia |
| **bradykinin** *A peptide that causes contraction of smooth muscle and dilation of blood vessels.* | bradichinina |
| **brain** *A common term for cerebrum.* | cervello |
| **brain death** *Cessation of cerebral functioning.* | morte cerebrale |
| **brain stem** *An organ that consists of the medulla oblongata, pons and midbrain.* | tronco cerebrale |
| **brainstem herniation** *Movement of the brainstem into the incisura because of increased intracranial pressure.* | formazione di ernia del tronco cerebrale |
| **branchial** *Referring to or resembling the gills of a fish.* | branchiale |
| **break** *A common term for a fracture in a bone.* | frattura ossea |
| **breast** *Mammary tissue including the areola.* | petto |
| **breast feeding** *The process of giving milk to a baby via the nipple.* | allattamento al seno |
| **breath** *One respiration.* | respiro |
| **breath sounds** *The noise heard upon auscultation with a stethoscope.* | suoni e rumori respiratori |
| **breath test (for alcohol)** *A check of alcohol level by testing exhaled air.* | analizzatore del respiro |
| **breech birth** *Delivery with the feet or buttocks coming first.* | parto podalico |
| **breech presentation** *Position of the feet or buttocks near the cervix.* | presentazione di podice |
| **bregma** *Located at the convergence of the coronal and sagittal sutures.* | bregma |
| **bright** *Giving out a lot of light.* | brillante |
| **bring, to** *To carry or transport something.* | portare |
| **brisk** *Rapid or fast.* | vivace |
| **broad ligament of uterus** *Supports the uterus on both sides.* | legamento largo dell'utero |
| **Brodie's knee** *Also referred to as chronic hypertrophic synovitis of the knee.* | sinovite cronica ipertrofica |
| **broken (arm)** *Fracture of the arm.* | braccio rotto |
| **bromidrosis** *Foul smelling perspiration.* | bromidrosi |
| **bromism** *Poisoning caused by excessive intake of bromine.* | bromismo |
| **bronchial carcinoma** *A general term for a malignancy of the bronchi.* | carcinoma bronchiale |
| **bronchial** *Referring to the bronchus.* | bronchiale |
| **bronchiectasis** *The presence of abnormally wide bronchi or branches.* | bronchiettasia |
| **bronchiole** *A small branch that a bronchus divides into.* | bronchiolo |
| **bronchiolitis** *Inflammation of the pulmonary bronchioles.* | bronchiolite |

| English | Italian |
|---|---|
| **bronchitis** *Inflammation of the mucous membranes of the bronchioles that causes bronchospasm and cough.* | bronchite |
| **bronchogenic** *Referring to the bronchi.* | broncogeno |
| **bronchography** *Roentgenography of the bronchi after administration of contrast media.* | broncografia |
| **bronchopneumonia** *Pneumonia that starts in the distal bronchioles.* | broncopolmonite |
| **bronchoscopy** *Use of a scope to visualize the bronchi.* | broncoscopia |
| **bronchospasm** *Bronchial smooth muscle spasm.* | broncospasmo |
| **bronchus** *The major air channels that bifurcate from the distal trachea.* | bronco |
| **brow presentation** *The term used to describe which part of the body (forehead) is being delivered first in childbirth.* | presentazione di fronte |
| **brown** *Coffee-colored.* | bruno |
| **Brown-Séquard syndrome** *Unilateral spinal cord lesions, proprioception loss and weakness occur ipsilateral to the lesion, while pain and temperature loss occur contralateral.* | sindrome di Brown-Séquard |
| **brucellosis** *A gram-negative bacteria in cattle that causes persistent fever in humans.* | brucellosi |
| **Brudzinski sign** *Involuntary flexion of the knees and hips after flexion of the neck while supine; seen in meningitis.* | segno di Brudzinski |
| **bruise** *Common term for ecchymosis.* | contusione |
| **bruit** *An abnormal sound heard through a stethoscope indicating turbulent blood flow.* | rumore, soffio |
| **brush** *Implement used for cleaning or for taking a tissue sample.* | spazzola |
| **brush biopsy** *The process of tissue sampling using a brush.* | biopsia del spazzola |
| **bubo** *An inflamed, swollen lymph node in the axilla or inguinal region.* | bubbone |
| **bubonic plague** *A form of plague exhibited by the formation of buboes.* | peste bubbonica |
| **buccal** *Referring to the cheek.* | diretto verso la guancia |
| **buccinator muscle** *Pulls the mouth posteriorly.* | muscolo buccinatore |
| **Budd-Chiari syndrome** *Hepatomegaly, severe portal hypertension and ascites related to thrombosis of the hepatic vein.* | sindrome di Budd-Chiari |
| **bug** *Insect.* | picollo insetto |
| **bulbar palsy** *Paralysis due to changes in the motor center of the medulla oblongata.* | paralisi bulbare |
| **bulbocavernosus reflex** *Brisk contraction of the ischiocavernosus and bulbocavernosus muscles when the glans penis is compressed.* | riflesso bulbocavernoso |
| **bulge** *A protuberance on a flat surface.* | rigonfiamento esterno |
| **bulimia** *Pathologic increase in hunger.* | bulimia |
| **bulky** *Voluminous or substantial.* | grosso, voluminoso |
| **bulla** *A large cutaneous serous filled vesicle.* | bolla |
| **bullous pemphigoid** *A benign disease of the aged characterized by large bullae forming on the torso and extremities.* | pemfigoide bolloso |
| **Bumke's pupil** *Dilation of the pupil in response to anxiety.* | pupilla di Bumke |
| **bundle branch block** *A cardiac dysrhythmia produced by a blockage of a branch of the bundle of His.* | blocco di branca |
| **bundle of His** *The atrial contraction rhythm is facilitated by this bundle to the ventricles.* | fascio di His |
| **bunion** *Swelling of the bursa of the metatarsal head of the first metatarsal.* | borsite e periborsite dell'alluce |
| **burn** *An injury caused by exposure to heat.* | ustione |
| **burr or bur** *A rotary cutting instrument.* | strumento da taglio |
| **burr hole** *A treatment of subdural hematoma that involves drilling a hole into the cranium to release the hematoma.* | fori di trapanazione |
| **bursitis** *Inflammation of the bursa.* | borsite |
| **burst, to** *To rupture.* | fare scoppiare |

| English | Italian |
|---|---|
| **buttocks (buttock)** *The bilateral region covering the gluteal muscles.* | natiche (natica) |
| **Buzzard maneuver** *Testing of the patellar reflex while the client firmly touches the floor with their toes in a sitting position.* | manovra di Buzzard |
| **bypass** *An alternate route, typically referring to an arterial bypass.* | scavalcamento |
| **byssinosis** *A disease caused by inhalation of cotton dust; a type of pneumoconiosis.* | bissinosi |
| **cachexia** *Generalized weakness and severe wasting.* | cachessia |
| **cadaver** *A dead body.* | cadavere |
| **caduceus** *An ancient herald's wand with two serpents twined around that is a symbol of the medical arts.* | caduceo |
| **caisson disease** *Decompression sickness.* | malattia dei cassoni |
| **calcaneal spur** *A bony protrusion on the calcaneus.* | sperone calcaneare |
| **calcaneus** *Commonly called the heel bone.* | calcagno |
| **calcareous** *Referring to something containing lime or calcium.* | calcareo |
| **calciferol** *It is formed when egesterol is exposed to ultraviolet light; a D vitamin.* | calciferolo |
| **calcification** *Deposition of calcium salts causing hardening of an organic tissue.* | calcificazione |
| **calcitonin** *A thyroid hormone that lowers serum calcium levels.* | calcinazione |
| **calcium** *A chemical element that is an essential component in teeth and bone.* | calcio |
| **calcium channel blocker** *A medication used to treat angina, supraventricular arrhythmias and hypertension; it works by blocking calcium influx into myocytes and vascular smooth muscle cells.* | bloccante i canali del calcio |
| **calculus** *A stone of minerals that can lead to the blockage of the bile duct or ureters.* | calcolo |
| **calf** *Muscles of the posterior portion of the lower leg.* | polpaccio |
| **calibrate, to** *To adjust an instrument using a standard.* | calibrare |
| **calibration** *The process of calibrating an instrument.* | calibrazione |
| **callosity** *Callus; thickened hardened skin.* | callosità |
| **callus** *Thickened hardened skin.* | callo |
| **calorie** *A unit of heat.* | caloria |
| **calvaria** *The portion of the skull that is composed of the superior aspects of the occipital, parietal and frontal bones.* | calvaria; volta cranica |
| **calyx** *A cup shaped organ or cavity.* | calce |
| **canaliculus** *A term for various small channels.* | canalicolo |
| **cancel, to** *To stop or revoke.* | cancellare |
| **cancellous** *A bony mesh-like structure with many pores.* | struttura reticolare spongiosa |
| **cancer; carcinoma** *A disease of uncontrolled abnormal cell growth.* | cancro |
| **cancroid** *A tumor occurring in the stomach, small or large bowel.* | cancroide |
| **cancrum oris** *Gangrenous stomatitis.* | stomatite gangrenosa |
| **candle** *A cylindrical piece of wax with a central wick.* | candela |
| **canine teeth** *Located between the incisors and premolars.* | dente canino |
| **canker sore** *An ulceration, usually of the mouth or lips.* | ulcerazione della bocca; stomatite aftosa |
| **cannabis** *A plant from the Cannibidaceae family that is known for its psychotropic effects.* | canapa |
| **cannula** *A tube inserted into the body.* | cannula |
| **cantering rhythm** *Gallop rhythm.* | ritmo di galoppo |
| **capillary** *A vessel that connects arterioles to venules.* | capillare |

| English | Italian |
|---|---|
| **capillary fragility test** *Application of a blood pressure cuff high enough to restrict venous return and after five minutes count the number or petechiae produced.* | prova di fragilità capillare |
| **capillary nevus** *A growth of skin that involves the capillaries.* | nevo capillare |
| **capitate bone** *The bone at the base of the palm that articulates with the third metacarpal.* | osso capitato del carpo |
| **Caplan nodules** *These are pulmonary nodules noted in people with rheumatoid arthritis who were exposed to coal dust.* | nodulo di Caplan |
| **capsule** *A membranous sheath that covers an organ or structure.* | capsula, tunica |
| **capsule** *Medication in the form of a capsule.* | capsula per medicamenti |
| **capsulitis** *Inflammation of a capsule.* | capsulite |
| **capsulotomy** *Incision of a capsule as in with eye surgery.* | capsulotomia |
| **caput** *The head.* | capo |
| **caput succedaneum** *Edema that occurs in the scalp of an infant during child-birth.* | caput succedaneum |
| **carbohydrate** *A group of organic compounds including sugar and starch.* | carboidrati |
| **carbon dioxide gas** *A gas expelled during exhalation.* | gas monossido di carbonio |
| **carbon monoxide poisoning** *This tasteless, odorless gas causes constitutional symptoms but can lead to death upon inhalation.* | avvelenamento da monssido di carbonio |
| **carboxyhemoglobin** *A compound formed from hemoglobin when it is exposed to carbon monoxide.* | carbossiemoglobina |
| **carcinogenic** *That which causes cancer.* | cancerogeno |
| **carcinoid** *A tumor occurring in the stomach, intestine and colon.* | carcinoide |
| **carcinoma** *A malignant growth.* | carcinoma, cancro |
| **carcinomatosis** *Dissemination of cancer throughout the body.* | carcinomatosi |
| **cardia** *The superior aspect of the stomach at the opening of the esophagus.* | cardias |
| **cardiac** *Referring to the heart.* | cardiaco |
| **cardiac arrest** *Cessation of function of the heart.* | arresto cardiaco |
| **cardiac failure** *Decreased cardiac output of the heart.* | insufficienza cardiaca congestizia |
| **cardiac output** *Amount of blood pumped by the heart in liters per minute.* | gittata cardiaca |
| **cardiac pacing** *Electromechanical stimulation of the heart.* | stimulazione cardiaca |
| **cardiology** *A specialty of medical practice involve treatment and prevention of heart disease.* | cardiologia |
| **cardiomyopathy** *Chronic cardiac muscle disease.* | miocardiopatia |
| **cardiopulmonary resuscitation** *Use of artificial means to support respiration and circulation.* | rianimazione cardiorespiratoria |
| **cardiovascular** *Referring to the heart or circulatory system.* | cardiovascolare |
| **carditis** *Inflammation of the heart.* | cardite |
| **caregiver** *A person who provides care to another.* | chi presta soccorso medico |
| **caries** *Referring to decay or death of a tooth.* | carie |
| **carina** *The protrusion of the lowest tracheal cartilage.* | carena |
| **carneous** *Synonym of fleshy.* | carnoso |
| **carotene** *A hydrocarbon that can be converted to vitamin A.* | carotene |
| **carotid body** *Carotid artery receptors that are sensitive to blood chemistry changes.* | glomo carotideo |
| **carotid bruit** *An abnormal noise heard over the carotid artery that may be a sign of stenosis or aortic valvular disease.* | soffio carotide |

| English | Italian |
|---|---|
| **carotid sinus reflex** *Bradycardia as a result of pressure on the carotid sinus.* | riflesso del seno carotideo |
| **carotid sinus syncope** *Dizziness and syncope that results from hyperactivity of the carotid sinus reflex.* | sincope del seno carotideo |
| **carotid** *Referring to the large artery on each side of the neck.* | arteria carotide |
| **carpal tunnel syndrome** *Paresthesia that results from compression of the median nerve.* | sindrome del tunnel carpale |
| **carpometacarpal** *Referring to the carpus and metacarpus.* | carpometacarpico |
| **carpopedal spasm** *A spasm of the carpus and the foot.* | spasmo carpopedale |
| **carpus** *The joint between the hand and wrist.* | carpo |
| **caruncle** *A small fleshy protuberance.* | caruncola |
| **casein** *The principal protein in milk, a phospholipid.* | caseina |
| **Casoni's test** *Hydatid fluid is injected intradermally; subsequent formation of a larger papule indicates hydatid disease.* | prova di intradermoreazione di Casoni |
| **cast; plaster cast** *Use of plaster of paris to immobilize an extremity.* | corsetto gessato |
| **castor bean** *A bean that can yield the poisonous compound ricin.* | semi di ricino |
| **castration** *Excision of the gonads.* | castrazione |
| **casualty** *A person who is killed or seriously injured.* | persona che ha subito un infortunio |
| **cat cry syndrome** *A hereditary congenital disorder exhibited by microcephaly, hypertelorism, and cognitive deficits.* | sindrome del grido di gatto |
| **cat scratch fever** *An infectious disease characterized by local inflammation a the site of the scratch, local lymph adenopathy and fever.* | malattia da graffio di gatto |
| **catabolism** *The reduction of complex molecules to more simple ones in living organisms.* | catabolismo |
| **catalepsy** *A condition exhibited by rigidity and the person maintains the same position if he is moved by another.* | catalessia |
| **cataphoresis** *The use of an electric field to move charged particles in fluid.* | cataforesi |
| **cataplexy** *A condition exhibited by rigidity and immobility.* | cataplessia |
| **cataract** *An opacity of an eye lens or the capsule.* | cataratta |
| **catarrh** *Inflammation of a mucous membrane.* | catarro |
| **catatonia** *Seen in schizophrenia, it is a state of stupor or excitability and abnormal movements.* | catatonia |
| **catch a cold** *To come down with a viral upper respiratory tract infection.* | prendersi un raffreddore |
| **catharsis** *The act of cleansing or purging, usually referring to thought.* | catarsi |
| **cathartic** *To be cleansed or evacuated, referring to thought or the cleansing of the bowels.* | catartico |
| **catheter** *A flexible tube inserted into the body.* | catetere |
| **cat's eye pupil** *A pupil in the shape of an oval.* | dell'occhio di gatto |
| **cauda equina syndrome** *Neurologic condition manifested by pain, paresthesia and weakness but no bowel/bladder dysfunction.* | sindrome della coda equina |
| **caudal** *Referring to a cauda.* | caudale |
| **caudate** *Referring to the caudate nucleus.* | caudato |
| **causative** *Something that induces an effect.* | responsabile |
| **caustic** *Abrasive or corrosive.* | caustico |
| **cautery** *Application of an electric current to cut something.* | cauterio |
| **cavernous hemangioma** *A tumor composed of connective tissue with blood filled areas.* | emangioma cavernoso |
| **cavernous sinus** *Large venous sinus located adjacent to the sphenoid bone and posterior to the petrosal sinuses.* | seno cavernoso |

| English | Italian |
|---|---|
| **cavernous sinus thrombosis** *A blood clot in the base of the brain.* | trombosi del seno cavernoso |
| **cavity** *Pouch or chamber.* | cavità |
| **cecum** *The portion of the bowel between the ileum and and the ascending colon.* | ceco |
| **celiac** *Referring to the abdominal cavity.* | celiaco |
| **cell body** *The portion of the cell containing the nucleus.* | corpo cellulare |
| **cell membrane** *The semipermeable structure surrounding the cytoplasm of a cell.* | membrana cellulare |
| **cell** *The smallest functional unit of an organism.* | cellulare |
| **cell wall** *The peripheral border of the cell.* | parete cellulare |
| **cellulitis** *Infection characterized by diffuse, subcutaneous inflammation.* | inflammazione del tessuto cellulare |
| **cellulose** *A polysaccharide that occurs naturally in fibrous products.* | cellulosa |
| **center** *A point equidistant from all sides.* | centre |
| **centigrade** *A scale with 100 gradations, usually referring to a temperature scale.* | centigrado |
| **centimeter** *One hundredth of a meter.* | centimetro |
| **central nervous system (CNS)** *The brain and spinal cord.* | sistema nervoso centrale |
| **centrifuge** *Machine used to separate substances of different weights.* | centrifuga |
| **centripetal** *The movement toward the center.* | centripeto |
| **cephalic** *Towards the head.* | cefalico |
| **cercaria** *Larval trematode worm that live in a molluscan.* | cercaria |
| **cerebellum** *The part of the brain in the posterior portion of the skull that controls muscle coordination and movement.* | cervelletto |
| **cerebral malaria** *A severe form of malaria manifested by seizures and a decreased level of consciousness.* | malaria cerebrale |
| **cerebral palsy** *A condition exhibited by motor incoordination and speech changes that is the result of brain injury occurring ante-, intra- or post- partum.* | paralisi cerebrale |
| **cerebral** *Referring to the cerebrum.* | cerebrale |
| **cerebration** *Operating activity of the cerebrum.* | cerebrazione |
| **cerebrospinal fluid (CSF)** *The fluid between the pia mater and arachnoid membrane.* | liquor cerebrale |
| **cerebrovascular accident (stroke)** *A decrease in level of consciousness and paralysis caused by a cerebrovascular thrombosis, hemorrhage or vasospasm.* | infarto rosso o ictus cerebrale |
| **cerumen** *Waxy substance found normally in the external ear canals.* | cerume |
| **cerumen impaction** *External ear canal full of wax resulting in hearing loss until the impaction is removed.* | zaffo di cerume |
| **Cervical insufficiency (formerly incompetent cervix)** *Painless changes in the cervix that result in recurrent second semester pregnancy loss.* | incompetenza cervicale |
| **cervical pleura** *The dome-like cap of the pleura.* | pleura cervicale |
| **cervical** *Referring to the neck or the cervix.* | cervicale |
| **cervicectomy** *Excision of the cervix uteri.* | cervicectomia |
| **cervicitis** *Inflammation of the cervix.* | cervicite |
| **cervix uteri** *The narrow end of the uterus.* | cervice |
| **cesarean section** *Incision of the abdominal and uterine walls in order to deliver a fetus when natural delivery is not possible.* | taglio cesareo |
| **cestode** *A class of parasitic flatworms.* | cestodi |
| **chalazion** *A chronic granuloma of a meibomian gland.* | calazio |
| **chancre** *The initial ulcer that is seen with primary syphilis.* | sifiloma |

| English | Italian |
|---|---|
| **chancroid** *A sexually transmitted disease caused by Haemophilus ducreyi that is exhibited by ulcers without indurated margins.* | ulcera molle o venerea |
| **check for, to** | controllare per |
| **cheek** *Lateral facial tissue.* | guancia |
| **chelation** *The process used to bind a compound with metal typically used in the treatment of poisoning.* | chelazione |
| **cheilitis** *Inflammation of the lip.* | cheilite |
| **chemoreceptor** *A sense organ that responds to stimuli.* | chemiorecettore |
| **chemosis** *Swelling of conjunctival tissue adjacent to the cornea.* | chemosi |
| **chemotaxis** *The response of an organism to chemical agents.* | chemiotassi |
| **chemotherapy** *Use of medication (chemical agents) in the treatment of disease. This term is commonly used to refer to the treatment of cancer patients with medication.* | chemioterapia |
| **chest** *Thorax.* | torace |
| **chest leads (precordial)** *Leads going from the skin to an electrocardiographic device.* | derivazione precordiali |
| **chest wall** *Thoracic wall.* | parete toracica |
| **chest x-ray** *Roentography of the thorax.* | raggio X di torace |
| **chew, to** *Masticate.* | masticare |
| **Cheyne-Stokes respirations** *A breathing pattern characterized by alternating apnea with hyperpnea.* | respiro di Cheyne-Stokes |
| **chiasma** *The optic chiasma is the area inferior to the hypothalamus where the optic nerves cross.* | chiasma |
| **chicken pox, varicella** *A viral disease characterized by extremely pruritus blisters over the entire body.* | varicelle |
| **chigger** *A parasitic mite of the genus Trombicula.* | acaro dei Thrombiculidae |
| **child** *A person aged 1 to 8 years old. (male, female)* | bambino, bambina |
| **childbirth** *Parturition; the process of labor and delivery of an infant.* | parto |
| **childhood** *The time between infancy and puberty.* | fanciullezza |
| **chill** *Sensation of coldness.* | freddo |
| **chimera** *A mixture of genetically distinct tissues.* | chimera |
| **chin** *Mentum; the anterior projection of the lower jaw.* | mento |
| **chiropodist** *A doctor trained in the treatment of feet.* | podiatra |
| **chiropractic** *Referring to the medical practice of adjusting malaligned joints.* | chiropratica |
| **chiropractor** *A medical practitioner who is involved with the treatment of disease by manipulating malaligned joints.* | chiropratico |
| **chlamydiosis** *A disease caused by the species Chlamydia.* | infettato da Chlamydia |
| **chloasma** *Brown or black macula that occur on the face during pregnancy or when there is ovarian dysfunction.* | cloasma |
| **chloroform** *A colorless, sweet smelling liquid formerly used as a general anesthetic.* | cloroformio |
| **chloroma** *A malignant tumor associated with myelogenous leukemia.* | cloroma |
| **choanae** *The two openings between the nasal cavity and the nasopharynx.* | coana |
| **choanal atresia** *A congenital condition characterized by blockage of the nasal passages by tissue.* | atresia di coana |
| **choice** *Selection or decision.* | scelta |
| **choke, to** *To retch, cough or fight for breath.* | togliere il respiro |
| **cholagogue** *A compound used to stimulate flow of bile from the liver.* | colagogo |
| **cholangiogram** *Radiologic imaging of the gallbladder and bile ducts.* | colangiogramma |
| **cholangitis** *Inflammation of the bile ducts.* | colangite |
| **cholecystectomy** *Surgical excision of the gallbladder.* | colecistectomia |

| English | Italian |
|---|---|
| **cholecystenterostomy** *Creation of a surgical anastomosis between the intestine and the gallbladder.* | colecistoenterostomia |
| **cholecystitis** *Inflammation of the gallbladder.* | colecistite |
| **cholecystolithiasis** *The presence of gallstones in the gallbladder.* | colecistolitiasi |
| **choledocholithotomy** *Creation of an incision in the bile duct for the purpose of removing a stone.* | coledocolitotomia |
| **cholelithiasis** *Presence or creation of gallstones.* | colelitiasi |
| **cholemia** *Bile or bile products in the blood.* | colemia |
| **cholera** *An infectious disease exhibited by vomiting and diarrhea and caused by Vibrio cholerae.* | colera |
| **cholestatic hepatitis** *Liver inflammation caused by obstruction of bile flow from the liver to the duodenum.* | epatite colostatica |
| **cholesteatoma** *A cystic mass that has a lining made of keratinizing material and cholesterol.* | colesteatoma |
| **cholesterol** *A compound or its derivatives are found in cell membranes and precursors to hormones but high levels can cause atherosclerosis.* | colesterolo |
| **cholinergic** *Referring to the stimulation, activation or transmission of acetylcholine.* | colinergico |
| **cholinesterase** *An esterase used to cleave acetylcholine into choline and acetic acid.* | colinesterasi |
| **choluria** *Term indicating the presence of bile in the urine.* | coluria |
| **chondralgia** *Cartilaginous pain.* | condrodinia |
| **chondritis** *Cartilaginous inflammation.* | condrite |
| **chondroma** *Cartilaginous hyperplastic growth.* | condroma |
| **chondromalacia** *Excessive softening of the cartilages.* | condromalacia |
| **chondromalacia of the patella** *Softening of the articular cartilage of the patella.* | condromalacia patellare |
| **chondrosarcoma** *Cartilaginous tumor which exhibits rapid growth.* | condrosarcoma |
| **chorda** *A cord or sinew.* | corda |
| **chordee** *Downward bending of the penis.* | grifosi |
| **chorditis** *Inflammation of a vocal or spermatic cord.* | cordite |
| **chorea** *Involuntary, continuous rapid, jerking movements.* | corea |
| **chorionic villi** *Cord-like projections of a fertilized ovum.* | villi corionico |
| **choroid** *Similar to the chorion (fertilized ovum or zygote)* | coroideo |
| **choroiditis** *Inflammation of the choroid.* | coroidite |
| **choroidocyclitis** *Inflammation of the ciliary processes and choroid.* | coroidociclite |
| **chromatin** *A desocyribose nucleic acid that carries the genes of inheritance.* | cromatina |
| **chromosome** *A structure in the nucleus of living cells that carries genetic information.* | cromosoma |
| **chronic** *When referring to an illness, it means recurring or persistent.* | cronico |
| **chyle** *A combination of lymph fluid and fat that enters the blood via the thoracic duct.* | chilo |
| **chylomicron** *A one micron particle of emulsified fat.* | chilomicrone |
| **chylous** *Referring to chyle.* | chiloso |
| **chyme** *The gruel produced by gastric digestion.* | chimo |
| **cicatricial** *Referring to cicatrix.* | cicatriziale |
| **cicatrix (scar)** *New tissue in a healed wound.* | cicatrice |
| **cilia** *The hairs growing on the eyelid or a motile extension of a cell surface.* | ciglia |
| **ciliary body** *The connection between the iris and the choroid.* | corpo ciliare |
| **cinchonism** *The toxic effects induced by ingestion of cinchona bark; it is exhibited by tinnitus, deafness and cognitive changes.* | cinconismo |

| English | Italian |
|---|---|
| **circadian** *Referring to a 24 hour period.* | circadiano |
| **circadian rhythm** *Naturally recurring fluctuations in a 24 hour period.* | ritmo circadiano |
| **circumcision** *Surgical excision of the foreskin.* | circoncisione |
| **circumference** *The distance around an object or part.* | circonferenza |
| **circumflex nerve** *The axillary nerve that has an origin in the posterior branch of the brachial plexus.* | nervo circonflesso |
| **circumscribed** *To have well defined borders.* | circoscritto |
| **cirrhosis** *A liver disease characterized by destruction of liver cells and increased connective tissue.* | cirrosi |
| **cirsoid** *Similar to a tortuous vein, artery or lymph vessel.* | varicoso |
| **cisternal puncture** *A trans-occipitoatlantoid ligament puncture of the cisterna magna so CSF can be obtained.* | puntura cisterna |
| **clasp** *Holding onto something with one's hand.* | gancio |
| **clasp knife reflex** *An abnormal response seen in the setting of a pyramidal tract lesion in which there is a rapid decrease in resistance during passive movement of a joint.* | rigidità spastica |
| **claudication** *Intermittent claudication is a phrase used to describe pain experienced in the leg from arterial insufficiency.* | claudicazione |
| **claustrophobia** *An unreasonable fear of being in an enclosed environment.* | claustrofobia |
| **clavicle** *A bone that articulates with the sternum and scapula.* | clavicola |
| **clavus** *A corn or horny protrusion.* | callosità |
| **clawhand** *A hand deformity caused by ulnar nerve palsy exhibited by the hyperextension of the metacarpophalangeal joints and flexion of the interphalangeal articulations.* | mano ad artiglio |
| **clean catch urine specimen** *A urine specimen obtained by having a patient cleanse the perineal area prior to voiding in a collection device.* | esame delle urine (nel mezzo della corrente) |
| **clear** *Lucid.* | lucido |
| **clear** *Transparent.* | trasparente |
| **clear one's throat, to** *To cough lightly in attempt to speak more clearly.* | schiarirsi la voce |
| **clearance** *The process of removing something.* | sgombero |
| **cleavage** *A sharp division or demarcation.* | divisione |
| **cleft lip** *A congenital abnormal opening of the lip.* | labbro leporino |
| **cleft palate** *A congenital abnormal opening in the palate.* | protesi per palatoschisi |
| **cleidocranial dysostosis** *A congenital condition exhibited by abnormal ossification of the cranial bones and absence of clavicles.* | sindrome di Marie-Sainton; disostosi cranioclavicolare |
| **cleidotomy** *A procedure used in difficult deliveries in which the clavicle is broken to facilitate childbirth.* | cleidotomia |
| **click** *A sound heard by the sudden closure of a heart valve.* | suono breve |
| **clinic** *A building where patients are evaluated.* | clinico |
| **clinical record** *The ongoing medical summary.* | cartella clinica |
| **clinical examination** *Physical assessment data.* | esame clinico |
| **clitoris** *A small erectile body in the anterosuperior aspect of the vulva.* | clitoride |
| **clockwise** *Movement in the same direction as a normal clock.* | destrorso |
| **clonic** *Referring to a spasm that alternates in rigidity and relaxation.* | clonico |
| **closed** | chiuso |
| **closed reduction** *The realignment of a fracture without use of surgery.* | riduzione chiusa |
| **clot** *A thrombus or embolus.* | coagulo |
| **clubbing** *Increase in the mass of the soft tissue of the terminal phalanges.* | ippocratismo digitale |
| **cluster headache** *A unilateral, severe, recurrent headache.* | cefalea a grappolo |

| English | Italian |
|---|---|
| **cnemial** *Referring to the shin.* | cresta tibiale |
| **coagulation** *The formation of a clot.* | coagulazione |
| **coarctation of the aorta** *A stricture, as in narrowing of the aorta.* | coartazione dell'aorta |
| **coated tablet** *A pill covered with a substance to slow absorption or reduce gastric irritation.* | pillola rivestimento |
| **cobalt** *A metal that with causes polycythemia with increased ingestion.* | cobalto |
| **cocaine** *A highly addictive opiate derivative.* | cocaina |
| **cocaine addiction** *Physical habituation to cocaine.* | dipendenza da cocaina |
| **coccus** *A spherical shaped bacterium.* | cocco |
| **coccydynia** *Coccygeal pain.* | coccigodinia |
| **coccyx** *The small bone formed by the natural fusion of rudimentary vertebrae.* | coccige |
| **cochlea** *The essential organ of hearing which is in a spiral form.* | chiocciola |
| **cock-up splint** *A splint used to maintain the wrist in dorsiflexion; used for carpal tunnel syndrome.* | stecca di polso dorsiflessione |
| **cockroach** *A beetle-like insect with long legs and antennae.* | blatta |
| **cod** *A large marine fish, also called codfish.* | merluzzo |
| **codeine** *A morphine derived analgesic.* | codeina |
| **codon** *A series of three nucleotides that form a unit of genetic code.* | codone |
| **coffee-ground emesis** *Bloody vomitus with appearance of ground coffee.* | caffè macinato emesi |
| **cogwheel rigidity** *As in cogwheel rigidity which is a jerky passive movement after there was increased tone.* | rigidità a troclea dentata |
| **cognition** *The process of acquiring thought or understanding.* | conoscenza |
| **cognitive disorders** *Any disease process that involves altered cognition.* | disturbo cognitivo |
| **coitus** *Sexual intercourse between members of the opposite sex.* | coito |
| **cold** *Having a sense of being cold.* | freddo |
| **cold sore** *A perioral blister caused by herpes simplex.* | herpes simplex |
| **cold** *Viral upper respiratory tract infection.* | raffreddore comune |
| **colectomy** *Surgical removal of part of the colon.* | colectomia |
| **colic** *Acute abdominal pain.* | colica |
| **colitis** *Inflammation of the colon.* | colite |
| **collagen** *The principal supportive protein bone, skin, tendon and cartilage.* | collageno |
| **collapse** *A physical or mental breakdown.* | collasso |
| **collarbone** *Common term for the clavicle.* | clavicola |
| **collodion** *A product of the breakdown of colloid.* | collodio |
| **colloid** *A solution used for infusion, such as albumin or hetastarch, that are more likely to remain in the intravascular space than crystalloids.* | colloidale |
| **coloboma** *A congenital defect that involves a fissure of the eye.* | coloboma |
| **colon** *The portion of the large intestine that goes from the cecum to the rectum.* | colon |
| **colonoscopy** *Inspection the color, ideally to the cecum, with a lighted scope.* | coloscopia |
| **color blindness** *The inability to distinguish colors.* | cecità per i colori |
| **color chart** *A card used to check for color blindness.* | cartelle colori |
| **color of conjunctiva** *A point of assessment to check for pallor.* | colori di congiuntiva |
| **colostomy bag** *A pouch attached to the skin with a mild adhesive that collects stool emitted from a colostomy.* | sacco colostomia |
| **colostomy** *Surgically creating an opening in the colon that is extended to outside the abdominal wall.* | colostomia |

| English | Italian |
|---|---|
| **colostrum** *The fluid secreted by the mammary glands a few days around parturition.* | colostro |
| **colpitis**; *vaginitis Inflammation of the vagina.* | vaginite |
| **colpocele** *A hernia into the vagina.* | colpocele |
| **colporrhaphy** *A surgical procedure that involves suturing the vagina.* | colporrafia |
| **colposcope** *A scope used to visualize the vagina.* | colposcopio |
| **colposcopy** *Use of a scope to visualize the vagina and cervix.* | colposcopia |
| **coma** *A state of unconsciousness.* | coma |
| **comatose** *Referring to a coma.* | comatoso |
| **comedone** *The medical term (singular) for blackheads.* | comedone |
| **commensal** *Living in or on another organism without being a detriment.* | commensale |
| **comment** *A remark providing an opinion.* | osservazione |
| **common** *That which is usual.* | comune |
| **compatible** *To coexist without problems.* | compatibile |
| **compendium** *A concise summary about a subject.* | compendio |
| **complaint** *Grievance.* | lamento |
| **complement fixation test** *A laboratory test for the presence of an antibody in the serum that involves inactivation of the complement in the serum.* | prova di fissazione del complemento |
| **complete blood count** *An assay that includes white blood cell, red blood cell, platelet count, hemoglobin, hematocrit and white blood cell differential.* | esame morfologico completo |
| **compliance** *The act of going along with a plan.* | compiacenza |
| **comply, to** *Adhere to.* | essere compiacente |
| **compound** *A substance formed by covalent union of two or more atoms.* | composti |
| **compound fracture** *Open fracture.* | frattura composta |
| **comprehension** *Understanding.* | insieme |
| **compression** *Squeezing together.* | compressione |
| **concavity** *The state of being concave.* | concavità |
| **concentration** *The quantity of a substance per unit volume.* | concentrazione |
| **concentric** *Referring to circles or arcs that share the same center.* | concentrico |
| **conception** *The act of an egg being fertilized by sperm.* | concepimento |
| **concha** *A part of the body that is spiral shaped. Nasal concha are the small bones in the sides of the nasal cavity.* | conca |
| **concretion** *A hard solid mass.* | concrezione |
| **concussion** *Head trauma resulting in temporary loss of consciousness.* | commozione cerebrale |
| **condom** *A covering for the penis or the vagina (female condom) used during sexual intercourse that is meant to reduce the chance of pregnancy or infection.* | preservativi |
| **condyle** *A rounded protrusion of a bone.* | condilo |
| **condyloma** *A warty papule near the anus or vulva.* | condiloma acuminato |
| **cone** *A light sensitive cell in the retina.* | cono |
| **confabulation** *The fabrication of experiences to compensate for memory loss.* | conffabulazione |
| **confidence** *Self-assurance.* | confidenza |
| **confinement** *As in confined to bed.* | confinamento |
| **conflict** *Dispute or disagreement.* | conflitto |
| **confusion** *Disorientation.* | confusione |
| **congenital** *A disease or anomaly present from birth.* | congenito |
| **congenital heart disease** *A cardiac disorder present prior to birth.* | malattia di cuore congenito |

| English | Italian |
|---|---|
| **congenital syphilis** *Passed to the child in utero, the child may have failure to thrive, fever and a flattened bridge of the nose.* | sifilide congenita |
| **congestive** | congestizio |
| **congestive heart failure** *A diminished cardiac output leading to passive engorgement.* | insufficienza cardiaca congestizia |
| **conjugate diameter** *A pelvic inlet measurement used to determine whether a woman is capable of delivering a fetus vaginally.* | diametro coniugata |
| **conjunctiva** *The membrane that lines the eyelid.* | congiuntiva |
| **conjunctival reflex** *Closure of the eyes in response to irritation of the conjunctiva.* | riflesso congiuntivale |
| **conjunctivitis** *Inflammation of the conjunctiva.* | congiuntivite |
| **consanguinity** *The relationship by blood.* | consanguineità |
| **conscious** *Being award and being able to respond to one's surroundings.* | conscio |
| **consensual light reflex** *Constriction of the pupil of one eye in sync with the other pupil upon exposure to light.* | accomodazione consensuale |
| **conservative** *Control rather than elimination of a disease.* | conservativo |
| **consistent** *Compatible with something or congruous with.* | compatibile con |
| **consolidation** *An area of fixed secretions in the lung.* | solidificazione |
| **constipation** *A condition exhibited by difficulty in having a bowel movement due to hard stools.* | stitichezza |
| **constriction** *Circumferential tightening* | costrizione |
| **contact** *The touching of two bodies or a person who has been exposed to a contagious disease.* | contagio |
| **contact lens** *A lens that fits over the cornea to correct refractive errors.* | lenti a contatto |
| **contagious** *Description of a disease that can be spread by direct or indirect contact.* | contagioso |
| **contaminate, to** *To make impure by exposing to an polluted agent.* | contaminazione |
| **content** *What something is made up of.* | contento |
| **contraceptive** *A device or medication used to prevent pregnancy.* | contraccezione |
| **contradictory** *Two elements that are inconsistent.* | contraddittorio |
| **contraindication** *A situation in which two elements are inconsistent.* | contraddizione |
| **contusion** *An area of broken capillaries in the skin causing discoloration; commonly called a bruise.* | contusione |
| **convenient** *Opportune or well-timed.* | conveniente |
| **conversion reaction** *When referring to a psychiatric condition it is the exhibition of physical symptoms as a manifestation of mental disease.* | reazione conversione |
| **convex** *Having an exterior curved the outside of a sphere.* | convesso |
| **convulsion** *An involuntary series of tonic and clonic movements.* | convulsioni |
| **cool** *Chilly or cold.* | raffreddare |
| **cope, to** *To deal with a difficult situation.* | lottare |
| **copper** *A chemical element with atomic number of 29.* | rame |
| **copra itch** *A pruritus noted in people working with copra (dried kernel from a coconut).* | prurito copra |
| **copulation** *Sexual relations.* | copulazione |
| **cor pulmonale** *Heart disease that is secondary to lung disease.* | cuore pulmonare |
| **coracoid** *A prominence on the scapula to which the biceps is attached.* | apofisi coracoide |
| **cord compression** *Pressure being applied to the spinal cord.* | compressione di midollo spinale |
| **cord presentation** *The presence of the umbilical cord at the cervix during active labor.* | presentazione del cordone ombelicale |
| **core** *Central part of a structure.* | parte centrale |
| **cornea** *The transparent segment located at the anterior part of the eye.* | cornea |

| English | Italian |
|---|---|
| **corneal** *Referring to the cornea.* | corneale |
| **corneal reflex** *Closure of the eyelids when the cornea is touched lightly with a soft material. Also called the lid reflex.* | riflesso corneale |
| **corneal transplant** *Surgical replacement of a cornea with a donor cornea.* | trapianto corneale |
| **coronal suture** *The line of intersection of the frontal bone and the two parietal bones.* | sutura coronario |
| **coronary angiography** *Roentgenographic visualization of the coronary vessels after injection of dye.* | angiografia delle coronarie |
| **coronary occlusion** *A blockage in a coronary artery.* | occlusione coronarica |
| **coronary vessel** *Referring to a coronary artery.* | arteria coronaria |
| **coroner** *A person who investigates sudden or suspicious deaths.* | coroner |
| **coronoid** *Crown-shaped.* | coronoide |

| English | Italian |
|---|---|
| **corpulence** *Fatness.* | corpulenza |
| **corpus callosum** *A point of connection between the two cerebral hemispheres.* | corpo calloso |
| **corpus luteum** *A structure that is discharged from an ovary; it degenerates if it is not impregnated.* | corpo luteo |
| **corpuscle** *A red or white blood cell.* | corpuscolo |
| **cortex** *An external layer.* | corteccia |
| **cortical** *Referring to the cortex.* | corticale |
| **corticosteroid** *A hormone developed in the adrenal cortex.* | corticosteroide |
| **corticotropin** *A hormone of the adrenal cortex.* | corticotropina |
| **cortisol** *An adrenal cortical hormone, also called hydrocortisone.* | cortisolo |
| **cortisone** *An adrenal cortical hormone responsible for carbohydrate regulation.* | cortisone |
| **coryza** *An acute condition exhibited by copious nasal discharge.* | corizza |
| **cost** *The fee or penalty.* | costo, prezzo |
| **costochondritis** *Inflammation of the rib and or its cartilage.* | costocondrite |
| **cotton wool** *Raw cotton.* | cotton grezzo |
| **cotton wool spots** *Condition characterized by blue or white discoloration on the retina related to nerve ischemia.* | essudati cotonosi |
| **cough** *Forceful expulsion of air from the lungs.* | tosse |
| **cough, hacking** *A dry, episodic cough.* | tosse secca, debole e frequente |
| **count, to** *To determine a number.* | contare |
| **cowpox; vaccinia** *A viral disease of cows that was used for an original smallpox vaccine.* | vaiolo bovino |
| **cow's milk** | latte di mucca |
| **coxalgia** *Pain in the hip.* | mal di lombi; coxalgia |
| **crab louse** *Phthirus pubis is formal name for a louse that infests pubic hair and causes intense itching.* | phthirus pubis |
| **crack one's knuckles** *Moving the fingers side to side or with flexion in such a manner to cause a popping or crackling sound.* | nocca scoppiettante |
| **crackles or rales** *A crackling noised noted while auscultating the lungs.* | rantoli crepitanti |
| **cradle** *A bed for an infant.* | culla |
| **cramp** *A painful contraction of muscles.* | crampo |
| **cranial mononeuropathy III** *Dysfunction of the third cranial nerve causes double vision and eyelid drooping.* | mononeuropatia craniale III |
| **cranial mononeuropathy VI** *A disorder of the sixth cranial nerve causes double vision.* | mononeuropatia craniale VI |
| **cranial** *Referring to the skull.* | craniale |
| **cranioclast** *An instrument used to crush a fetal skull.* | cranioclasto |
| **craniopharyngioma** *A tumor that originates in the hypophyseal stalk.* | craniofaringioma |
| **craniosynostosis** *Closure of the sutures of the skull that occurs prematurely.* | craniostosi |
| **craniotabes** *Softening of the skull bones causing widened sutures; this occurs in rickets.* | craniotabe |
| **craniotomy** *Surgical creation of a hole in the skull.* | craniotomia |
| **cranium** *The skeleton of the head.* | cranio |
| **craving** *An unusually strong urge for something.* | desiderio insaziabile |

| English | Italian |
|---|---|
| **craw-craw** *A pruritic papular skin eruption sometimes caused by Onchocerca.* | craw-craw |
| **creatine** *A compound involved with muscle contraction.* | creatina |
| **creatinine** *A compound excreted in the urine that is produced by the metabolism of creatine.* | creatinina |
| **Credé's maneuver** *Manual pressure over the bladder to assist in expression of urine in an atonic bladder.* | metodo di Crede |
| **cremasteric reflex** *Retraction of the testicle and scrotum upon stroking of the ipsilateral inner thigh.* | riflesso cremasterico |
| **crenotherapy** *A form of treatment from mineral springs.* | crenoterapia |
| **crepitus** *A noise heard when one auscultates the lungs that is similar to the sound of rubbing hair between one's fingers. It is also considered the sound of two broken bones rubbing together.* | crepitio |
| **cretinism** *A chronic condition caused by diminished thyroid hormone secretion.* | cretinismo |
| **crevice** *A narrow opening.* | crepa; fessura |
| **cribriform** *Like a sieve; the olfactory nerves pass through the cribriform plate of the ethmoid bone.* | bucato |
| **cricoid cartilage** *The ring-shaped cartilage of the larynx.* | cartilagine cricoidea |
| **cripple** *A person with a physical disability; not used in polite society.* | invalido |
| **crisis** *A turning point in the treatment of a disease.* | crisi |
| **Crohn's disease** *An inflammatory bowel disease.* | malatti di Crohn |
| **cross-infection** *Transfer of infection between individuals, each with a different organism.* | infezione crociata |
| **cross-matching (blood)** *Evaluation of blood to determine compatibility between the donor and recipient prior to transfusion.* | prova crociata di compatibilità |
| **cross-section** *A transverse section through a specimen or structure.* | sezione trasversale |
| **croup** *An acute laryngeal condition that is accompanied by a hoarse, barking cough.* | croup |
| **cruciform** *Shaped like a cross.* | forma di croce |
| **crural; femoral** *Referring to the femur or leg.* | crurale |
| **crush syndrome** *Rhabdomyolysis occurring as a result of muscle injury from mechanical stress.* | sindrome di compressione |
| **crust** *Dried serous exudate covering a wound.* | crosta |
| **crutch** *Long metal or wooden stick used for support while walking.* | gruccia |
| **cryesthesia** *Abnormal sensitivity to cold.* | crioestesia |
| **cryosurgery** *The application of extreme cold to destroy tissue.* | criochirurgia |
| **cryotherapy** *The use of cold for therapeutic purposes.* | crioterapia |
| **cryptococcal meningitis** *A meningeal infection associated with AIDS.* | meningite criptococcica |
| **cryptorchism** *A condition characterized by the failure of the testes to descend into the scrotum.* | criptorchidismo |
| **cryptosporidiosis** *A parasitic related diarrhea seen in AIDS.* | criptosporidiosi |
| **crystalloid** *A substance that can pass through a semipermeable membrane; not a colloid.* | cristalloide |
| **crystalluria** *The presence of crystals in the urine.* | cristalluria |
| **CSF** *Abbreviation for cerebrospinal fluid.* | liquido cerebrospinale |
| **CT scan** *Computerized axial tomography.* | stratigrafia computerizzata |
| **cubital fossa** *The bend at the elbow.* | fossa cubitale |
| **cuffed endotracheal tube** *A cannula that has an balloon on the tip that can be inflated with air and placed into the trachea.* | tubo endotracheale con palloncino |
| **culdoscopy** *Examination of the female pelvic viscera with a scope inserted through the posterior vaginal fornix.* | culdoscopia |
| **culture** *The growth of bacteria in artificial medium.* | coltura |

| English | Italian |
|---|---|
| **culture broth** *A medium used to grow bacteria.* | terreno di coltura |
| **cumulative effect** *A consequence of successive additions.* | effetto cumulativo |
| **cuneiform** *The three bones between the navicular bone and the metatarsals.* | cuneiforme |
| **curare** *A toxic botanical substance used at one time in poison darts in South America. Curare derivatives have been used in general anesthesia.* | curaro |
| **curative** *A remedy capable of healing completely.* | curativo |
| **cure** *A remedy for a medical illness.* | cura di una malattia |
| **curettage** *Removal of tissues from a cavity.* | curettage |
| **curette** *The instrument used during a curettage.* | cucciaio per raschiamento |
| **current** *Flow or stream.* | corrente |
| **currently** *Presently.* | attualmente |
| **Cushing's syndrome** *Characterized by truncal obesity, moon face, acne, abdominal striae, hypertension, decreased carbohydrate tolerance, protein catabolism, psychiatric disturbances, and osteoporosis.* | morbo di Cushing |
| **cushion** *A pillow or stuffed pad used to sit on.* | cuscino |
| **cut** *An incision.* | insezione |
| **cutaneous** *Referring to the skin.* | cutaneo |
| **cuticle** *The dead skin at the base of the toenail or fingernail, also called the eponychium.* | cuticola |
| **cyanocobalamin** *Also called B12; used to treat pernicious and other macrocytic anemias.* | cianocobalamina |
| **cyanosis** *Bluish discoloration of the skin and mucous membranes.* | cianosi |
| **cyclical vomiting** *Periods of recurrent vomiting with no apparent pathologic cause and the person has a normal state of health between the episodes.* | ciclo di vomito |
| **cyclitis** *Inflammation of the ciliary body.* | ciclite |
| **cyclodialysis** *The surgical creation of a communication between the anterior chamber of the eye and the suprachorodial space for the purpose of treating glaucoma.* | ciclodialisi |
| **cycloplegia** *Paralysis of the ciliary muscle.* | cicloplegia |
| **cyclothymia** *Manic-depressive tendencies.* | ciclotimia |
| **cyclotomy** *Surgically creating an opening in the ciliary body.* | ciclotomia |
| **cystadenoma** *Adenoma associated with cysts of neoplastic origin.* | adenoma cistico |
| **cystectomy** *Surgical removal of a cyst or the bladder.* | cistectomia |
| **cystic** *Referring to a cyst.* | cistico |
| **cystic duct** *The duct connecting the gallbladder to the common bile duct.* | ducto cistico |
| **cystic fibrosis** *A congenital disorder exhibited by abnormal thick mucous which leads to problems in the intestines, pancreas and lungs.* | fibrosi cistica |
| **cysticercosis** *The state of being infected with a type of tapeworm.* | cisticercosi |
| **cystinosis** *A congenital disorder of increased cystine that leads to renal insufficiency, rickets and dwarfism.* | cistinosi |
| **cystinuria** *The presence of cystine in the urine.* | cistinuria |
| **cystitis** *Inflammation of the urinary bladder.* | cistite |
| **cystocele** *Protrusion of the urinary bladder through the vaginal wall.* | cistocele |
| **cystography** *Roentgenographic visualization of the urinary bladder after insertion of contrast media.* | cistografia |
| **cystolithiasis** *Presence of a calculus in the urinary bladder.* | cistolitiasi |
| **cystoscope** *A device used to visualized the urinary bladder.* | cistoscopio |

| English | Italian |
|---|---|
| **cystoscopy** *Direct visualization of the urinary bladder with a cystoscope.* | cistoscopia |
| **cytology** *The study of cells, their function and structure.* | citologia |
| **cytoplasm** *The protoplasm of the cell except for the nucleus.* | citoplasma |
| **cytotoxic** *Referring to being harmful to cells.* | citotossico |
| **cytotoxin** *That which is harmful to cells.* | citotossina |
| **dacryoadenitis** *Inflammation of the lacrimal gland.* | dacrioadenite |
| **dacryocystitis** *Inflammation of a lacrimal sac.* | dacriocistite |
| **dacryocystorhinostomy** *Surgical reaction of a communication between the lacrimal sac and nasal cavity.* | dacriocistorinostomia |
| **dacryolith** *A stone in the lacrimal sac or duct.* | dacriolito |
| **dandruff** *Dead skin found in the hair.* | forfora |
| **dark adaptation** *Adjustment to low light by reflex dilation of the pupil.* | adattamento scotopico |
| **date of admission** *Beginning date of hospitalization.* | data di ingresso ospedale |
| **date of birth** | data di nascita |
| **daughter** | figlia |
| **De Quervain tenosynovitis** *Inflammation of the tendons of the wrist including the abductor pollicis longus and extensor pollicis brevis.* | malattia di De Quervain |
| **dead** *Deceased.* | morto |
| **dead space** *The area in the respiratory tract where air is not exchanged.* | spazio morto |
| **deadline** *Cutoff date.* | scadenza |
| **deaf** *Absence of the sense of hearing.* | sordo |
| **deaf-mute** *Inability to hear or speak.* | sordomuto |
| **deafness** *Having impaired hearing.* | sordità |
| **death** *The action of dying.* | morte |
| **debility** *Physical weakness.* | debolezza |
| **debridement** *Trimming the dead tissue adjacent to a wound.* | sbrigliamento |
| **decade** *Ten years.* | decina |
| **decapitate, to** *The physical separation of the head from the body.* | decapitare |
| **decerebrate rigidity** *Rigid extension of the arms which is an abnormal posture associated with increased intracranial pressure.* | rigidità decerebrato |
| **decerebrate** *The removal of the brain.* | decerebrare |
| **decibel** *A unit used in the measurement of sound.* | decibel |
| **decidua** *The mucous membrane lining the uterus during pregnancy.* | decidua |
| **deciduous teeth** *The first teeth.* | denti deciduo |
| **decline** *As in a decrease in status or health.* | declino |
| **decompensation** *The inability of an organ to respond to functional overload.* | scompenso |
| **decompression** *The surgical procedure relieving pressure on a part.* | decompressione |
| **decrease** *Becoming smaller or fewer.* | diminuzione |
| **decubitus ulcer** *A wound caused by laying in one position for too long; also referred to as a pressure ulcer.* | piaga da decubito |
| **decussation** *An area of intersection.* | decussazione |
| **deep** *Having significant depth.* | profondo |
| **deep tendon reflex** *Reflexes exhibited by the stretching of a tendon.* | riflesso tendine profondo |
| **deep vein thrombosis (DVT)** *A blood clot that forms within a vein, typically in the lower extremities.* | trombosi venoso profonda |
| **deer tick** *Ixodes scapularis.* | zecca cervo |
| **defecation** *The discharge of feces from the rectum.* | defecazione |
| **defect** *A shortcoming or imperfection.* | imperfezione |

| English | Italian |
|---|---|
| **defibrillator** *A device used to convert an abnormal cardiac rhythm (ventricular fibrillation) into a normal rhythm with use of electrical stimulation.* | defibrillatore |
| **deficiency** *Insufficiency or deficit.* | mancanza |
| **deformity** *A malformation or imperfection.* | deformità |
| **deglutition** *The process of swallowing.* | deglutizione |
| **dehydration** *The status of having a decrease in total body water.* | disidratazione |
| **delirium** *An acute mental state exhibited by altered thought processes and restlessness.* | delirio |
| **delirium tremens** *A condition seen when alcohol is withdrawn which is exhibited by restlessness, hallucinations and tremors.* | delirium tremens |
| **delivery** *The process of giving birth.* | parto |
| **deltoid** *A term referring to "three". The deltoid muscle has its origin at three areas: clavicle, acromion, and spine of the scapula.* | deltoide |
| **delusion** *A belief that is contradictory to rational thought.* | delirio |
| **delusional** *Referring to a delusion.* | delirante |
| **demanding** *Requiring a lot of skill or requiring a lot of others.* | esigente |
| **demarcation** *Having a fixed boundary.* | demarcazione |
| **dementia** *A chronic brain disorder exhibited by memory loss, personality changes and faulty reasoning.* | demenza |
| **demography** *The study of the structure of human populations.* | demografia |
| **demulcent** *Something that relieves irritation or inflammation.* | lenitivo |
| **demyelinating disease** *A condition characterized by the loss of myelin.* | malatti di memielinizzazione |
| **dendrite** *Impulses are transmitted along a dendrite to a nerve cell body.* | dendrite |
| **denervation** *The removal of nerve supply.* | denervazione |
| **dengue** *A mosquito-borne viral disease exhibited by fever and joint pain.* | dengue |
| **density** *The denseness of an object.* | densità |
| **dental** *Referring to teeth.* | dentale |
| **dental calculus** *Calcium phosphate and carbonate adhered to the teeth.* | tartaro dentario |
| **dental caries** *Decay of teeth.* | carie dentaria |
| **dentatum** *Also referred to as dentate nucleus of cerebellum.* | nucleo dentato |
| **dentist** *A professional capable of treating diseases of the teeth and gums.* | medico dentista |
| **dentition** *The natural teeth.* | dentizione |
| **denture** *A frame that holds artificial teeth.* | dentiera |
| **deny, to** *To reject or repudiate.* | negare |
| **deoxyribonucleic acid (DNA)** *The carrier of genetic information.* | acido desossiribonucleico |
| **depilatory** *An agent used to remove hair.* | depilatorio |
| **depressed** *Melancholy.* | depresso |
| **depressed skull fracture** *Concave fracture deformity of the skull.* | frattura depressa del cranio |
| **depression** *A medical condition exhibited by profound despondency.* | depressione |
| **deprivation** *The lack of a necessity.* | deprivazione |
| **dermatitis** *Non-specific inflammation of the skin.* | dermatite |
| **dermatography** *A description of the skin.* | dermatografia |
| **dermatologist** *A physician specializing in dermatology.* | dermatologo |
| **dermatology** *The medical profession involving the treatment of skin conditions.* | dermatologia |
| **dermatome** *The area of sensation of the skin supplied by a single posterior spinal root.* | dermatomo |

| English | Italian |
|---|---|
| **dermatomycosis** *An infection of the skin by Trichophyton, Microsporum or Epidermophyton fungi.* | dermatomicosi |
| **dermatomyositis** *Inflammation of the skin, subcutaneous tissue and adjacent muscle.* | dermatomiosite |
| **dermatophyte** *A fungal parasite living on the skin.* | dermatofito |
| **dermatosis** *Any skin disease.* | dermatosi |
| **dermis** *The "true skin" that lies beneath the epidermis.* | derma |
| **dermographia** *A raised, pale line with hyperemic borders is elicited upon scratching the skin with a dull instrument, in this condition.* | dermografismo |
| **dermoid cyst** *An abnormal growth containing hair follicles, skin and sebaceous glands.* | cisto dermoide |
| **descending** *Moving toward the inferior portion.* | discendente |
| **desensitize, to** *To gradually expose a person to an offending agent to prevent an abnormal response upon a secondary exposure.* | desensibilizzare |
| **desiccation** *The act of drying up.* | essicctivo |
| **desmoid** *A tumor typically found in the abdomen which contains. muscle and connective tissue.* | desmoide |
| **despite** *Notwithstanding.* | malgrado |
| **desquamation** *The shedding of skin in flakes or sheets.* | desquamazione |
| **deterioration** *Worsening in one's medical condition.* | deterioramento |
| **detoxification** *The process of removing toxins from the body.* | disintossicazione |
| **detrimental** *Harmful.* | dannoso |
| **detritus** *Particulate matter produced by the decomposition of an organic substance.* | detrito |
| **detrusor urinae** *Smooth muscle fibers that extend from the urinary bladder to the pubis.* | muscolo pubovescicale |
| **deuteranomaly** *Abnormal color vision sometimes called "green weakness".* | deuteranomalia |
| **deviated septum** *Characterized by deviation of the nasal septum.* | setto deviazione |
| **deviation** *Away from the norm. (deviation to the right)* | deviazione (caduta verso destra) |
| **devic disease** *Also known as neuromyelitis optica; it is a demyelinating disorder associated with a transverse myelopathy and optic neuritis.* | neuromielite ottica di Devic |
| **dexter**; *right; straight; erect* | destro |
| **dextran** *A high glucose polymer used as a plasma substitute.* | destrano |
| **dextrocardia** *Location of the heart in the right hemithorax.* | destrocardia |
| **dhobie itch** *So called because the contact dermatitis is caused by the soap used by laundry workers in India who are called "dhobie".* | inguinocrurale pruriginosa dei lavandai |
| **diabetes insipidus** *Caused by a deficiency in vasopressin, it is exhibited by great thirst and large volume urine output (and normal blood sugar).* | diabete insipido |
| **diabetes mellitus** *A disease exhibited by a deficiency of the pancreatic hormone insulin.* | diabete mellito |
| **diabetic** *A person who has diabetes mellitus.* | diabetico |
| **diabetic neuropathy** *Pain and burning initially in the feet, associated with diabetes mellitus.* | neuropatia diabetico |
| **diagnostic** *A specific symptom or characteristic.* | diagnostico |
| **diapedesis** *The outward passage of blood elements through an intact vessel wall.* | diapedesi |
| **diaper** *Undergarment worn to absorb urine in incontinent persons.* | pannolino assorbente |
| **diaper rash** *Macular rash in the inguinal/perineal region related to exposure to urine.* | dermatite da pannolino |
| **diaphoretic** *Exhibited by profuse perspiration.* | diaforetico |

| English | Italian |
|---|---|
| **diaphragm** *The muscular separation between the thoracic and abdominal cavities.* | diaframma |
| **diaphragmatic hernia** *Protrusion of visceral contents through the diaphragm.* | ernia diaframmatica |
| **diaphysis** *The central part of a long bone.* | diafisi |
| **diarrhea** *Increase in frequency and a loose consistency of the stools.* | diarrea |
| **diarthrosis** *An articulation allowing free movement.* | diartrosi |
| **diastase** *Amylase.* | diastasi |
| **diastole** *The period of dilatation of the heart; between the first and second heart sounds.* | diastole |
| **diathermy** *The use of heat produced from high-frequency electric currents to medically or surgically treat someone.* | diatermia |
| **diathesis** *A medical tendency to develop a specific condition.* | diatesi |
| **die, to** *To stop living, to expire.* | morire |
| **diet** *The kinds of food a person eats.* | dieta |
| **dietitian** *A professional who works with diet and nutrition.* | dietista |
| **differential diagnosis** *A term used to refer to the various options for diagnoses.* | diagnosi differenziale |
| **differential leukocyte count** *The percentage of different types of leukocytes.* | differenziale conteggio dei leucociti |
| **digestion** *The process of enzymatic breakdown of food in the alimentary canal.* | digestione |
| **digit** *Finger or toe.* | dito della mano o di un piede |
| **digitalis** *Cardiac medication derived from the leaf of Digitalis purpurea.* | digitalis |
| **dilatation** *The process of becoming wider or larger.* | dilatazione |
| **dilator** *An instrument that dilates.* | dilatatore |
| **dilution** *The process of making a weaker solution.* | diluizione |
| **dimercaprol** *A medication used as a binding agent for heavy metal poisoning.* | dimercaprolo |
| **dioptre** *Referring to refraction or transmitted and refracted light.* | diottria |
| **dioxide** *A compound containing two oxygen atoms.* | biossido |
| **diphtheria** *A contagious bacterial disease characterized by a grey membrane on the pharynx along with respiratory or cutaneous symptoms; caused by Corynebacterium diphtheriae.* | difterite |
| **diplegia** *The paralysis of both arms or both legs.* | diplegia |
| **diplococcus** *A bacterium that occurs in pairs including pneumococcus and Neisseria gonorrhoeae and Neisseria meningitidis.* | diplococcus |
| **diploid** *A nucleus containing two complete sets of chromosomes.* | diploide |
| **diplopia** *Double vision.* | diplopia |
| **dipsomania** *Compulsion to drink alcoholic beverages.* | dipsomania |
| **dirty** *Unclean.* | sporco |
| **disability** *Decreased or impaired mental or physical ability.* | incapacità lavorativa |
| **disaccharide** *A type of sugar that yields two monosaccharides upon hydrolysis.* | disaccaride |
| **disappearance** *An instance of something/someone gone missing.* | scomparsa |
| **disarticulation** *The separation or amputation of a joint.* | disarticolazione |
| **discharge, ear** *Otic secretions.* | essudazione orecchio |
| **discharge, nasal** *Nasal secretions.* | essudazione nasale |
| **discharge, postpartum vaginal** *The secretions noted after delivery.* | essudazione dopo il parto vaginale |
| **discharge, vaginal** *Vaginal secretions.* | leucorrea |

| English | Italian |
|---|---|
| **discharge date** *The day a patient is released from the hospital.* | data di licenziamento ospedal |
| **discomfort** *A feeling of physical or mental unease.* | disagio |
| **discrete** *Separate and distinct.* | separato, distinto |
| **disease** *Malady or disorder.* | malattia, infermità |
| **disease outcome** *The response obtained from treatment.* | esito di malattia |
| **disequilibrium** *The absence of stability.* | squilibrio fisico |
| **disinfectant** *A substance that kills bacteria.* | disinfettante |
| **dislocation** *The displacement of a bone when referring to an articulation.* | lussazione |
| **disorder** *Impairment.* | disordine |
| **disorientation** *Mental confusion.* | disorientamento |
| **displacement** *Movement from normal position.* | spostamento dall abituale posizione |
| **disrobe, to** *To remove clothing.* | spogilare |
| **dissecting aneurysm** *A condition in which blood is present between the layers of an artery.* | aneurisma disseccante |
| **dissection** *Autopsy or postmortem exam.* | preparato anatomico ottenuto per dissezione |
| **dissemination** *To be spread or dispersed widely.* | disseminazione |
| **dissolution** *Disintegration.* | dissolvimento |
| **distal** *Situated away from the center of the body.* | distale |
| **distended bladder** *Urinary bladder filled beyond the normal capacity.* | vescica urinaria esteso |
| **distension** *Swollen.* | distensione |
| **distichiasis** *Presence of two rows of eyelashes on one eyelid which are turned inward toward the globe.* | distichiasi |
| **distribution** *The manner in which something is shared or spread out.* | distribuzione |
| **diuresis** *Increased excretion of urine.* | diuresi |
| **diuretic** *Medication which causes an increased excretion of urine.* | diuretico |
| **diurnal** *Occurring during the day.* | diurno |
| **diverticulitis** *Inflammation of the diverticulum.* | diverticolite |
| **diverticulosis** *Presence of diverticulum.* | diverticolosi |
| **diverticulum** *A sac or pouch created by herniation of a mucous membrane in the alimentary canal.* | diverticolo |
| **diver** *A person who swims in deep water.* | subacqueo |
| **dizygotic twins** *Twins from two separate zygotes (non-identical twins).* | gemelli dizigotici |
| **dizziness** *Sensation of losing one's balance.* | trastornos del equilibrio |
| **DNA** *Deoxyribonucleic acid. The hereditary material in humans and almost all other organisms.* | acido desossiribonucleico |
| **DNR** *Do not resuscitate. The term used to indicate a person should not have life sustaining measures taken if they were to have cardiopulmonary arrest.* | non rianimare |
| **donor** *Referring to a person who donates tissue or an organ.* | donatore |
| **dopa reaction** *A dopa-oxidase reaction, changing dopa into melanin.* | reazione dopa |
| **dopamine** *An intermediate product in the creation of norepinephrine.* | dopamina |
| **dorsal** *Referring to the back or back surface.* | dorsale |
| **dorsal root** *A description of the site of ganglion found on the dorsal root of each spinal nerve.* | radice dorsale |
| **dorsiflexion** *Backward bending of the foot or hand.* | dorsiflessione |
| **dorsum** *The back part.* | dorso |
| **dosage** *The amount and frequency a medication is given.* | dosaggio |
| **dose** *The quantity of a medication.* | dose |
| **dose, maintenance** *The chronic dose given after the initial bolus.* | dose di mantenimento |

| English | Italian |
|---|---|
| **dosing interval** *The number of times per unit a medication is given.* | intervallo di dosaggio |
| **double** *Twice the size, quantity or strength.* | doppia |
| **douche** *Cleansing of a canal; unless otherwise specified it refers to cleansing of the vaginal canal.* | doccia |
| **Douglas' pouch** *A recess in the peritoneum between the rectum and the uterus. Also called the rectouterine pouch.* | tasca di Douglas |
| **down** *In a lower position.* | lanugine |
| **Down's syndrome** *A congenital chromosomal defect (trisomy 21) that causes diminished intellectual function, short stature and a broad face.* | sindrome di Down |
| **drainage tube** *A cannula used to allow outflow of fluids.* | tubo drenaggio |
| **drape** *The fabric used as a sterile covering in the OR.* | drappo di sala operatoria |
| **drastic** *Having significant effect.* | drastico |
| **dream** *The thoughts or images occurring during sleep.* | sogno |
| **dressing** *The gauze applied to a wound. (dry dressing)* | medicazione (medicazione a secco) |
| **dribble, to** *To slowly, drip-by-drip, release urine for example.* | gocciolare |
| **drill** *Cylindrical metal tool uses for creating a hole in bone in surgery.* | trapano |
| **drink, to** *To imbibe.* | bere |
| **drinking water** *Water clean enough to ingest orally.* | acqua potabile |
| **drop** *A single bit of fluid as in a drop seen while giving IV fluids.* | goccia |
| **drop by drop** *Expression meaning little by little.* | goccia a goccia |
| **drop foot gait** *A gait characterized by dragging the foot, as there is no ankle dorsiflexion; usually associated with steppage gait.* | camminata piede cadente |
| **drop foot** *The symptom in a person with a nerve injury causing impaired ankle dorsiflexion.* | piede cadente |
| **dropper** *A device used to administer medicines one drop at a time.* | contagocce |
| **drops per minute** *Refers to iv fluid rate.* | gocce al minuto |
| **drowning** *The process of dying from submerging in and inhaling water.* | morte per annegamento |
| **drowsiness** *Sleepiness.* | sonnolenza |
| **drug** *A medication, sometimes with negative connotation.* | farmaco; medicamento |
| **drug dependence** *Addiction to a substance.* | farmaco-dipendenza |
| **drug eruption** *A diffuse rash caused by a medication.* | eruzione di droga |
| **drug reaction** *Typically refers to an adverse effect of medication.* | reazione della droga |
| **drunk** *Inebriated.* | ubriaco |
| **dry** *Absence of moisture.* | secco; asciutto |
| **dry cough** *A cough without sputum production.* | tosse secca |
| **dual diagnosis** *Term used to describe the presence of alcohol/drug addiction associated with a psychiatric diagnosis such as depression.* | abitudine alla droga e disturbo di salute mentale |
| **duct** *Hollow tubular tissue used to carry fluid from a secretory organ.* | cotto; canale; tubo |
| **ductus arteriosus** *A fetal artery that communicates between the pulmonary artery and the descending aorta.* | dotto arterioso pervio |
| **dumping syndrome** *Characterized by rapid bowel evacuation after eating in patients with prior gastric surgery.* | sindrome da rapido svuotamento |
| **duodenal** *Referring to the duodenum.* | duodenale |
| **duodenal ulcer** *A defect in the lining of the first portion of the small bowel, typically caused by H. pylori.* | ulcera duodenale |
| **duodenectomy** *Excision of the duodenum.* | duodenectomia |
| **duodenitis** *Inflammation of the duodenum.* | duodenite |
| **duodenum** *The portion of the small bowel between the stomach and jejunum.* | duodeno |
| **duplication** *The process of duplicating something.* | duplicazione |
| **Dupuytren's contracture** *A disease of the palmar fascia causing a flexion contracture of the fourth and fifth fingers.* | morbo di Dupuytren |

| English | Italian |
|---|---|
| **dura mater** *The outermost covering of the brain and spinal cord.* | dura madre |
| **dust** *Dry earthen particles found on the ground and surfaces.* | polvere |
| **dwarf** *Abnormally small person.* | sottosviluppato |
| **dysaphia** *Altered sense of touch.* | disafia |
| **dysarthria** *Difficulty in articulation of speech.* | disartria |
| **dysbarism** *Condition caused by a change in pressure, noted most commonly among scuba divers.* | disbarismo |
| **dyschezia** *Pain experienced during defecation.* | dischezia |
| **dyschondroplasia** *The formation of cartilaginous and bony tumors near the epiphyses.* | discondroplasia |
| **dyscoria** *A discordance in pupillary reaction.* | discoria |
| **dyscrasia** *An abnormal condition, mostly referring to the blood.* | discrasia |
| **dysdiadocokinesia** *The inability to arrest one motor response and substitute its opposite.* | disdiadococinesia |
| **dysentery** *A severe form of diarrhea with blood and mucous in the stool.* | dissenteria |
| **dysesthesia** *1. Impairment of the sense of touch. 2. The presence of persistent pain upon receiving a light touch.* | disestesia |
| **dysfunction** *Abnormal function in a gland or body organ.* | disfunzione |
| **dyshidrosis** *Disregulation of sweating* | disidrosi |
| **dyshidrotic eczema** *A dermatitis characterized by vescicobullous lesions.* | dermatite di disidrosi |
| **dyskinesia** *Abnormal movement.* | discinesia |
| **dyslalia** *The absence of comprehensible speech articulation.* | dislalia |
| **dyslexia** *Difficulty in learning or reading written language with no effect on intelligence.* | dislessia |
| **dysmenorrhea** *Pain during menstruation.* | dismenorrea |
| **dyspareunia** *Pain during sexual intercourse.* | dispareunia |
| **dyspepsia** *Indigestion.* | dispepsia |
| **dysphagia** *Difficulty in swallowing.* | disfagia |
| **dysphasia** *Difficulty in speaking caused by cerebral dysfunction.* | disfasia |
| **dysplasia** *The increase in organ size due to an increase in the number of abnormal cell types.* | displasia |
| **dyspnea** *Difficult breathing.* | dispnea |
| **dystocia** *Difficult birth caused by fetal position, narrow pelvis or lack of opening of the cervix.* | distocie |
| **dysuria** *Difficulty or pain upon urination.* | disuria |
| **ear** *The organ of hearing and balance.* | orecchio |
| **ear infection** *General term referring to otitis media or otitis externa.* | infezione orecchio |
| **ear, external** *Auris externa.* | orecchio esterno |
| **ear, inner** *Auris interna.* | orecchio interno |
| **ear, middle** *Auris media.* | orecchio medio |
| **ear-drum** *Common term for tympanic membrane.* | membrana del timpano |
| **earache** *Pain associated with the ear.* | otalgia; dolore all'orecchio |
| **earlobe** *The soft, fleshy inferior portion of the pinna.* | lobo dell'orecchio |
| **eat, to** *To consume food.* | mangiare |
| **eating disorder** *General term for pathologic eating habits.* | disturbo alimentare |
| **ecchondroma** *Hyperplastic growth of cartilage on the surface of other cartilage.* | eccondroma |
| **ecchymosis** *Skin discoloration caused by bleeding beneath the epidermis.* | ecchimosi |

| English | Italian |
|---|---|
| **Echinococcus** *A tapeworm of the family Taeniidae that can cause hydatid cysts.* | echinococco |
| **echocardiography** *The use of ultrasound waves to visualize the heart and its structures.* | ecocardiografia |
| **echolalia** *The meaningless repetition of the words spoken by another person.* | ecolalia |
| **eclampsia** *A maternal condition characterized by convulsions and hypertension that can lead to maternal and fetal death.* | eclampsia |
| **ecmnesia** *Memory loss for recent events but retained memory of remote events.* | ecmnesia |
| **ectasia** *Expansion or distension.* | ectasia |
| **ectoderm** *The outermost layer of the three layers of the embryo.* | ectoderma |
| **ectopic** *Abnormal position.* | ectopico |
| **ectopic pregnancy** *A pregnancy that is not intrauterine.* | gravidanza ectopica |
| **ectrodactylia** *A congenital anomaly exhibited by absence of one digit or part of a digit.* | ectrodattilia |
| **ectropion** *Eversion of the eyelid, usually the lower lid.* | ectropion |
| **eczema** *A medical condition exhibited by pruritic, red, scaly patches on the scalp, cheeks and extensor surfaces.* | eczema |
| **edema** *Extravascular fluid accumulation.* | edema |
| **edematous** *Referring to the presence of edema.* | edematoso |
| **education** *Instruction or guidance.* | educazione |
| **effector** *An organ that responds to a stimulus.* | effettore |
| **efficacious** *Effective.* | efficace |
| **effort** *Attempt or endeavor.* | sforzo |
| **effusion** *The accumulation of fluid in a body cavity.* | effusione |
| **egg** | uovo |
| **egocentric** *Thinking of self without considering the feelings or thoughts of others.* | egocentrico |
| **ehrlichiosis** *A tickborne infectious disease.* | ehrlichiosi |
| **ejaculation** *The emission of semen at the moment of sexual climax in a male.* | eiaculazione |
| **elastic bandage** *A stretch gauze used for compression of an extremity.* | bendaggio elastico |
| **elastin** *A connective tissue-based glycoprotein.* | elastina |
| **elbow** *The joint between the humerus and radius/ulna.(right elbow, left elbow)* | gomito |
| **elderly** *Advanced in years.* | anziano |
| **elective** *Non-urgent and not life-saving.* | elettivo |
| **electrocardiogram** *Display of a person's heart beat that can be used in the diagnosis of cardiac disorders.* | elettrocardiogramma |
| **electroconvulsive therapy (ECT)** *The electrical stimulation of the brain to treat mental disorders.* | terapia elettroconvulsivante |
| **electrode** *A device used to facilitate conduction of electricity to or from a body.* | elettrodo |
| **electroencephalogram (EEG)** *A display of brain waves used in the diagnosis of brain disorders, especially epilepsy.* | elettroencefalogramma |
| **electrolyte** *The ionized constituents including potassium, sodium, chloride and others.* | elettrolito |
| **electromyography** *The display of the electrical activity of muscle.* | elettromiografia |
| **electron microscope** *A device that uses electron beams and lenses to give high magnification.* | microscopio elettrone |
| **electrophoresis** *The movement of charged particles in a fluid that is under the influence of an electric field. This is used in testing for various maladies in the form of serum protein electrophoresis.* | elettroforesi |

| English | Italian |
|---|---|
| **elephantiasis** *A condition caused by nematode parasites leading to lymphatic obstruction and limb or scrotal swelling.* | elefantiasi |
| **elixir** *A medical solution.* | elisir |
| **emaciation** *Abnormally thin and weak.* | emaciazione |
| **embolectomy** *The removal of an embolus.* | embolectomia |
| **embolus** *A blood clot, air bubble or fatty deposit that cause obstruction of a vessel.* | embolo |
| **embryo** *The term used to describe a fertilized ovum in the first 8 weeks of development.* | embrione |
| **embryology** *The study of the embryo.* | embriologia |
| **emergence** *Coming into prominence.* | apparizione |
| **emergency** *An urgent, life-threatening situation.* | emergenza |
| **emergency room** *A ward used for initial treatment of critical patients.* | sala pronto soccorso |
| **emesis** *Vomiting.* | vomito |
| **emesis basin** *A small bowl used to catch vomitus.* | basino di memtismo |
| **emetic** *An agent that induces vomiting.* | emetico |
| **emmetropia** *The normal correlation between eye refraction and the axial length of the eyeball.* | emmetropia |
| **emollient** *Having softening or soothing qualities.* | emolliente |
| **emotion** *An intense feeling.* | emozione |
| **empathy** *To be concerned for and share the feelings of another.* | empatia |
| **emphysema** *Abnormal enlargement of the airspaces distal to the terminal bronchioles.* | enfisema |
| **empty** *Containing nothing.* | vuote |
| **empty sella syndrome** *Compressed or flattened pituitary related to herniating arachnoid, surgery or radiotherapy.* | sindrome della sella turcica vuota |
| **empyema** *A collection of purulent material in a body cavity, usually referring to a thoracic empyema.* | empiema |
| **emulsion** *The dispersion of one liquid into another, but it is not dissolved.* | emulsione |
| **enarthrosis** *The type of joint in which a spherical bone is set into the socket of another bone.* | enartrosi |
| **encephalic** *Referring to the brain.* | encefalico |
| **encephalitis** *Inflammation of the brain.* | encefalite |
| **encephalocele** *The protrusion of the brain through a defect in the skull.* | encefalocele |
| **encephalography** *Roentgenography of the brain.* | encefalografia |
| **encephalomacia** *Abnormal softness of the brain.* | encefalomalacia |
| **encephalomyelitis** *Inflammation of the brain and spinal cord.* | encefalomielite |
| **encephalopathy** *Degeneration of cerebral function.* | encefalopatia |
| **enchondroma** *An abnormal increase in cartilage growth on the inside of bone or of other cartilage.* | encondroma |
| **encopresis** *Involuntary defecation.* | encopresi |
| **end organ** *The encapsulated end of a sensory nerve.* | corpuscolo terminale |
| **end point** *The last stage of a process.* | punto estremo |
| **end stage** *Terminal stage. End stage cancer means there is no cure possible and death is imminent.* | ultimo stadio |
| **endarteritis** *Tunica intima inflammation.* | endoarterite |
| **endemic** *When a disease is commonly found in a location or in a people group.* | endemico |
| **endocarditis** *Inflammation of the endocardium.* | endocardite |
| **endocervicitis** *Inflammation of the mucosal lining of the cervix.* | endometrite cervicale |
| **endocrine gland** *A gland that secrete hormones and other substances into the blood.* | ghiandola endocrino |

| English | Italian |
|---|---|
| **endocrine** *Referring to glands that secrete hormones and other chemicals into the blood.* | endocrino |
| **endocrinology** *The study of endocrine glands and hormones.* | endocrinologia |
| **endoderm** *The innermost layer of the embryonic germ cell layers.* | entoderma |
| **endogenous** *Originating from within.* | endogeno |
| **endolymph** *The fluid collection the labyrinth of the ear.* | endolinfa |
| **endometrioma** *An isolated benign mass containing endometrial tissue.* | endometrioma |
| **endometriosis** *Presence of uterine mucosal tissue in the pelvis in abnormal locations.* | endometriosi |
| **endometritis** *Inflammation of the endometrium.* | endometrite |
| **endometrium** *The mucous membrane lining of the uterus.* | endometrio |
| **endoneurium** *The tissue in a peripheral nerve that separates the individual nerve fibers.* | endonervio |
| **endoplasmic reticulum** *A framework of tubules within the cytoplasm of eukaryotic cells.* | reticolo endoplasmico |
| **endorphin** *Hormone secreted that activates the body's opiate receptors and acts as an analgesic.* | endorfine |
| **endoscope** *A device used to view the interior of a hollow organ (sigmoidoscope, gastroscope)* | endoscopio |
| **endothelioma** *A mass that propagates from the endothelium of blood vessels, lymphatics or serous cavities.* | endotelioma |
| **endotracheal** *Within the trachea.* | endotracheale |
| **endow, to** *To supply or provide for.* | provvedere |
| **enema** *A procedure involving insertion of fluid into the rectum.* | clisma |
| **enkephalin** *Peptide found in the brain that has similar effects as the endorphins.* | encefaline |
| **enlargement** *Becoming bigger.* | ingrossamento |
| **enophthalmos** *Posterior displacement of the eyeball in the orbit.* | enoftalmo |
| **enormous** *Very large.* | enorme |
| **enostosis** *The abnormal bony growth inside a bone or on the cortex.* | enostosi |
| **ensure, to** *To make certain of.* | garantire |
| **ENT** *Abbreviation for ears, nose and throat.* | Orecchio, naso, gola |
| **enteral feeding** *Nutrition supplied via the alimentary canal.* | alimentazione enterico |
| **enterectomy** *Surgical resection of part of the intestine.* | enterectomia |
| **enteric** *Referring to the intestines.* | enterico |
| **enteritis** *Inflammation of the intestines.* | enterite |
| **enterobiasis** *An infection caused by worms from the genus Enterobius.* | infestazione da vermi del genere Enterobius |
| **enterococcus** *A gram positive cocci that occurs naturally in the intestine but is pathogenic elsewhere in the body.* | enterococco |
| **enterolith** *A calculus of the intestine.* | enterolito |
| **enteroptosis** *Inferior displacement of the intestines in the abdomen.* | enteroptosi |
| **enterotomy** *A surgical opening of the intestines.* | enterotomia |
| **entrapment neuropathy** *Weakness or numbness caused by compression of a peripheral nerve.* | neuropatia intrappolamento |
| **enucleation** *Surgical removal of a globe.* | enucleazione |
| **enuresis** *Involuntary urination.* | enuresi |
| **enzyme** *A compound that acts as a catalyst for reactions within cells as assists with digestion outside of cells.* | enzima |
| **eosinophil** *A cell with eosin stain used to designate a type of leukocyte that is elevated during allergic reactions.* | eosinofilo |
| **eosinophilia** *An increased number of eosinophils in the blood.* | eosinofilia |

| English | Italian |
|---|---|
| **ependyma** *The glial lined covering of the cerebral ventricles and the central portion of the spinal cord.* | ependima |
| **ependymoma** *A tumor composed of cells that line the ventricles of the brain.* | ependimoma |
| **ephedrine** *A chemical used to treat asthma because it expands bronchial passages and used to control spinal anesthesia associated shock because it constricts blood vessels.* | efedrina |
| **ephemeral fever** *A fever lasting no more than 24-48 hours.* | febbre effimero |
| **epiblepharon** *A condition exhibited by the eyelashes pressing against the eyeball.* | epiblefaron |
| **epicardium** *The serous membranous, innermost lining of the pericardium.* | epicardio |
| **epicondyle** *A protrusion at the distal end of the humerus.* | epicondilo |
| **epicondylitis** *Inflammation of the epicondyle.* | epicondilite |
| **epicranium** *The skin, fibrous layer (aponeurosis), and muscles lining the scalp.* | epicranio |
| **epidemic** *Ubiquitous development of an infectious disease.* | epidemico |
| **epidemiology** *The study of the incidence, development and control of disease.* | epidemiologia |
| **epidermis** *The skin cells overlying the dermis.* | epidermide |
| **epidermophytosis** *A fungal skin infection caused by an organism from the genus Epidermophyton.* | epidermofitosi |
| **epididymitis** *Inflammation of the duct that moves sperm from the testis to the vas deferens.* | epididimite |
| **epididymo-orchitis** *Inflammation of the epididymis and the testis.* | orchiepididimite |
| **epidural** *The space around the dura of the spinal cord.* | epidurale |
| **epidural anesthesia** *Medication into this space produces analgesia for surgical procedures.* | anestesia epidurale |
| **epidural hematoma** *Formation of a collection of blood outside the dural layer of the brain; usually caused by trauma.* | ematoma epidurale |
| **epigastrium** *The section of the abdomen that overlies the stomach.* | epigastrio |
| **epiglottis** *Tissue at the base of the tongue that covers the trachea when one swallows.* | epiglottide |
| **epilation** *Removal of hair and the roots.* | depilazione |
| **epilepsy** *A condition associated with abnormal brain activity and exhibited by sudden, recurrent convulsions, sensory disturbances and loss of consciousness.* | epilessia |
| **epileptic seizure** *A convulsion related to abnormal brain activity (as opposed to being precipitated by hypoglycemia.)* | convulsione epilettico |
| **epileptiform** *Being similar to epilepsy.* | epilettiforme |
| **epileptogenic** *That which induces seizures.* | epilettogeno |
| **epinephrine** *A hormone secreted by the adrenal gland.* | adrenalina |
| **epiphysis cerebri** *A small structure situated on the mesencephalon between the two sections of the thalamus.* | epifisi cerebrale |
| **epiphysitis** *Inflammation of the end of a long bone that is separated from the shaft by a cartilaginous disc.* | epifisite |
| **episcleritis** *Inflammation of the tissue lying above the sclera.* | episclerite |
| **episiotomy** *A surgical incision of the vagina used to aid childbirth.* | episiotomia |
| **epispadias** *A congenital condition characterized by the urethral meatus being at the superior aspect of the penis* | epispadia |
| **epistaxis** *Bleeding emanating from the nose.* | epistassi |
| **epithelial** *Referring to the epithelium.* | epiteliale |
| **epithelial cast** *Debris found in the urine composed of columnar renal epithelium.* | cilindro renale epiteliale |

| English | Italian |
|---|---|
| **epithelioma** *A malignant tumor composed of epithelial cells.* | epitelioma |
| **epithelium** *The tissue lining the skin and the gastrointestinal tract that is derived from the embryonic ectoderm and endoderm..* | epitelio |
| **epitrochlea** *The medial condyle of the humerus.* | epitrocleare |
| **equal** *The same or uniform.* | equivalente |
| **equilibrium** *When opposing forces are in balance.* | equilibrio |
| **equipment** *Apparatus or instrument.* | equipaggiamento |
| **ergometer** *A device that measures energy expenditure.* | ergometro |
| **ergonomics** *The study of workplace design that focuses on reducing work-related injuries.* | ergonomia |
| **ergosterol** *A compound converted to vitamin D2 upon exposure to ultraviolet light.* | ergosterolo |
| **erosion** *The gradual destruction of surface tissue.* | erosione |
| **error** *Mistake or inaccuracy.* | errore |
| **eructation** *Belch or burp.* | eruttazione |
| **erysipelas** *An acute infection caused by Streptococcus pyogenes that causes fever along with swelling and inflammation. The infection frequently effects the face or one leg.* | erisipela |
| **erythema mutliforme** *A skin condition exhibited by purpuric lesions and bullae usually on the distal parts of extremities but can affect the face and trunk.* | eritema multiforme |
| **erythema nodosum** *The presence of red or purple nodules on the pretibial area.* | eritema nodoso |
| **erythroblast** *A nucleus containing immature erythrocyte.* | eritroblasto |
| **erythroblastosis fetalis** *A hemolytic disease of the newborn.* | eritroblastosi fetale |
| **erythrocyanosis** *A condition exhibited by purple patches with asymmetric swelling, pruritus and burning.* | eritrocianosi |
| **erythrocyte** *Called a red blood cell, it transports oxygen and carbon dioxide to and from the tissues.* | eritrocito |
| **erythrocytopenia** *Low level of erythrocytes in the blood stream.* | eritropenia |
| **erythrocytosis** *A higher than normal level of erythrocytes in the blood stream.* | eritrocitosi |
| **erythropoiesis** *The production of red blood cells.* | eritropoiesi |
| **eschar** *Dry, hard, dead tissue commonly seen with a chronic pressure ulcer or anthrax.* | escara |
| **eserine** *Physostigmine.* | eserina |
| **esophageal** *Referring to the esophagus.* | esofageo |
| **esophagectomy** *Surgical removal of the esophagus.* | esofagectomia |
| **esophagitis** *Inflammation of the esophagus.* | esofagite |
| **esophagoscopy** *Visual inspection the esophagus utilizing a scope.* | esofagoscopia |
| **esophagus** *The muscular tube that connects the throat to the stomach.* | esofago |
| **esotropia** *Medial deviation of the eyes at primary gaze.* | strabismo interno o convergente |
| **essential** *Crucial or necessary.* | essenziale |
| **estrogen** *A hormone involved with developing and maintaining female sexual characteristics.* | estrogeno |
| **ethanol** *Synonym for ethyl alcohol.* | etanolo |
| **ethmoid bone** *A bone at the root of the nose which has perforations for the olfactory nerves to transit.* | osso etmoide |
| **etiology** *The underlying cause of a problem.* | eziologia |
| **eunuch** *A man who has been castrated.* | eunuco |
| **euthanasia** *Killing someone painlessly who is thought to have a terminal condition.* | eutanasia |
| **evacuation** *The emptying of an organ of fluids or gas.* | evacuazione |

| English | Italian |
|---|---|
| **evaluation** *Assessment or evaluation.* | valutazione |
| **eventration** *Protrusion of the intestines from the abdomen.* | sventramento |
| **eversion** *To turn outward.* | eversione |
| **every** *Each or all possible.* | ogni |
| **every day** *Each day.* | ogni giorno |
| **every other day** *On alternate days.* | ogni altro giorno |
| **evident** *Obvious.* | evidente |
| **evisceration** *The removal of bowels from the body.* | eviscerazione |
| **evoked potential** *Electrical impulses that can be noted after stimulation of sensory organs.* | potenziali evocati |
| **evulsion** *Forcible extraction.* | avulsione |
| **exacerbation** *Worsening of an existing problem.* | esacerbazione |
| **examination** *Assessment or evaluation.* | esame |
| **exanthema** *A rash that accompanies a disease or fever.* | esantema |
| **excess** *Surplus or overabundance.* | eccesso |
| **exchange transfusion** *Treatment of hyperbilirubinemia in neonates.* | transfusione sostitutiva |
| **excipient** *An inactive substance used to deliver an active substance.* | eccipiente |
| **excisional biopsy** *Surgical removal of tissue for pathologic examination.* | biopsia escissionale |
| **excoriation** *Superficial loss of skin.* | escoriazione |
| **excrement** *Feces.* | escremento |
| **excreta** *Fecal material.* | escreti |
| **exenteration** *Complete surgical removal of an organ.* | eviscerazione |
| **exercise-induced dyspnea** | dispnea indotta da esercizio |
| **exercised induce angina** *Chest pain noted during exertion related to coronary artery disease.* | angina indotta da esercizio |
| **exfoliation** *The shedding of scales.* | esfoliazione |
| **exhumation** *To remove a dead body from a grave.* | esumazione |
| **exogenous** *Referring to external factors.* | esogeno |
| **exomphalos** *Umbilical hernia.* | exonfalo |
| **exostosis** *A bony prominence growing from the surface of a bone.* | esostosi |
| **exotoxin** *A toxin released from a living cell.* | esotossine |
| **exotropia** *A type of strabismus that is characterized by the eyes turned outward.* | exotropia |
| **expansion** *Enlargement or increase in size.* | espansione |
| **expect, to** *To suppose or presume.* | prevedere |
| **expectorant** *A substance that promotes the secretion of sputum.* | espettorante |
| **expectoration** *The presence of sputum that has been coughed out.* | espettorazione |
| **expiration date** *The date when a medication should no longer be used.* | data di scadenza |
| **expiratory** *Referring to exhalation of air from the lungs.* | espiratorio |
| **expiratory reserve volume** *Amount of air left in the lung after a maximal exhalation, in liters.* | volume di riserva espiratoria |
| **exploratory laparotomy** *Abdominal surgery with the intent of examining the abdominal contents.* | laparotomie explorative |
| **expulsion** *Evacuation or elimination.* | espulsione |
| **expulsion of placenta** *Passage of the placenta out the cervix after childbirth.* | espulsione della placenta |
| **extend, to** *To expand or stretch out.* | estendere |
| **extension** *Going from a bent to straight position.* | estensione |
| **extensor plantar response** *Great toe extension indicating a positive Babinski sign.* | riposta plantare dell'estensore |

| English | Italian |
|---|---|
| **extensor** *Referring to the extension of an extremity or part of an extremity.* | estensore |
| **external ear canal** *Auditory canal.* | condotto uditivo esterno |
| **external** *Outside of the body.* | esterno |
| **extirpate, to** *To totally destroy.* | estirpare |
| **extracapsular** *Situated outside a capsule.* | extracapsulare |
| **extracellular** *Outside the cell.* | extracellulare |
| **extract** *A substance in a concentrated form.* | estratto |
| **extrapyramidal tract** *Motor nerves that are not part of the pyramidal tract.* | sistema motorio extrapiramidale |
| **extrasystole** *Either a premature atrial or ventricular contraction.* | extrasistole |
| **extravasation** *Referring to a situation in which blood or fluid goes out of a vessel it is normally flowing into.* | stravaso |
| **extremity** *Refers to one arm or one leg.* | estremità |
| **extrinsic** *Coming from outside or external sources.* | estrinseco |
| **extubation** *The removal of a tube that was in a body orifice.* | disintubazione |
| **exudate** *The fluid, cells, and debris found in the tissues or a cavity (like pleural space) during inflammation.* | essudato |
| **eye drops** *Liquid applied to eyes for various medical problems.* | collirio |
| **eyebrow** *Supercilium.* | sopracciglio |
| **eyeglasses** *Eye wear used for cosmetic or prescription purposes.* | lenti da vista |
| **eyeground** *The fundus that is visualized with an ophthalmoscope.* | fondo dell'occhio |
| **eyelash** *Each of the short hairs on the eyelid.* | ciglia |
| **eyelid** *Palpebra.* | palpebra |
| **eyesight** *A person's ability to see.* | vista |
| **face** *Anterior aspect of the head from the forehead to the chin.* | faccia |
| **face presentation** *Referring to the part of the body coming out of the cervix first during childbirth.* | presentazione di faccia |
| **facet** *A small flat surface of a bone.* | faccetta |
| **facial nerve** *Cranial nerve VII that supplies the face and tongue.* | nervo facciale |
| **facial paralysis** *Lack of movement or sensation in the distribution of the facial nerve.* | paralisi facciale |
| **facial reflex or bulbomimic reflex** *Pressure on the eyeballs causes contraction of facial muscles on the side contralateral to the side of the lesion in the patient in a coma. In coma from a metabolic problem the reflex is present bilaterally.* | riflesso bulmomimic |
| **facies** *A facial expression that is typical for a particular disease.* | espressione del viso |
| **faint** *Weak and dizzy.* | fiacco |
| **fair** *Equitable.* | giusto |
| **falciform** *Referring to something that is curved. The falciform ligament attaches the liver to the diaphragm.* | falciforme |
| **fallopian tubes** *Either of a pair of long narrow ducts located in a female's abdominal cavity that transport the male sperm cells to the egg.* | tube di falloppio |
| **Fallot, tetrology of** *Congenital cardiac defects including ventricular septal defect, pulmonic valve stenosis or infundibular stenosis, and dextroposition of the aorta.* | tetralogia di Fallot |
| **falx cerebri** *A fold in the dura that separates the two cerebral hemispheres.* | falce cerebri |
| **familial** *Referring to the family* | familiare |
| **family** | famiglia |
| **family history** *A review of past medical history of related persons.* | storia di famiglia |
| **family planning** *Birth control.* | programmazione della famiglia |

| English | Italian |
|---|---|
| **Fanconi's syndrome** *An idiopathic refractory anemia exhibited by pancytopenia, bone marrow hypoplasia and congenital anomalies.* | sindrome di Fanconi |
| **faradism** *The gradual increasing and decreasing of the amplitude of electricity.* | faradismo |
| **farmer's lung** *Coined because farmers are susceptible to this disease by inhaling fungi from hay; also called Aspergillosis.* | pneumopatia granluomatosa interstiziale |
| **fart, to** *Slang term for releasing flatus.* | scoreggiare |
| **fascia** *The fibrous sheath enclosing a muscle or organ.* | fascia |
| **fascicle** *A bundle of nerve or muscle fibers.* | fascicolo |
| **fasciculation** *Involuntary contraction of muscle fibers.* | fascicolazione |
| **fasciitis** *Inflammation of a fascia.* | fascite |
| **fasciotomy** *Incision into a fascia.* | fasciotomia |
| **fasting** *Absence of caloric intake for a specified period.* | digiuno |
| **fat** *A greasy or oiling substance naturally occurring in the body.* | grasso |
| **fat embolism** *A deposit of fat that obstructs a vessel.* | embolia grassa |
| **fatal** *Lethal.* | mortale |
| **fatigue** *Tiredness and exhaustion.* | fatica |
| **fatty** *Greasy or oily.* | adiposo |
| **fatty acid** *A carboxylic acid occurring as a an ester in fats and oils.* | acido grasso |
| **favus** *Tinea capitis caused by Trichopyton schoenleini.* | tigna favosa |
| **fear** *Fright or trepidation.* | paura |
| **febrile** *Presence of an supraphysiologic temperature.* | febbrile |
| **fecal impaction** *The presence of hard excrement in the rectum that requires manual removal.* | fecaloma |
| **feces** *Excrement.* | feci |
| **fecundity** *The capability of producing offspring quickly and frequently.* | fecondità |
| **feeble-minded** *Antiquated term used to describe a person unable to make seemingly simple decisions because of a cognitive impairment.* | oligofrenico |
| **feeding behavior** *How a child is tolerating breast or cup feeding.* | comportamento di alimentazione |
| **feel better, to** *To have improved health symptomatically.* | per sentirsi meglio |
| **feel, to** *To perceive or discern.* | toccare |
| **Felty syndrome** *Rheumatoid arthritis with leukopenia and splenomegaly.* | sindrome di Felty |
| **female** *Feminine.* | femminile |
| **feminine pad** *Gauze specially designed to absorb menstrual flow.* | tampone |
| **femoral artery** *Continuation of the external iliac to the popliteal artery.* | arteria femorale |
| **femoral nerve** *Supplies the motor function of the quadriceps and the sensation over the anterior and medial thigh.* | nervo femorale |
| **femoral triangle** *An area that is bordered by the sartorius muscle, the adductor longus muscle and the inguinal ligament.* | triangolo femorale |
| **femur** *The long bone in the thigh.* | femore |
| **fenestration** *Usually referring to a surgical window.* | fenestrazione |
| **fertility** *The ability of a person to contribute to contraception.* | fertilità |
| **fertilization** *The melding of male and female gametes to form a zygote.* | fecondazione |
| **fester, to** *To become infected.* | suppurare in superficie |
| **festinating gait** *Walking with increased speed involuntarily; often seen in Parkinson's disease.* | andatura festinazione |

| English | Italian |
|---|---|
| **fetal alcohol syndrome** *A condition caused by alcohol use by the mother during pregnancy and exhibited by poor intrauterine growth, decreased muscle tone, delayed development and widened palpebral fissures.* | sindrome alcolica fetale |
| **fetal distress** *Term used to describe an abnormal heart rate or rhythm in a fetus indicating the need for urgent childbirth.* | afflizione fetale |
| **fetal heart tone** *Refers to the cardiac rate and pattern of the fetus.* | frequenza cardiaca fetale (FCF) |
| **fetal cardiac monitor** *Device used to monitor fetal heart rate and rhythm.* | monitoraggio cardiaco fetale |
| **fetal movements** *Sensations by the mother of fetal activity.* | movimento fetale intrauterina |
| **fetal position** *Refers to how the fetus lies within the uterus.* | posizione fetale |
| **fetal** *Referring to the fetus.* | fetale |
| **fetichism** *The glorification of an inanimate object.* | feticismo |
| **fetor** *A foul odor.* | fetore |
| **fetus** *Medical term for the infant prior to birth.* | feto |
| **fever** *A temperature above the normal range.* | febbre |
| **fibrillation** *Uncoordinated, ineffective contraction as in atrial fibrillation.* | fibrillatura |
| **fibrin** *An insoluble protein formed when fibrinogen is acted upon by thrombin.* | fibrina |
| **fibroadenoma** *A benign breast mass composed of fibrous and glandular tissue.* | fibroadenoma |
| **fibroblast** *A collagen producing cell in connective tissue.* | fibroblasto |
| **fibrochondritis** *The inflammation of a structure composed of cartilage and fibrous tissue.* | fibrocondrite |
| **fibroelastosis** *The abnormal increase in growth of fibrous and elastic tissue.* | febroelastosi |
| **fibroid** *A benign mass, typically uterine, composed of fibrous and muscle tissue.* | fibroide |
| **fibromyoma** *A mass containing fibrous and muscle tissue.* | fibromioma; leiomioma |
| **fibrosarcoma** *A sarcoma composed primarily of malignant fibroblasts.* | fibrosarcoma |
| **fibrosis** *Connective tissue that is scarred and thickened after injury.* | fibroso |
| **fibrositis** *Fibrous connective tissue that is inflamed.* | fibrosite |
| **fibula** *The smaller of two bones in the lower leg.* | fibula |
| **Fifth disease** *Erythema infectiosum is a viral disease caused by parovirus B19.* | quinta malattia |
| **filaria** *A parasitic nematode worm that is transmitted by flies and mosquitos causing filariasis.* | filaria |
| **file** *Patient record or folder.* | archivio |
| **filiform** *Threadlike.* | filiforme |
| **filum terminale** *The thin structure at the end of the conus medullaris which connects the spinal cord with the coccyx.* | filo terminale |
| **fimbria** *A slender projection at the end of the fallopian tube near the ovary.* | fimbria |
| **finger** *Any of the five digits on the hand.* | dito della mano |
| **finger agnosia** *The inability to distinguish which finger is being touched.* | agnosia digitale |
| **finger nose test** *A test for dysmetria in which a person reaches out to touch their own nose with an extended finger with their eyes closed.* | prove indice-naso |
| **fingerstick device** *A device used to project a lancet into the skin so a drop of blood can be obtained for analysis.* | dispositivo di prelievo |
| **fingertip** *Distal aspect of a finger.* | polpastrello |

| English | Italian |
|---|---|
| **fingernail** *Thin horny plate over the dorsal aspect of the end of finger.* | unghia di un dito |
| **finger-thumb reflex** *Opposition and adduction of the thumb with flexion at the MCP joint and extension at the interphalangeal joint when there is flexion of the 3rd, 4th, and 5th finger. This is present normally and absent with with pyramidal lesions.* | riflesso del dito pollice |
| **Finkelstein test** *Pain elicited with thumb flexion and wrist flexion is indicative of De Quervain tenosynovitis.* | prova di Finkelstein |
| **firm** *Hard or unyielding.* | fermo |
| **first aid** *The initial treatment after an injury.* | pronto soccorso |
| **fish** *A cold-blooded vertebrate with gills and fins.* | pesce |
| **fissure** *A general term for a cleft or deep groove. An anal fissure, for example, is a small ulcer adjacent to the anus.* | fessura |
| **fist** *When a person has their fingers clenched tightly to the palm.* | pugno |
| **fistula** *An abnormal communication between two organs or an organ and the skin, as in rectovaginal fistula.* | fistola |
| **fixation** *1. An obsessive interest. 2. The securing of a body part.* | fissazione |
| **flaccid** *Limp. A term applied to an extremity one cannot move actively.* | flaccido |
| **flagellation** *1. The protrusion found on flagella. 2. Massage administered by tapping a body part with fingers.* | flagellazione |
| **flagellum** *A slender appendage that allows protozoa to swim.* | flagello |
| **flail chest** *The term used when one has multiple rib fractures causing a segment of the chest wall to move incongruently with the rest of the chest wall.* | parete toracica flaccida (respiro paradosso) |
| **flame photometer** *A device used to measure the intensity of light.* | fotometro a fiamma |
| **flap** *A term used to describe a piece of tissue partially excised and placed over an adjacent surface. (cross arm flap)* | lembo (lembo da braccio a braccio) |
| **flare-up** *A sudden worsening one's condition.* | riesacerbazione |
| **flask** *A narrow-necked container.* | fiasco |
| **flat** *Level or even; without bulges.* | piatto |
| **flatfoot** *Common term for pes planus.* | piede piatto |
| **flatten, to** *To make even.* | appiattire |
| **flatulence** *The gas expulsed from the anus.* | flatulenza |
| **flatus** *Term for air that is expelled from the anus.* | flatulenza |
| **flatworm** *A class of worms that includes parasitic flukes and tapeworms.* | verme piatto |
| **flea** *A small wingless insect that feeds on blood of mammals.* | pulce |
| **flesh** *The tissue between the skin and bones.* | carne |
| **flexor** *A muscle that bends an extremity or part of an extremity.* | muscolo flessore |
| **flexure** *The action of bending.* | flessura |
| **flight of ideas** *Streams of unrelated ideas noted in a manic phase.* | fuga delle idee |
| **floating** *Buoyant or suspended.* | flottante |
| **flow** *Movement in a continuous stream.* | flusso |
| **fluid intake** *The amount of oral consumption plus the amount of intravenous fluids administered.* | assunzione di liquidi |
| **fluke** *Parasitic nematode worm; an example is Schistosoma.* | verme trematode |
| **fluoresceine** *A fluorane dye used to check for corneal ulcers.* | fluoresceina |
| **fluorescent antibody test (FTA test)** | antitreponemico fluorescente |
| **fluorescent screen** *A screen used to view x-rays.* | schermo fluorescente |
| **fluoridation** *The addition of fluorine to something.* | fluorurazione |
| **fluorine** *A chemical that causes severe burns if exposed to the skin.* | fluoro |
| **fluoroscopy** *The continuous viewing of roentgenographic images with a fluorescent screen.* | radioscopia |

| English | Italian |
|---|---|
| **flush, to** *Term used to describe an irrigation procedure, as in flushing an NG tube.* | lavaggio |
| **flushing** *Transient erythema due to heat, stress or disease.* | colore |
| **flutter** *Used to describe a cardiac rhythm disturbance, as in atrial flutter.* | flutter |
| **foam** *A mass of small bubbles in a liquid.* | schiuma |
| **Foley catheter** *A drainage tube placed in the urinary bladder via the urethra.* | catetere urinario di Foley |
| **folic acid** *Also called pteroylglutamic acid; a deficiency can cause megaloblastic anemia.* | acido folico |
| **follicle stimulating hormone (FSH)** *An anterior pituitary gland hormone responsible for production of sperm or ova.* | FSH ormone follicolo stimolante |
| **follicular** *Referring to a small secretory gland.* | follicolare |
| **fontanelle or fontanel** *The space between the bones in the skull that are separate at birth.* | fontanella |
| **food** *Nutrition.* | nutrimento |
| **food intake** *Quantitative record of nutritional intake.* | assunzione di cibo |
| **food poisoning** *Poisoning where the active agent is in the food.* | intossicazione alimentare |
| **foot** *The lower extremity distal to the ankle.* | piede |
| **foot and mouth disease** *A contagious viral disease exhibited by oral and digital vesicles.* | afta epizootica |
| **foot drop** *Caused by palsy of the nerve controlling foot dorsiflexion.* | piede cadente |
| **foramen** *An opening in a bone.* | forame |
| **foramen magnum** *The hole in the skull that the spinal cord passes through.* | forame magno |
| **foramen ovale** *A hole in the atrial septal wall in a fetus.* | forame ovale |
| **forced vital capacity** *Vital capacity measured as the patient is exhaling as rapidly as possible.* | capacità vitale forzata |
| **forced expiratory volume per second (FEV1)** *The amount of air exhaled with maximal effort, measured in liters, over one second.* | volume espiratorio massimo in 1 secondo |
| **forceps** *A surgical instrument, commonly called tweezers.* | forcipe |
| **forearm** *Segment of the arm from the elbow to wrist.* | avambraccio |
| **forearm crutch** *A long stick with a place for a hand-grip to aid in ambulation when there is lower extremity weakness.* | stampella avambraccio |
| **forebrain** *The part of the brain that includes the thalamus, hypothalamus and cerebral hemispheres.* | prosencefalo |
| **forehead** *Section of the face from the hairline to the eyebrows.* | fronte |
| **foreign body** *Term used to describe an object found in a body orifice that is not part of the body.* | corpo estraneo |
| **forensic** *Referring to the scientific method of studying crime.* | forense |
| **foreskin** *Also called prepuce, the skin that naturally covers the glans but can be rolled back.* | prepuzio |
| **former** *Prior.* | previo |
| **formulary** *A list of medicines that are permissible to prescribe.* | formulario |
| **fornix** *A vaulted structure.* | fornice |
| **forwards** *Towards the front.* | in avanti |
| **fossa** *A shallow depression.* | fossa |
| **fourchette** *The fork shaped fold of skin where the labia minora meet superior to the perineum.* | forchetta |
| **fovea** *The area on the retina where the visual acuity is optimal.* | fossa, fovea |
| **Foville's syndrome** *Caused by a lesion within the pons, there is ipsilateral facial and abducens nerve paralysis and contralateral hemiplegia.* | sindrome di Foville |
| **fracture** *A broken bone.* | frattura |

| English | Italian |
|---|---|
| **fracture, avulsion** *A broken bone associated with a ligament or tendon pulling a piece of the bone away.* | frattura da avulsione |
| **fracture, closed** *A broken bone where there is no break in the skin.* | frattura semplice |
| **fracture, comminuted** *A broken bone where one segment overrides the other.* | frattura comminuta |
| **fracture, depressed** *The presence of concavity associated with a fracture as in a depressed skull fracture.* | frattura depressa |
| **fracture, greenstick** *A spiral fracture.* | frattura a legno verde |
| **fracture, open** *A fracture in which there is a break in the skin and bone is exposed.* | frattura aperta |
| **fracture, pathologic** *A fracture due at least in part to another condition, such as a fracture at a location where there is bone cancer.* | frattura pathologica |
| **fracture, stress** *A fracture associated with overuse.* | frattura sforzo |
| **fragilitas ossium** *A condition exhibited by excessively brittle bones. Also called osteogenesis imperfecta.* | osteogenesi imperfetta |
| **framboesia; yaws** *An endemic tropical disease caused by Treponema pertenue.* | framboesia |
| **free** *Lacking or absent.* | libero |
| **free from** *Without or clear of.* | libero da |
| **freezing (as in ambient temperature)** *Below 0 Celsius.* | congelamento |
| **fremitus** *A vibration that is appreciated with palpation.* | fremito |
| **frenulum** *The tissue that connects the inferior portion of the tongue to the base of the mouth.* | frenulo |
| **frequency** *Rate of occurrence.* | frequenza |
| **friable** *Easily reduced to powder.* | friabile |
| **friction** *Grating or rasping.* | attrito, sfegamento |
| **friction rub** *A noise heard during cardiac auscultation in patients with pericarditis, for example.* | rumore di sfegamento |
| **frog** *A tailless amphibian that is short with long hind legs for jumping.* | rana |
| **frog in the throat, to have** *An expression describing hoarseness.* | avere la raucedine |
| **frontal** *Referring to the anterior aspect, as in frontal lobe.* | frontale |
| **frontal sinus** *A paranasal sinus on both sides of the lower part of the frontal bone.* | seno frontale |
| **frost itch** *A pruritus noted when exposed to cold weather.* | prurito da freddo |
| **frostbite** *Local tissue destruction after exposure to cold.* | congelamento |
| **froth** *Covered with a mass of small bubbles.* | schiuma |
| **froth at the mouth, to** *To have a mass of saliva with small bubbles in it coming out of the mouth.* | schiuma alla bocca |
| **frozen** *Past participle of to freeze. Freeze: turn a liquid into a solid.* | gelato |
| **frozen shoulder** *Common term for adhesive capsulitis.* | tenosinovite scapolo-omerale cronica; spalla congelata |
| **fructosuria** *Presence of fructose in the urine.* | fruttosuria |
| **FTA test** *Fluorescent treponemal antibody test for syphilis.* | antitreponemico fluorescente |
| **full-term** *A normal length pregnancy.* | completamente a termine |
| **fulminant** *Sudden and severe.* | fulminante |
| **function** *An activity natural to a person or thing.* | funzione |
| **fundus oculi** *Portion of the interior eyeball in the posterior aspect which can be viewed by an ophthalmoscope.* | fondo dell'occhio |
| **fundus of the stomach** *Referring to the part of the stomach above the cardiac notch.* | fondo gastrico |
| **fungicide** *An agent that destroys fungus.* | fungicida |
| **fungus** *A spore-producing organism that feeds on organic matter.* | fungo |

| English | Italian |
|---|---|
| **funiculus of the spinal cord** *The white matter of the spinal cord that is further defined by location.* | cordone anteriore del midollo spinale |
| **funiculus, lateral** *The lateral white column of the spinal cord between the anterior and posterior nerve roots.* | funicolo laterale |
| **funiculitis** *Inflammation of the funiculi.* | funicolite |
| **funnel chest** *Anterior thorax funnel shaped depression, also called pectus excavatum.* | torace a imbuto |
| **furuncle** *A painful erythematous nodule with a central core.* | forunucolo |
| **furunculosis** *The presence of multiple furuncles.* | foruncolosi |
| **fusiform** *Spindle-shaped.* | fusiforme |
| **gag reflex** *Contraction of the pharynx muscles when the back of the pharynx is stimulated by touch.* | riflesso faringeo |
| **gait** *The way one walks.* | andatura |
| **galactocele** *A milk-filled cyst in the mammary gland.* | galattocele |
| **galactorrhea** *Excessive production of milk.* | galattorrea |
| **galactose** *A sugar that is a constituent of lactose.* | galattosio |
| **galactosemie** *1. Galactose in the blood. 2. A congenital condition exhibited by impaired carbohydrate metabolism.* | galattosemia |
| **gallbladder** *The organ adjacent to the liver that stores bile and secretes it into the duodenum.* | cistifellia |
| **gallop** *An abnormal heart sound.* | galoppo |
| **gallstone** *Calculus produced in the bile duct or gallbladder.* | calcoli biliari |
| **galvanism** *The use of electric currents for medical treatment.* | galvanismo |
| **galvanometer** *A device used to measure small electric currents.* | galvanometro |
| **gamete** *A germ cell that is able to unite with another germ cell of the opposite gender to form a zygote.* | gamete |
| **gamma globulin** *A blood serum protein with little electrophoretic mobility.* | gammaglobulina |
| **gamma ray** *A type of electromagnetic radiation.* | raggi gamma |
| **ganglionectomy** *The removal of a benign swelling on a tendon sheath.* | gangliectomia |
| **gangrene** *Tissue death from either impaired blood flow or an infection.* | gangrena |
| **gaping** *Wide open.* | sbadiglio |
| **gargle, to** *To rinse one's mouth out and exhale through the liquid.* | gargarizzare |
| **gargoylism** *A congenital defect, also known as Hurler syndrome, it is characterized by skeletal anomalies, mental retardation and gargoyle-like facial features.* | gargoilismo |
| **gas gangrene** *A life and limb threatening disorder caused associated with tissue death and caused by an anaerobic bacterium in the genus of Clostridium.* | gangrena gassosa |
| **gastrectomy** *Complete or partial surgical resection of the stomach.* | gastrectomia |
| **gastric lavage** *Instillation and removal of large quantities of saline into the stomach in order to treat poisoning.* | lavaggio gastrico |
| **gastric** *Referring to the stomach.* | gastrico |
| **gastric secretions** *Fluids secreted from gastric mucosa.* | secrezioni gastriche |
| **gastrin** *Hormones that stimulates gastric secretions.* | gastrina |
| **gastritis** *Inflammation of the stomach.* | gastrite |
| **gastrocele** *Protrusion of part of the stomach in the form of a hernia.* | archenteron |
| **gastrocnemius** *A large muscle in the lower leg, responsible for ankle plantar flexion, that is attached to the distal femur and achilles tendon.* | muscolo gastrocnemio |
| **gastrocolic reflex** *Peristalsis of the colon produced by food entering the stomach.* | riflesso gastrocolico |
| **gastroduodenal ulcer** *A lesion in the mucosal lining of the stomach or duodenum.* | ulcera gastroduodenale |

| English | Italian |
|---|---|
| **gastroenteritis** *A bacterial or viral infection that leads to vomiting and diarrhea.* | gastroenterite |
| **gastroenterostomy** *A surgical opening in the stomach or intestine.* | gastroenterostomia |
| **gastrointestinal tract** *The alimentary canal from the distal esophagus to the cecum.* | tratto gastrointestinale |
| **gastrojejunostomy** *A surgical procedure that directly connects the stomach to the jejunum.* | gastrodigiunostomia |
| **gastropexy** *Securing the stomach to the abdominal wall.* | gastropessia |
| **gastroscopy** *Use of an endoscope to directly visualize the stomach.* | gastroscopia |
| **gastrostomy** *A surgical creation of an opening in the stomach.* | gastrostomia |
| **gauge** *The size or thickness of something. An 18gauge needle.* | calibro |
| **gauze** *A fabric used for dressing changes.* | garza |
| **gavage syringe** *A syringe used for irrigation.* | siringa sonda gastrica |
| **gavage** *The instillation of food into the stomach with use of a tube.* | alimentazione per sondaggio gastrico |
| **gavage tube** *A tube used for instillation of liquids into the stomach.* | tubo sonda gastrica |
| **gaze** *Steady, intent look.* | sguardo |
| **gel** *A jellylike substance.* | gel |
| **gene** *A unit of heredity that is passed on from parent to child.* | gene |
| **general** *Common or expected.* | generale |
| **general appearance** *The overall look of a patient.* | aspetto generale |
| **genetic counseling** *A discussion of the concerns related to genetic testing.* | consulenza genetica |
| **genetic** *Referring to genes or heredity.* | genetico |
| **geniculate** *Bent at a sharp angle.* | genicolato |
| **geniculate body** *Protrusions on the thalamus that relay visual and auditory signals to the brain.* | corpo genicolato |
| **geniculate ganglion** *The sensory ganglion of the facial nerve.* | ganglio genicolato |
| **geniculate neuralgia** *Severe intermittent pain in the external ear and deep in the ear.* | neuralgia genicolato |
| **genital ambiguity** *A disorder of sexual development in which the genitalia are not sufficiently developed to tell clearly if the person is male or female.* | genitali ambigui |
| **genital herpes** *A sexually transmitted infection caused by herpes simplex.* | herpes genitale |
| **genital wart** *The common term for Condylomata acuminata.* | verruca genitale |
| **genitalia** *Genitals.* | genitale |
| **genitourinary** *Referring to the urinary system through the organs or urine excretion.* | genitourinario |
| **genome** *A full set of genetic information for an organism.* | genoma |
| **gentian violet** *An antiseptic derived from rosaniline.* | violetto di genziana |
| **genu valgum** *A condition exhibited by the knees turning inward, commonly referred to as knock-knee.* | ginocchio valgo |
| **genu varum** *A condition exhibited by the knees turning outward, commonly referred to as bowleg.* | ginocchio varo |
| **GERD gastroesophageal reflux disease** *A condition characterized by gastric contents being regurgitated into the esophagus or mouth.* | malattia da reflusso gastroesofageo |
| **geriatrics** *The study of the health of old people.* | geriatria |
| **germ** *Microorganism.* | germe |
| **German measles** *(rubella) A contagious viral infection.* | rosolia |
| **gerontology** *The study of old persons.* | gerontologia |
| **Gerstmann syndrome** *Finger agnosia, agraphia and acalculia caused by a lesion between the occipital region and angular gyrus.* | sindrome di Gerstmann |

| English | Italian |
|---|---|
| **gestation** *The development of a fetus from conception until birth.* | gestazione |
| **giant** *Huge or massive.* | gigantesco |
| **giardiasis** *A flagellate protozoa, Giardia lamblia, that causes diarrhea.* | giardiasi |
| **giddiness** *A tendency to fall or dizziness.* | capogiro |
| **gingival** *Referring to the gums.* | gengiva |
| **gingivitis** *Inflammation of the gums.* | gengivite |
| **ginglymus** *A joint that allows movement in one direction only.* | ginglimo |
| **glabella** *The area of the forehead above and between the eyebrows.* | glabella |
| **glance** *A brief look at something.* | occhiata |
| **glans penis** *The distal aspect of the penis.* | glande del pene |
| **glare** *An angry stare.* | sguardo furioso |
| **Glasgow coma scale** *A scale used to grade one's level of consciousness with a score of 3 being totally unresponsive and a score of 15 being normal.* | scala di Glasgow del coma |
| **glaucoma** *A condition characterized by increased intraocular pressure.* | glaucoma |
| **glenoid** *Referring to the fossa that is a shallow depression, such as the hollow of the scapula where the humeral head sets.* | glenoideo |
| **glioma** *A neural malignant tumor of glial cells.* | glioma |
| **gliomyoma** *A mass with gliomatous and myomatous characteristics.* | gliomioma |
| **globus pallidus** *A portion of the lentiform nucleus in the brain.* | globus pallidus |
| **glomerulonephritis** *Inflammation of the renal glomeruli, usually from hemolytic streptococcus.* | glomerulonefrite |
| **glomerulus** *A grouping of capillaries where waste is filtered from the blood.* | glomerulo |
| **glomus tumor** *A reddish-blue painful papule that occurs on the distal aspects of the digits.* | tumore di glomus |
| **glossal** *Referring to the tongue.* | linguale |
| **glossectomy** *Surgical resection of the whole or part of the tongue* | glossectomia |
| **glossitis** *Inflammation of the tongue.* | glossite |
| **glossodynia** *Tongue pain.* | glossodinia |
| **glossopharyngeal** *The name for cranial nerve IX that supplies the tongue and pharynx.* | glossofaringeo |
| **glottis** *Essentially the vocal structure, including the true vocal cords and the opening between them.* | glottide |
| **glove** *A covering for hand protection.* | guanto |
| **glove anesthesia** *Absence of sensation of the hand and wrist.* | anestesia del guanto |
| **glucagon** *A pancreatic enzyme responsible for breakdown of glycogen to glucose.* | glucagone |
| **glucose tolerance test** *The oral administration of a carbohydrate load and then evaluation of the blood sugar at timed intervals.* | test di tolleranza al glucosio |
| **glue** *Plastic cements* | colla |
| **glue sniffing addiction** *Habituation of plastic cement fumes inhalation which includes toluene, xylene and benzene.* | dipendenza di l'annusar colla |
| **gluteal** *Referring to the gluteus.* | gluteale |
| **gluteal fold** *The horizontal crease between the buttock and upper thigh.* | piega glutea |
| **gluteal or gluteus muscle** *A paired set of three muscles, the gluteus maximus, medius and minimus, that all have origins in the ilium and insertions in the femur. (buttocks)* | muscolo gluteo |
| **gluteal reflex** *After the skin of the buttocks are stimulated the gluteal muscles contract.* | riflesso gluteale |
| **glycemia** *The amount of glucose in the blood.* | glicemia |
| **glycerin** *A byproduct in the manufacture of soap that is used as a laxative.* | glicerina |

| English | Italian |
|---|---|
| **glycogen** *A compound that stores glucose and when it undergoes hydrolysis forms glucose.* | glicogeno |
| **glycogenesis** *The production of glycogen from glucose.* | glicogenesi |
| **glycolysis** *The production of energy and pyruvic acid when glucose is broken down by enzymes.* | glicolisi |
| **glycoprotein** *A protein that has a carbohydrate attached to its polypeptide chain.* | glicoproteina |
| **glycosuria** *Presence of glucose in the urine.* | glicosuria |
| **gnathic** *Referring to the jaws.* | zigomatico |
| **gnosia** *Ability to recognize things and people.* | gnosia |
| **goblet cell** *Aids in the secretion of respiratory and intestinal mucous.* | cellula calice |
| **goggles** *Close fitting, protective eyeglasses.* | occhiali di protezione |
| **goiter** *Swelling of the thyroid gland.* | gozzo |
| **gold** *Precious metal with atomic number of 79.* | oro |
| **gonad** *A testis or an ovary.* | gonade |
| **gonadal dysgenesis** *The lack of complete development of the gonads.* | disgenesi gonadico |
| **gonadotrophin** *Pituitary hormone that promotes gonadal activity.* | gonadotropina |
| **gonococcus** *A diploccocal bacteria that is the causative agent in gonorrhea, formally Neisseria gonorrhoeae.* | gonococco |
| **gonorrhea** *A sexually transmitted disease that is exhibited by purulent discharge from the vagina or penis.* | gonorrea |
| **gonorrheal arthritis** *A type of arthritis caused by the gram negative diplococcus Neisseria gonorrhoeae.* | artrite gonococcico |
| **gonorrheal ophthalmia** *An acute purulent conjunctivitis that can occur in neonates within 2-5 days of birth.* | oftalmia blenorragica |
| **Goodpasture' syndrome** *Glomerulonephritis, preceded by hemoptysis. The nephritis can quickly progress to death from renal failure.* | sindrome di Goodpasture; pneumopatia interstiziale ed emorragica con nefrite |
| **goose bumps** *Cutis anserina.* | pelle d'oca; cutis anserina |
| **gouge** *A chisel with a concave blade used in surgery.* | sgorbia |
| **gout** *Monosodium urate crystal deposition disease.* | gota |
| **gown** *A sterile gown used during surgical procedures.* | abito sterile |
| **grade** *A level of rank or quality.* | grado |
| **Graefe's sign** *Also called lid lag, a sign characterized by the upper eyelid not closing over the globe. This is seen commonly in exophthalmic goiter.* | segno di Graefe |
| **graft** *A piece of tissue surgically transplanted.* | trapianto |
| **gram** *A unit of mass, 1/1000th of a kilogram.* | grammo |
| **granular layer** *A deep layer of the cerebellum.* | strato granulare |
| **granulation tissue** *Vascular connective tissue forming granular protrusions on the surface of a healing wound.* | tessuto granulazione |
| **granulocyte** *A white blood cell with cytoplasmic secretory granules.* | granulocito |
| **granuloma** *A mass of granulation tissue.* | granuloma |
| **grasp reflex** *Flexion of the fingers or toes when stimulated.* | riflesso in prensione forzata |
| **Graves' disease** *A form of hyperthyroidism exhibited by a goiter and exophthalmos.* | morbo di Grave |
| **gravida** *Pregnant.* | gravida, incinta |
| **gray matter** *The section of the brain and spinal cord composed of branching dendrites and nerve cell bodies.* | materia grigia |
| **greater than normal** *Above normal.* | maggiore del normale |
| **grief** *Deep sorrow.* | angoscia |
| **grip strength** *Quantitative measurement of the force of a hand grip.* | forza prensile |

| English | Italian |
|---|---|
| **groan** *A deep inarticulate sound made due to pain or despair.* | gemito |
| **groggy** *Drowsy.* | stordito |
| **groin pull** *A muscle strain in the inguinal region.* | storcersi inguinale |
| **groin** *The genital region.* | regione inguinale |
| **gross** *Distended; not well defined.* | grosso |
| **ground itch** *Marked pruritus caused by a hookworm larvae, known otherwise as cutaneous larva migrans.* | dermatie vescicolosa da embrione di anchilostoma |
| **growth** *The increase in physical size.* | crescita |
| **growth hormone-releasing factor** *Released by the hypothalamus, it induces the release of somatotropin.* | fattore di rilascio dell'ormone della crescita |
| **grunting** *A low guttural sound used to describe a person with profound respiratory difficulty.* | grugnito |
| **guaiac** *A substance derived from guaiacum trees used to test for trace amounts of blood, in stool for instance.* | guaiaco |
| **guarding** *A symptom used to describe a patient resisting an examination because of severe pain; often seen in patients with peritonitis.* | sorveglianza |
| **Guillain-Barré syndrome** *An acute autoimmune disorder that causes nerve inflammation subsequently muscle weakness.* | sindrome di Guillain-Barré |
| **guinea worm** *A parasitic nematode worm that, in cases of infection, lives under the skin, formally called Dracunculus medinensis.* | verme della Guinea |
| **gum** *Gingiva.* | gengiva |
| **gum (chewing gum)** | gomma da masticare |
| **gumboil** *Swelling noted on the gingiva over a dental abscess.* | ascesso gengivale sottoperiosteo |
| **gumma** *A soft granulomatous tumor of the skin or cardiovascular system seen in tertiary syphilis.* | gomma |
| **gunshot wound** *An penetrating injury sustained from a bullet.* | ferita da arma da fuoco |
| **gustatory agnosia** *The loss of the sense of taste.* | agnosia gustativa |
| **gustatory** *Referring to sense of taste.* | gustativa |
| **guttural** *Having a harsh quality; coming from the back of the throat.* | gutturale |
| **gynecology** *The branch of medicine associated with the reproductive system of women.* | ginecologia |
| **gynecomastia** *Enlargement of the breasts.* | ginecomastia |
| **gyrus** *Convolutions of the brain where there is infolding.* | circonvoluzione |
| **habit** *A custom or inclination.* | abitudine |
| **hair (of body)** | corpo capelli |
| **hair (of head)** | capelli |
| **hair cell** *Epithelial cells with hairlike projections.* | cellula capello |
| **hair follicle** *Tubelike invagination of the epidermis that the hair shaft develops from.* | follicolo pilifero |
| **hairy** *A profuse amount of hair.* | peloso |
| **hairy tongue** *Lingua villosa, a benign condition associated with antibiotic used caused by candida albicans infection.* | linguetta pelosa |
| **half** *Divided in two.* | mezzo |
| **half-life** *The time a drug decreases its effect in half over time.* | emivita |
| **halitosis** *Foul odor emanating from the mouth.* | alitosi |
| **hallucination** *A perception that is not based on reality.* | allucinazione |
| **hallucinogen** *A substance that elicits hallucinations.* | allucinogeno |
| **hallux valgus** *Also called bunion, it is the lateral deviation of the great toe.* | alluce valgo |
| **hallux varus** *Medial deviation of the great toe.* | alluce varo |
| **hamartoma** *A nodule of superfluous tissue.* | amartoma |

| English | Italian |
|---|---|
| **hamate bone; uncinate bone** *The medial bone in the distal row of carpal bones adjacent to the fifth metacarpal.* | osso uncinato |
| **Hamman-Rich syndrome** *Idiopathic pulmonary fibrosis.* | sindrome di Hamman-Rich |
| **hammer toe** *A condition characterized by extension of the proximal phalanx and flexion of the second and distal phalanges.* | dito a martello |
| **Hampton maneuver** *Rolling a patient during gastrointestinal fluoroscopy in order to obtain an air contrast of the antrum and duodenum.* | manovra di Hampton |
| **hamstrings** *Tendons of the posterior thigh.* | tendine delimitante la fossa poplitea |
| **hand** *The upper extremity distal to the wrist.* | mano |
| **hangnail** *A loose piece of skin attached near the medial or lateral nail fold.* | lembo di cuticola ungueale |
| **Hanhart's syndrome** *Also referred to as micrognathia with peromelia. There is hypoplasia of the mandible, malformed or missing teeth, birdlike face and severe upper extremity deformities.* | sindrome di Hanhart |
| **Hansen's disease** *Leprosy* | malattia di Hansen; lebbra |

| English | Italian |
|---|---|
| **haploid** *Either a single set of chromosomes or a set of nonhomologous chromosomes.* | aploide |
| **hapten** *The molecular component that determines immunologic specificity.* | aptene |
| **hard** *Rigid or very firm.* | duro |
| **hard of hearing** *Decreased sense of hearing.* | duro di udito |
| **harmless** *Safe or benign.* | innocuo |
| **hay fever** *An allergy exhibited by pruritus of the eyes and nose, rhinorrhea and excessive lacrimal secretion.* | febbre da fieno |
| **hazy** *Cloudy.* | torbido |
| **head** | testa |
| **head trauma** *Any injury to the brain.* | lesione alla testa |
| **headache** *Cephalgia.* | cefalea |
| **healing** *The process of becoming healthy again.* | salubre |
| **health** *The state of being free of illness.* | salute |
| **health center** *A physical location where patients are treated.* | poliambulatorio; centro sanitario |
| **healthy** *In good health.* | sano |
| **hearing** *Auditory perception.* | udito |
| **hearing aid** *A device that fits in the ear used to amplify sound.* | apparecchio acustico |
| **heart** *Muscular organ that pumps blood thru the circulatory system.* | cuore |
| **heart beat** *A single contraction of the heart.* | battito cardiaco |
| **heart block** *An alteration in the cardiac electrical conduction system.* | blocco cardiaco di conduzione |
| **heartburn** *Synonym of pyrosis.* | pirosi esofagea |
| **heart lung machine** *Device used during cardiac surgery to replace the function of the heart and lungs while surgery is performed.* | macchina cuore -polmoni |
| **heart murmur** *An abnormal heart sound usually related to valvular disease.* | soffio cardiaco |
| **heart rate** *Number or cardiac contractions per minute.* | frequenza cardiaca |
| **heat** *The quality of being hot.* | calore |
| **heat exhaustion** *A condition that occurs secondary to prolonged exposure to high ambient temperature; it is exhibited by subnormal temperature, dizziness and nausea.* | collasso da calore |
| **heat stroke** *A condition caused by excessive exposure to high ambient temperature; it is exhibited by dry skin, thirst, vertigo, muscle cramps and nausea. The three forms are heat exhaustion, heat cramps and sunstroke.* | colpo di calore |
| **heavy** *Possessing great weight.* | pesante |
| **hebephrenia** *A type of schizophrenia exhibited by hallucinations and inappropriate laughter.* | ebefrenia |
| **Heberden's node** *Hard nodules formed at the distal interphalangeal joints in osteoarthritis.* | noduli di Heberden |
| **hedonism** *Devoting oneself to being happy.* | edonismo |
| **heel** *Proximal portion of the plantar aspect of the foot.* | calcagno |
| **heel-shin test (heel to knee to toe test)** *A test of position sense and coordination; one moves the heel of one foot from the knee on the other foot down to the foot.* | prove calcagno-ginocchio |
| **height** *Distance between the bottom of the foot and top of the head.* | altezza |

| English | Italian |
|---|---|
| **Heimlich maneuver** *A forceful upward thrust to the diaphragm to dislodge an airway obstruction.* | manovra di Heimlich |
| **heliotherapy** *Treatment of disease with sunlight.* | elioterapia |
| **helium** *An inert gas that is the lightest of the noble gases.* | elio |
| **helminth** *A fluke, tapeworm or nematode.* | elminto |
| **helminthiasis** *Being infected by a helminth.* | elmintiasi |
| **hemagglutinin** *An antibody that facilitates the agglutination of blood.* | emoagglutinina |
| **hemangioma** *A benign tumor composed of blood vessels.* | emangioma |
| **hemarthrosis** *Presence of intra-articular blood.* | emartro |
| **hematemesis** *Vomiting blood.* | ematemesi |
| **hematin** *The insoluble iron protoporphyrin component of hemoglobin.* | ematina |
| **hematocele** *A mass or area of swelling caused by the accumulation of blood.* | ematocele |
| **hematochezia** *Presence of blood in the excrement.* | ematochezia |
| **hematocrit** *The measurement of the volume of red blood cells compared to the total volume of blood; recorded in percent.* | ematocrito |
| **hematoma** *A mass containing blood.* | ematoma |
| **hematometra** *The accretion of blood in the uterus.* | ematrometra |
| **hematomyelia** *Accumulation of blood in the spinal cord.* | ematomielia |
| **hematoporphyrin** *A derivative of heme that does not contain iron.* | ematoporfirina |
| **hematosalpinx** *Presence of blood in the fallopian tube.* | emosalpinge |
| **hematuria** *The presence of blood in the urine.* | ematuria |
| **heme** *A constituent of hemoglobin that is an insoluble iron protoporphyrin.* | eme |
| **hemeralopia** *Night blindness.* | emeralopia |
| **hemianopsia** *Blindness over half the field of vision.* | emianopsia |
| **hemiballismus** *Severe motor restlessness unilaterally, usually from a subthalamic lesion.* | emiballismo |
| **hemicolectomy** *Surgical removal of part of the colon.* | emicolectomia |
| **hemicrania** *1. Pain on one side of the head. 2. Incomplete anencephaly.* | emicrania |
| **hemiparesis** *Unilateral muscle weakness (half the body).* | emiparesi |
| **hemiplegia** *Paralysis of one side of the body.* | emiplegia |
| **hemisphere** *Referring to either the right or left portion of the cerebrum.* | emisfero |
| **hemizygote** *A cell with only one set of genes.* | emizigote |
| **hemochromatosis** *A hereditary condition exhibited by iron deposition in the tissue and leading to liver disease, bronze discoloration of the skin and diabetes.* | emocromatosi |
| **hemoconcentration** *Decrease in the total fluid content of the blood, leading at times to a falsely elevated hematocrit.* | emoconcentrazione |
| **hemocytometer** *A device used for counting cells from a blood sample.* | emocitometro |
| **hemodialysis** *The process of filtering blood outside the body to remove toxins normally excreted by functioning kidneys.* | emodialisi |
| **hemoglobin** *An iron containing protein used for the transport of oxygen in blood.* | emoglobina |
| **hemoglobinuria** *Presence of free hemoglobin in the urine.* | emoglobinuria |
| **hemolysis** *Breakdown of hemoglobin.* | emolisi |
| **hemolytic** *Something that causes hemolysis.* | emolitico |
| **hemolytic anemia** *Reduced number of erythrocytes due to shortened survival and inability of the bone marrow to compensate.* | anemie emolitico |
| **hemopericardium** *Abnormal presence of blood in the pericardium.* | emopericardio |
| **hemoperitoneum** *Abnormal presence of blood in the peritoneum.* | emoperitoneo |

| English | Italian |
|---|---|
| **hemophilia** *A hereditary bleeding disorder characterized by hemarthroses and deep tissue bleeding as a result of absence of a coagulation factor such as factor VIII.* | emofilia |
| **hemophiliac** *A person with hemophilia.* | emofilico |
| **hemophilic arthropathy** *The permanent joint disease caused by recurrent bleeding into the joint.* | artropatia emofilico |
| **hemophthalmia** *Bleeding within the eye.* | emoftalmo |
| **hemopneumothorax** *Accumulation of blood and air in the pleural space.* | emopneumotorace |
| **hemopoiesis** *The production of blood cells from stem cells.* | emopoiesi |
| **hemopoietic** Referring to *a hormone secreted by the kidneys that stimulates the bone marrow to produce erythrocytes.* | emopoietico |
| **hemoptysis** *Expectoration of blood.* | emottisi |
| **hemorrhage** *Bleeding from a damaged blood vessel.* | emorragia |
| **hemorrhoidectomy** *Surgical excision of a hemorrhoid.* | emorroidectomia |
| **hemorrhoids** *Engorgement of the veins in the anus or rectum.* | emorroidi |
| **hemostasis** *The control of bleeding.* | emostasi |
| **hemothrorax** *The abnormal presence of blood in the pleural cavity.* | emotorace |
| **hence** *Thus.* | di qua, di qui, per cui |
| **Henoch purpura** *Exhibited by vomiting, diarrhea, abdominal pain and hematuria; a non-thrombocytopenic purpura.* | popora di Henoch |
| **Henri, syndrome of** *Congenital anomaly exhibited by different sized external orifices of the nostrils.* | sindrome di Henri |
| **heparin** *A polysaccharide that occurs naturally in the liver and is used as a medication to induce a hypocoagulable state.* | eparina |
| **hepatectomy** *Partial or complete surgical resection of the liver.* | epatectomia |
| **hepatic duct** *The right and left hepatic ducts join the cystic duct to form the common bile duct.* | dotto epatico |
| **hepatic flexure of the colon** *The junction of the ascending and transverse portion of the colon.* | flessione epatica del colon |
| **hepatic** *Referring to the liver.* | epatico |
| **hepatitis** *Inflammation of the liver.* | epatite |
| **hepatocyte** *A liver cell.* | epatocito |
| **hepatojugular reflex** *The presence of jugular venous distension with compression of the abdomen for at least 10 seconds.* | riflusso epatogiugulare |
| **hepatoma** *A tumor of the liver.* | epatoma |
| **hepatomegaly** *Enlargement of the liver.* | epatomegalia |
| **hepatosplenomegaly** *Enlargement of the spleen and the liver.* | epatosplenomegalia |
| **hereditary spherocytosis** *A familial hemolytic disease exhibited by abnormally thick erythrocytes.* | sferocitosi ereditaria |
| **hereditary** *That which is transmitted genetically* | ereditario |
| **hermaphrodite** *A person possessing gonadal characteristics of both sexes.* | ermafrodita |
| **hernia, femoral** *A bulge in the upper thigh/groin region because of bowel protruding through the muscle. Also called crural hernia.* | ernia femorale |
| **hernia, incarcerated** *An irreducible hernia.* | ernia strozzata |
| **hernia, inguinal** *Protrusion of abdominal-cavity contents through the inguinal canal.* | ernia inguinale |
| **hernia, lumbar** *Defect in the lumbar muscles or the posterior fascia, below the 12th rib and above the iliac crest.* | ernia lombare |
| **hernia, umbilical** *Protrusion of abdominal contents at the umbilicus.* | ernia ombelicale |
| **herniated disc** *Prolapse of the nucleus pulposus into the spinal cord.* | formazione di ernia del disco |
| **herniorrhaphy** *The surgical repair of a hernia.* | erniorrafia |

| English | Italian |
|---|---|
| **heroin** *A morphine derivative that is highly addictive.* | eroina |
| **herpangina** *An infectious disease caused by Coxsackie virus exhibited by vesicular lesion on the soft palate.* | angina erpetica |
| **herpes** *A skin condition exhibited by formation of clustered vesicular lesions; herpes simplex is at times referred to, albeit incompletely, as herpes.* | herpes, erpete |
| **herpes zoster; shingles** *A unilateral vesicular rash along one dermatome and caused by inflammation of a posterior nerve root by "the chicken pox virus".* | zona |
| **herpetic** *Referring to herpes.* | erpetico |
| **herpetiform** *Something that is characteristic of herpes.* | erpetiforme |
| **heterochromia iridis or syndrome of Eric** *Congenital anomaly in which the iris of each eye is of a different color.* | eterocromia dell'iride; sindrome di Eric |
| **heterogenous** *That which originates outside the organism.* | eterogeno |
| **heterotropia** *Synonym of strabismus.* | eterotropia |
| **heterozygous** *Having different alleles concerning a certain trait.* | eterozigotico |
| **hiatus hernia** *Protrusion of part of the stomach through the esophageal hiatus of the diaphragm.* | ernia iatale |
| **hiccup** *Involuntary spasm of the diaphragm with sudden closure of the glottis; this causes a characteristic cough.* | singhiozzo |
| **hidradenitis** *Inflammation of a sweat gland. When there is purulent discharge it is called hidradenitis suppurativa.* | idrosadenite |
| **hidrosis** *The production and secretion of sweat.* | sudorazione |
| **high** *Elevated.* | alto, elevato |
| **high blood pressure** *Elevated arterial blood pressure.* | alta pressione sanguigna |
| **high cholesterol** *Elevated serum cholesterol.* | colesterolo alto |
| **hilar** *Referring to a hilus.* | ilare |
| **Hillis-Müller maneuver** *A procedure to determine the descent of the head during active labor.* | manovra di Hillis-Müller |
| **hilum or hilus** *A depression where blood vessels and nerve fibers enter an organ.* | ilo |
| **hindbrain** *The brainstem which includes the pons, medulla oblongata and cerebellum.* | metencefalo |
| **hip** *The lateral eminence of the pelvis from the waist to the thigh; it is formed by the iliac crest and greater trochanter.* | anca; coscia |
| **hip joint** *The lateral eminence of the pelvis from the waist to the thigh; it is formed by the iliac crest and greater trochanter.* | articolazione dell'anca |
| **hip replacement** *Both joint surfaces are replaced by high density material such as plastic or metal.* | sostituzione dell'anca |
| **hippocampus** *The area at the base of the cerebral ventricles thought to be the center of memory and emotion.* | ippocampo |
| **Hippocratic oath** *An vow taken by doctors, indicating they will treat people properly.* | giuramento di Ippocrate |
| **hirsutism** *Abnormal growth on hair on a person's face and body.* | irsutismo |
| **histamine** *A chemical responsible for the reaction exhibited when a person has an allergic reaction.* | istamina |
| **histidine** *An amino acid precursor to histamine.* | istidina |
| **histiocyte** *A phagocytic cell found in connective tissue.* | istiocito |
| **histochemistry** *Study of intracellular distribution of chemicals, reaction sites and enzymes.* | istiocitochimica |
| **histology** *The study of the structure and composition of minute structures.* | istologia |
| **histoplasmosis** *A fungal pulmonary infection from bat and bird excrement.* | istoplasmosi |

| English | Italian |
|---|---|
| **HIV** *Abbreviation for human immunodeficiency virus.* | HIV virus dell'immuno deficienza umana |
| **hoarse** *A rough, harsh sounding voice.* | rauco |
| **Hodgkin's disease** *Also called Hodgkin's lymphoma, it is a cancer that begins in the lymphocytes.* | morbo di Hodgkin |
| **hollow** *An indentation.* | cavo |
| **homeless** *Having nowhere to live.* | senza casa |
| **homeopathy** *A treatment of disease by use of minute doses of toxic substances that would normally be harmful.* | omeopatia |
| **homeostasis** *The tendency of an organism to maintain a stable and uniform state.* | omeostasi |
| **homicide** *When one person kills another.* | omicida |
| **homograft** *A graft of tissue from the same species as the recipient.* | omotrapianto |
| **homolateral** *Ipsilateral.* | omolaterale |
| **homologous** *Referring to something derived from the same species but different genotype.* | omologo |
| **homosexual** *A person sexually attracted to someone of the same gender.* | omosessuale |
| **homozygous** *Having identical alleles for a particular trait.* | omozigotico |
| **hookworm** *A parasitic infection of the family Strongylidae that can cause anemia.* | anchilostoma |
| **hordeolum** *Inflammation of the sebaceous gland of the eye.* | orzaiolo |
| **hormone** *A substance produced in the body that effects a specific organ.* | ormone |
| **horn** *A keratinized outgrowth.* | corno |
| **Horner syndrome** *A lesion of the cervical sympathetic chain causes ipsilateral myosis, ptosis and facial anhidrosis.* | sindrome di Horner |
| **horseshoe kidney** *Anomalous renal development.* | rene a ferro di cavallo |
| **hospital** *Acute care medical/surgical facility.* | ospedale |
| **hospital discharge** *To leave the hospital.* | scarico dell'ospedale |
| **hot** *Very warm.* | molto caldo |
| **hot flash** *A symptom of menopause manifested as a sudden sensation of fever.* | vampate di calore |
| **housemaid's knee** *Also referred to as prepatellar bursitis.* | ginocchio delle lavandaie; borsite prepatellare |
| **HPV human papillomavirus** *The virus that causes genital warts.* | virus del papilloma umano |
| **Hueter's maneuver** *The application of downward and forward pressure on the tongue while passing an gastric tube.* | manovra di Hueter |
| **human** *Homo sapien.* | umano |
| **humerus** *The long bone in the upper arm.* | omero |
| **humor, aqueous** *The gelatinous fluid circulating between the cornea and lens.* | umor acqueo |
| **humor, vitreous** *The fluid circulating between the lens and retina.* | umor vitreo |
| **hunchback** *Synonym of kyphosis.* | cifosi |
| **hunger** *A sense of discomfort caused by a lack of food.* | fame |
| **Huntington's chorea** *A neurodegenerative disease characterized initially by behavioral changes and later by a movement disorder. Called Huntington's disease now.* | corea degenerativa di Huntington |
| **Hutchinson's mask** *The sensation the face is covered in cobwebs, associated with tabes dorsalis.* | faccia di Hutchinson |
| **Hutchinson's pupil** *Dilation of a pupil related to third nerve palsy on the side of the lesion as seen in herniation.* | pupilla di Hutchinson |

| English | Italian |
|---|---|
| **hyaline** *Having a glassy, transparent appearance.* | ialino |
| **hyaloid** *Transparent.* | ialino, vitreo |
| **hybrid** *An animal or plant produced from two different species.* | ibrido |
| **hydatid cyst** *A cyst produced by and containing tapeworm larvae.* | cisti idatidea |
| **hydatiform** *Referring to a hydatid cyst.* | idatidiforme |
| **hydrarthrosis** *An accumulation of water-like fluid in a joint cavity.* | idrartro |
| **hydration** *Used to describe fluid balance.* | idratazione |
| **hydrocele** *The accumulation of fluid in a body sac.* | idrocele |
| **hydrocephalus** *The excessive accumulation of cerebral spinal fluid in the brain causing enlargement of the head.* | idrocefalo |
| **hydrochloric acid** *A solution with a low pH formed by dissolving hydrogen chloride in water.* | acido cloridrico |
| **hydrochloride** | cloridrato |
| **hydrocortisone** *A natural steroid hormone secreted by the adrenal cortex and used in a synthetic formulation for treatment of various medical conditions.* | idrocortisone |
| **hydrolysis** *A reaction with water causing a compound to breakdown.* | idrolisi |
| **hydronephrosis** *Enlargement of a kidney due to interruption of outflow of urine from that kidney.* | idronefrosi |
| **hydrophobia** *Abnormal fear of water.* | idrofobia |
| **hydropneumothorax** *Abnormal accumulation of fluid and air in the pleural space.* | idropneumotorace |
| **hydrops** *The abnormal collection of fluid in a cavity.* | idrope |
| **hydrops fetalis** *The total body accumulation of fluid in a fetus; the result of a hemolytic reaction in a Rh neg mother.* | idrope fetalis |
| **hydrosalpinx** *Collection of fluid in a fallopian tube.* | idrosalpinge |
| **hydrothorax** *Accumulation of fluid within the thoracic cavity.* | idrotorace |
| **hygroma** *A cyst or bursa filled with fluid.* | igroma |
| **hygroscopic** *The tendency to absorb moisture from the air.* | igroscopico |
| **hymen** *A membrane in the vagina.* | imene |
| **hymenotomy** *Surgically creating an opening in the hymen.* | ementomia |
| **hyoid bone** *A horseshoe shaped bone located between the chin and thyroid cartilage.* | osso ioide |
| **hyperacidity** *An abnormally high acid level.* | iperacidità |
| **hyperactivity** *Abnormal increase in activity.* | iperattività |
| **hyperalgesia** *Greater than normal sensitivity to pain.* | iperalgesia |
| **hyperbaric** *Use of gas at a higher than normal pressure.* | iperberico |
| **hyperbaric chamber** *A device used to treat decompression illness.* | sala iperbarico |
| **hyperbilirubinemia** *Higher than normal level of bilirubin in the blood.* | iperbilirubinemia |
| **hypercalcemia** *Higher than normal level of calcium in the blood.* | ipercalcemia |
| **hypercapnia** *Higher than normal level of carbon dioxide in the blood stream.* | ipercapnia |
| **hypercholesterolemia** *Higher than normal level of cholesterol in the blood.* | ipercolesterolemia |
| **hyperchromia** *An excessive level of hemoglobin in erythrocytes.* | ipercromia |
| **hyperemia** *An increase in blood for the area of concern.* | iperemia |
| **hyperesthesia** *Higher than normal skin sensitivity.* | iperestesia |
| **hyperextension** *Extension of an articulation beyond the normal range.* | iperestensione |
| **hyperflexion** *Flexion of an articulation beyond the normal range.* | iperflessione |
| **hyperglycemia** *Higher than normal level of glucose in the blood.* | iperglicemia |
| **hypergonadism** *A condition of excessive gonadal activity and subsequently precocious sexual development.* | ipergonadismo |
| **hyperhidrosis** *Excessive perspiration.* | iperidrosi |

| English | Italian |
|---|---|
| **hyperkalemia** *Higher than normal level of potassium in the blood stream.* | iperkaliemia |
| **hyperkeratosis** *Excessive thickening of the outer layer of skin.* | ipercheratosi |
| **hyperkinesis** *Excessive activity and inability to concentrate.* | ipercinesia |
| **hyperlipidemia** *Higher than normal level of lipids in the blood stream.* | iperlipemia |
| **hypermetropia** *Farsightedness.* | ipermetropia |
| **hypermnesia** *Unusually good memory.* | ipermnesia |
| **hypermyotonia** *Excessive muscle tone.* | ipertonia musculare |
| **hypernatremia** *Elevated level of sodium in the blood.* | ipernatremia |
| **hypernephroma** *A renal tumor that mimic adrenal cortical tissue.* | ipernefroma |
| **hyperonychia** *Hypertrophic nails.* | iperonichia |
| **hyperopia** *Farsightedness.* | iperopia |
| **hyperosmia** *Increased sense of smell.* | iperosmia |
| **hyperparathyroidism** *Excessive level of parathyroid hormones in the blood stream causing weak bones and hypocalcemia.* | iperparatiroidismo |
| **hyperphagia** *Excessive food ingestion.* | iperfagia |
| **hyperphoria** *Upward deviation of the visual axis of the eye.* | iperforia |
| **hyperpituitarism** *Excessive eosinophilic hormone resulting in acromegaly or excessive basophilic hormone resulting in pituitary compression and ultimately hypopituitarism.* | iperpituitarismo |
| **hyperplasia** *Excessive growth of normal cells.* | iperplasia |
| **hyperpnea** *Abnormal increase in rate and depth of respiration.* | iperpnea |
| **hyperpyrexia** *Fever.* | iperpiressia |
| **hyperreflexia** *Abnormally brisk and vigorous reflex.* | iper-reflessia |
| **hypersensitivity** *Abnormal increase in sensitivity.* | ipersensibilità |
| **hypersplenism** *Excessive splenic activity resulting in decreased peripheral blood elements and sometimes splenomegaly.* | ipersplenismo |
| **hypertension** *Higher than normal blood pressure.* | ipertensione arteriosa |
| **hyperthermia** *Fever.* | ipertermia |
| **hyperthyroidism** *Increased thyroid activity resulting in exophthalmos and increased metabolic rate.* | ipertiroidismo |
| **hypertonia** *Excessive tone or tension.* | ipertonia |
| **hypertonic** *Increased osmotic pressure.* | ipertonico |
| **hypertrichosis** *Excessive hair growth.* | ipertricosi |
| **hypertrophy** *Pathologic organ enlargement.* | ipertrofia |
| **hyperuricemia** *Elevated level of uric acid in the blood.* | iperuricemico |
| **hyperventilation** *Rapid and deep respirations.* | iperventilazione |
| **hypervolemia** *Abnormally large amount of fluid in the blood stream.* | ipervolemia |
| **hyphema** *A blood collection in the front of the eye.* | ifema |
| **hypnotic** *Sleep inducing agent.* | ipnotico |
| **hypocalcemia** *Lower than normal level of calcium in the blood.* | ipocalcemia |
| **hypocapnia** *A decreased level of carbon dioxide in the blood.* | ipocapnia |
| **hypochlorhydria** *A state of decreased secretion of hydrochloric acid in the stomach.* | ipocloridria |
| **hypochondriac** *A person suffering from hypochondriasis.* | ipocondriaco |
| **hypochondriasis** *Abnormal increase in concern about one's own health.* | ipocondrìa |
| **hypochondrium** *The upper abdomen lateral to the epigastrium.* | ipocondrio |
| **hypochromic** *Referring to the abnormal decrease in hemoglobin content of erythrocytes.* | ipocromico |
| **hypodermic injection** *Subcutaneous injection.* | iniezione ipodermica |
| **hypoesthesia** *Abnormally decreased skin sensitivity.* | ipoestesia |

| English | Italian |
|---|---|
| **hypofibrinogenemia** *Diminished blood fibrinogen level.* | ipofibrinogenemia |
| **hypogastric** *Referring to the hypogastrium.* | ipogastrico |
| **hypogastrium** *The area of the central abdomen located below the stomach.* | ipogastrio |
| **hypoglossal nerve** *Twelfth cranial nerve pair.* | nervo ipoglosso |
| **hypoglycemia** *Abnormally low blood sugar.* | ipoglicemia |
| **hypogonadism** *Abnormal decrease in gonadal function with associated diminished growth and sexual development.* | ipogonadismo |
| **hypokalemia** *Diminished level of potassium in the blood stream.* | ipokaliemia |
| **hypokalemic periodic paralysis** *An inherited disorder that leads to muscle weakness related to a low serum potassium level.* | paralisi periodica ipokaliemica |
| **hypomania** *A moderate form of mania.* | ipomania |
| **hyponatremia** *Diminished level of sodium in the blood stream.* | iponatriemia |
| **hypoparathyroidism** *Abnormal decrease in parathyroid function.* | ipoparatiroidismo |
| **hypophoria** *Downward deviation of the visual axis of the eye.* | ipoforia |
| **hypophosphatasia** *A genetic defect of diminished alkaline phosphatase in the cells leading to bone demineralization.* | ipofosfatasia |
| **hypophysectomy** *Surgical removal of the pituitary gland.* | ipofisectomia |
| **hypophysis** *Pituitary gland.* | ipofisi |
| **hypopituitarism** *Diminished pituitary activity exhibited by obesity and persistence of adolescent characteristics.* | ipopituitarismo |
| **hypoplasia** *Incomplete development.* | ipoplasia |
| **hypopyon** *The presence of purulent fluid in the anterior chamber of the eye.* | ipopion |
| **hyposalivation** *Secretion of saliva below the normal rate.* | iposalivazione |
| **hypospadias** *Congenital condition exhibited by development of the urethral meatus on the inferior aspect of the penis.* | ipospadia |
| **hypostasis** *The formation of a deposit.* | ipostasi |
| **hypotension** *Abnormally low blood pressure.* | iipotensione |
| **hypothalamus** *Located inferior to the thalamus it controls visceral activities, water balance, temperature and sleep.* | ipotalamo |
| **hypothenar eminence** *The prominence on the palm at the base of the fingers adjacent to the ulna.* | eminenza ipotenar |
| **hypothermia** *Lower than normal temperature.* | ipotermia |
| **hypothyroidism** *Reduced functioning of the thyroid.* | ipotiroidismo |
| **hypotonia** *Reduced tone or activity.* | ipotonia |
| **hypoxia** *Diminished oxygen content.* | ipossia |
| **hysterectomy** *Surgical removal of the uterus.* | isterectomia |
| **hysteria** *A psychological condition exhibited by uncontrolled emotion or exaggerated manifestations.* | isteria |
| **hysterography** *1. Recording of uterine contractions. 2. Roentgenography of the uterus after administration of contrast media.* | isterografia |
| **hysteromyomectomy** *Surgical removal of a uterine myoma.* | isteromiomectomia |
| **hysteropexy** *Surgical fixation of the uterus by shortening of the round ligaments or by other means.* | isteropessi |
| **hysterosalpingography** *Roentgenography of the uterus and fallopian tubes after instillation of contrast media.* | isterosalpingografia |
| **hysterotomy** *Surgical opening of the uterus.* | isterotomia |
| **i.e.** *A latin derived abbreviation for "that is to say"(In latin: id est)* | id est; cioè |
| **iatrogenic** *A problem caused by medical treatment.* | iatrogeno |
| **ichthyosis** *A congenital anomaly exhibited by excessively dry, thick skin.* | ittiosi |
| **icterus** *Yellowing of the skin and sclerae because of excess bilirubin.* | ittero |

| English | Italian |
|---|---|
| **identical twins** *Twins from the same zygote.* | gemelli monozigotici |
| **idiopathic** *Relating to a disease with an unknown cause.* | idiopatico |
| **ileitis** *Inflammation of the ileum.* | ileite |
| **ileocecal valve** *The membranous folds between the ileum and cecum.* | valvola ileocecale |
| **ileocolitis** *Inflammation of the ileum and cecum.* | ileocolite |
| **ileocolostomy** *Creating a surgical opening between the ileum and colon.* | ileocolostomia |
| **ileoproctostomy** *Creating a surgical opening between the ileum and the rectum.* | ileoproctostomia |
| **ileostomy** *Surgical creation of an opening in the ileum that is placed at the skin surface.* | ileostomia |
| **ileum** *The portion of the small bowel from the jejunum to the cecum.* | ileo |
| **ileus** *A temporary obstruction in the intestine.* | ileo |
| **iliac crest** *The upper border of the ilium.* | cresta iliaca |
| **iliococcygeal** *Referring to the ilium and coccyx.* | iliococcigeo |
| **ilium** *The large bone at the superior aspect of the pelvis which is present bilaterally.* | osso iliaco |
| **illiterate** *Unable to read or write.* | illetterato |
| **immune** *Being resistant to an infection.* | immune |
| **immune response** *The body's reaction to what is perceived as a foreign substance.* | riposta immunitaria |
| **immunization** *A medication given to provide immunity.* | immunizzazione |
| **immunochemistry** *The study of immune response and biochemistry.* | immunochimica |
| **immunodeficiency** *An inadequate immune response.* | immunodeficienza |
| **immunoelectrophoresis** *A means of differentiating proteins and other compounds by comparing their mobility and antigenic specificities.* | immunoelettroforesi |
| **immunoglobulin** *Serum and cellular proteins of the immune system.* | immunoglobuline |
| **immunosuppression** *The inhibition of the immune response.* | immunosoppressione |
| **impaction, tooth** *A tooth that does not erupt because adjacent teeth prevent it.* | incuneamento di un dente |
| **impairment** *A specific disability.* | peggioramento |
| **imperforate** *Lack of an opening. An infant with an imperforate anus has a congenital defect with no anal opening.* | imperforato |
| **impervious** *Not affected by.* | impervio |
| **implant** *A device or prosthesis implanted in a person.* | impianto |
| **implementation** *The process of putting a plan into effect.* | implementazione |
| **impotence** *Inability to act or inability to achieve a penile erection.* | impotenza |
| **inanition** *Generalized weakness from lack of nutrition.* | inanizione |
| **inarticulate** *Indistinct speech.* | inarticolato |
| **incest** *Sexual relations between related people.* | incesto |
| **incipient** *Starting to happen.* | incipiente |
| **incision** *An intentional surgical cut in the skin.* | incisione |
| **incisor** *Sharp-edged tooth; humans have four incisors.* | incisivo |
| **incisura** *A notch or indentation usually on the edge of a bone.* | incisura |
| **incisure** *A notch or incision.* | depressione, incisione |
| **inclusion body** *Variably shaped bodies in the nuclei of cells found in infections such as rabies and herpes.* | corpo inclusione |
| **incoherent** *Absence of intelligible speech.* | incoerente |
| **incontinence** *Inability to control urination.* | incontinenza |
| **incoordination** *Absence of smooth, efficient body movement.* | incoordinazione |
| **increment** *An increase on a fixed scale.* | incremento |
| **incubator** *A warming device for infants.* | incubatrice |

| English | Italian |
|---|---|
| **incus** *The middle ear bone between the stapes and malleus.* | incudine |
| **indeed** *As a matter of fact.* | a dire il vero |
| **indigenous** *Naturally occurring.* | indigeno |
| **indigestion** *Inadequate digestion for various reasons.* | indigestione |
| **indolent** *1. Causing little pain. 2. Slow healing ulcer.* | indolore; torpido |
| **induce, to** *Facilitated. When referring to labor, it means medication was given to assist in delivery of the fetus.* | indurre |
| **induced abortion** *Surgical or medical evacuation of the fetus.* | aborto indotto |
| **induration** *An area that is abnormally hard.* | indurimento |
| **indwelling catheter** *Continuous use tube usually referring to a tube in the urinary bladder.* | catetere a permanenza |
| **inebriation** *Intoxication with drugs or alcohol.* | ebbrezza |
| **ineffective** *Unsuccessful or inefficient.* | inefficiente |
| **inertia** *The tendency to remain unchanged.* | inerzia |
| **inevitable** *Not preventable.* | inevitabile |
| **infancy** *Early childhood.* | infanzia |
| **infant** *Newborn.* | neonato |
| **infant, post-term** *A neonate born after the normal gestation.* | neonato postmaturo |
| **infant, pre-term** *A neonate born prior to normal gestation.* | neonato prematuro |
| **infant, term** *A neonate born at expected date.* | neonato a termine |
| **infantile** *Referring to babies or young children.* | infantile |
| **infarct** *Referring to dead tissue.* | infarto |
| **infarction** *Dead tissue, for example, myocardial infarction.* | infarto |
| **infectious** *Contagious.* | infettivo |
| **inferior** *The lower aspect.* | inferiore |
| **inferior pelvis strait** *The pelvic outlet.* | stretto inferiore della pelvi |
| **infestation** *The presence of large numbers, as in lice infestation.* | infestazione |
| **inflammation** *Localized redness, excessive warmth and swelling.* | infiammazione |
| **influenza** *Viral infection causing fever, muscle aches and catarrh.* | influenza |
| **infraspinous** *Below the scapular spine.* | infraspinoso |
| **infundibulum** *The connection between the hypothalamus and the posterior pituitary gland.* | infundibolo |
| **infusion** *The injection of fluid into tissue or a vein.* | infusione |
| **ingestion** *The intake of food or liquid orally.* | ingestione |
| **ingrown nail** *Also referred to as onychocryptosis.* | unghia incarnita |
| **inguinal** *Referring to the groin.* | inguinale |
| **inguinal ring (deep)** *Indirect inguinal hernias exit the abdominal cavity via the deep inguinal ring.* | anello inguinale profondo |
| **inhalation** *The act of breathing in.* | inalazione |
| **injection** *The act of a needle being inserted into a body.* | iniezione |
| **injure, to** *To hurt or to wound.* | ferire |
| **injury** *A wound, abrasion or contusion.* | lesione; ingiuria |
| **injury, closed head** *Brain trauma not associated with damage to the dura or skull.* | lesione alla testa chiusa |
| **injury, contrecoup of brain** *An injury to the brain on the side opposite of that which was struck.* | feerita di cervello contraccolpo |
| **injury, degloving** *Trauma that involves the ripping of skin and subcutaneous tissue from the underlying tissue.* | lesione scapsulamento |
| **injury, hyperextension-hyperflexion** *An injury, usually to the cervical spine, that involves rapid deceleration, causing pronounced extension and flexion.* | lesione iperestensione-iperflessione |

| English | Italian |
|---|---|
| **inner ear** *Made up of the cochlea and semicircular canals.* | otite interna |
| **innervation** *The presence of a nerve supply.* | innervazione |
| **innominate artery** *The first branch off the aortic arch that branches into the right common carotid and right subclavian arteries.* | arteria innominata |
| **innominate** *Referring to the innominate artery.* | innominata |
| **inoculation** *Injection with a vaccine to provide immunity.* | inoculazione |
| **inorganic** *Not coming from natural growth.* | inorganico |
| **insane** *A term not used in formal medical evaluations that when used by a layperson means a serious mental illness.* | alienato |
| **insanity** *Referring to a serious mental illness.* | alienazione mentale |
| **insensible** *Unable to perceive a stimulus.* | insensibile |
| **insertion** *The act of inserting something.* | inserzione |
| **inside** *Inner part, center.* | interno |
| **insidious** *A slow, gradual and harmful advancement.* | insidioso |
| **insomnia** *Sleeplessness.* | insonnia |
| **inspiration** *Drawing in a breath.* | inspirazione |
| **inspiratory reserve volume** *The amount of air that can be inhaled after a normal inhalation.* | volume di riserva inspiratoria |
| **inspissate, to** *To thicken or congeal.* | inspessire |
| **instep** *The medial aspect of the foot between the ankle and the ball of the foot.* | parte dorsale dell'arco del piede |
| **insulin** *A hormone produced by the pancreas and synthetically to control blood glucose levels.* | insulina |
| **insulinoma** *An islet cell tumor that causes abnormally high insulin secretion and thus hypoglycemia.* | insulinoma |
| **intake** *An amount of food taken into the body.* | assunzione |
| **integument** *Outer protective layer.* | tegumento |
| **intelligence quotient (IQ)** *A number representing a person's ability to problem solve compared to a matched-control.* | quoziente dell'intelligenza |
| **intensive** *Very thorough or vigorous.* | intensivo |
| **intensive care unit** *The unit where vigorous treatment of the acutely ill takes place.* | unità di cura intensiva |
| **intention tremor** *The tremulous movement noted when a person is beginning to perform a task but not seen at rest.* | tremore intenzionale |
| **interarticular** *Between the articular surfaces of a joint.* | interarticolare |
| **intercellular** *Between cells.* | intercellulare |
| **intermittent** *Occurring at irregular intervals.* | intermittente |
| **internal** *Situated on the inside.* | interno |
| **interosseous muscles** *Referring to the interosseous muscles of the hand.* | muscolo interosseo |
| **interstitial** *Referring to the interstices of tissue.* | interstiziale |
| **intertrigo** *Irritation present because adjacent surfaces rub together.* | intergrigine |
| **intertrochanteric** *Referring to the space within the trochanter.* | intertrocanterico |
| **interval** *An intervening time.* | intervallo |
| **interventricular** *Between the ventricles.* | interventricolare |
| **intestinal obstruction** *Blockage of the intestine by mass or volvulus.* | ostruzione intestinale |
| **intestinal** *Referring to the intestines.* | intestinale |
| **intestine** *A general term used for the section of bowel from the stomach to the anus.* | intestino |
| **intraabdominal abscess** *A collection of pus in the abdomen.* | ascesso intra-addominale |
| **intraabdominal** *Within the abdominal cavity.* | endoaddominale |
| **intraarticular** *Within a joint space.* | intra-articolare |
| **intracellular** *Within a cell.* | intracellulare |

| English | Italian |
|---|---|
| **intracerebral** *Within the cerebrum.* | intracerebrale |
| **intracranial** *Within the cranial vault.* | intracranico |
| **intradermal** *Within the dermis.* | intradermico |
| **intradural** *Within the dural space.* | intradurale |
| **intramedullary** *1. Within the medulla oblongata. 2. Within the bone marrow.* | intramidollare |
| **intramuscular** *Within a muscle.* | intramuscolare |
| **intraocular fluid** *Fluid within the globe.* | fluido intraoculare |
| **intraosseous** *Within a bone.* | intraosseo |
| **intraperitoneal** *Within the peritoneal cavity.* | intraperitoneale |
| **intrathecal** *Technically means within a sheath but this term is used when medication is instilled in the dura mater spinalis.* | intratecale |
| **intrauterine contraceptive device (IUD)** *A device used to physically prevent the implantation of a fertilized ovum.* | spirale |
| **intrauterine** *Within the uterus.* | intrauterino |
| **intravenous infusion** *Administration of fluid into a vein.* | infusione intravenoso; infusione endovenoso |
| **intravenous tubing** *The tubing used to administer fluids.* | tubo intravenoso |
| **intravenous** *Within a vein.* | intravenoso; endovenoso |
| **intubation** *Placement of a tube; commonly used to refer to endotracheal intubation.* | intubazione |
| **intussusception** *The inversion of one portion of the bowel into another.* | intussuscezione |
| **inulin** *A polysaccharide used in the testing of renal function.* | inulina |
| **inunction** *The application of lotion with friction.* | unzione |
| **involucrum** *A wrap or covering (referring to a sequestrum).* | involucro |
| **involutional** *The shrinkage of an organ when it is not in use, as in the uterus after childbirth.* | involutivo |
| **involved** *Difficult to comprehend.* | involuto |
| **iodine** *A chemical used as an antiseptic and a deficiency of it can lead to goiter.* | iodio |
| **iodism** *A condition caused by excessive iodine intake resulting in diarrhea, weakness, and convulsions.* | iodismo |
| **ion channel** *A selectively permeable cell membrane to certain ions.* | canale ionico |
| **ionizing radiation** *High energy radiation that produces ion pairs in matter.* | radiazioni ionizzanti |
| **ipsilateral** *On the same side.* | omolaterale |
| **iridectomy** *Surgical removal of part of the iris.* | iridectomia |
| **iridocyclitis** *Inflammation of the ciliary body and the iris.* | iridociclite |
| **iridoplegia** *Paralysis of part of the iris with subsequent lack of contraction or dilation of the pupil.* | iridoplegia |
| **iridotomy** *A surgical opening of the iris.* | iridotomia |
| **iris** *The colored membrane posterior to the cornea.* | iride |
| **iron** *An element found in hemoglobin.* | ferro |
| **iron-deficiency anemia** *A microcytic anemia.* | anemia da carenza di ferro |
| **irradiation** *The process of being irradiated.* | irradiazione |
| **irrelevant** *Not pertinent.* | estraneo, non pertinente |
| **irritable bowel syndrome** *A condition exhibited by chronic diarrhea or constipation and abdominal pain; it is sometimes associated with a labile emotional state.* | sindrome del colon irritabile |
| **ischemia** *Inadequate blood supply to a part of the body.* | ischemia |
| **ischemic contracture** *A muscle's resistance to passive stretch that is related to a decrease in arterial flow from any reason.* | contrattura ischemico |

| English | Italian |
|---|---|
| **ischemic heart disease** *Inadequate blood supply to the heart.* | cardiopatia ischemica |
| **ischemic optic neuropathy** *A general category of a cause of blindness with several subcategories.* | neuropatia ottica ischemica |
| **ischium** *The inferoposterior portion of the pelvis.* | ischio |
| **islet** *Tissue that is structurally separate from adjacent tissues.* | isola |
| **isoantibody** *A situation in which an antibody of person A reacts with an antigen of person B.* | isoanticorpo |
| **isolation** *To be kept separate or apart.* | isolamento |
| **isolation ward** *A ward where patients with infectious disease are housed.* | reparto di isolamento |
| **isthmus** *A narrow piece of tissue connecting two larger body parts.* | istmo |
| **itch** *A sensation that makes one want to scratch.* | dermatite pruriginosa |
| **jaundice** *Yellowing of the sclerae and skin because of excessive bilirubin in the blood.* | ittero |
| **jaundice of the newborn** *A form of jaundice seen in newborns in the first two weeks of life; also called icterus neonatorum.* | itterizia neonatale |
| **jaw** *Mandible.* | mandibola |
| **jaw reflex** *Contraction of the temporal muscles when a relaxed mandible is given a downward tap. Also, masseter reflex or jaw jerk.* | riflesso mandibola |
| **jejunectomy** *Surgical removal of the jejunum.* | digiunectomia |
| **jejunostomy** *Surgical creation of an opening in the jejunum.* | digiunotomia |
| **Jendrassik's maneuver** *A method of distracting a patient while checking the patellar reflex.* | manovra di Jendrassik |
| **Job syndrome** *Also known as hyperimmunoglobulin E syndrome, there are high levels if IgE, a leukocyte chemotactic defect, recurrent staph infections and cold abscess formation in the skin.* | sindrome di Job |
| **jock itch** *Pruritus caused by tinea cruris.* | tinea cruris |
| **joint** *Articulation of two adjacent bones.* | articolazione; giuntura |
| **jugular notch** *The notch on the upper border of the sternum.* | incisura giugulare |
| **jugular** *Referring to the neck, as in jugular vein.* | giugulare |
| **jugular vein (s)** *Includes the internal, external and anterior jugular veins.* | vena giugulare |
| **juvenile angiofibroma** *A noncancerous growth in the nose or pharyngeal region.* | angiofibroma giugulare |
| **juxta-articular** *Positioned near a joint.* | juxta-articolare; giusta-articolare |
| **juxtaglomerular apparatus** *Cells located in the tunica media of the afferent glomerular arterioles.* | apparecchio giustaglomerulare |
| **kala-azar** *A disease caused by Leishmania donovani that is exhibited by weight loss, fever, anemia and hepatosplenomegaly.* | kala-azar |
| **Kaposi sarcoma** *Typically seen in AIDS patients, it is characterized by cutaneous reddish-purple macules and plaques.Also called multiple idiopathic hemorrhagic sarcoma.* | acrosarcomatosi di Kaposi |
| **karyokinesis** *A part of mitosis involving the cell nucleus division.* | cariocinesi |
| **karyotype** *The arrangement of chromosomes in a single cell.* | cariotipo |
| **Kawasaki syndrome** *Begins with fever for 5 days, skin rashes, strawberry tongue, lymphadenopathy and swollen hands and feet. It is known to cause coronary artery aneurysms. Also called mucocutaneous lymph node syndrome.* | sindrome mucocutanea linfonodale |
| **keloid** *Hypertrophic scar tissue that forms after a minor cut or surgical procedure.* | cheloide |
| **keratectasia** *Obtrusion of the cornea.* | cheratectasia |
| **keratectomy** *Excision of a portion of the cornea.* | cheratectomia |
| **keratic** *Referring to the cornea.* | corneo |

| English | Italian |
|---|---|
| **keratin** *A protein found in the skin, hair, nails and enamel of the teeth.* | cheratina |
| **keratoma** *A protuberance of horny tissue.* | cheratoma |
| **keratomalacia** *Softening of the cornea.* | cheratomalacia |
| **keratosis** *A growth of keratin such as a wart or callosity.* | cheratosi |
| **kernicterus** *A condition associated with high bilirubin levels that causes yellow staining of cerebral tissues and subsequent neurologic dysfunction.* | ittero nucleare |
| **ketoacidosis** *Usually referring to diabetic ketoacidosis in which ketones are broken down, causing a decrease in blood pH.* | chetoacidosi |
| **ketone body** *One ketone with a decarboxylation product of acetone.* | corpo chetone |
| **ketonemia** *Presence of ketone in the blood.* | chetonemia |
| **ketonuria** *Presence of ketone in the urine.* | chetonuria |
| **ketosis** *The presence of an abnormally high level of ketones in the blood and body tissues.* | chetosi |
| **kick, to** *To strike an object with one's foot.* | dare un calcio a |
| **kidney** *One of two glandular organs that form urine.* | rene |
| **kinase** *An enzyme that facilitates movement of phosphate from ATP to another molecule.* | chinasi |
| **kineplasty** *An amputation done in a fashion to facilitate ambulation.* | cineplastica |
| **kinesis** *Movement of a part in response to a stimulus.* | cinesi |
| **kinky-hair syndrome** *Inborn error of copper metabolism, noted in the first few weeks of life. Exhibited by sparse kinky hair, failure to thrive and seizures. Also called Menke's syndrome or trichopoliodystrophy.* | malattia dei capelli riorti |
| **Klinefelter's syndrome** *Presence of an extra X chromosome, it is exhibited by longer legs, narrow shoulders, small testicles and gynecomastia.* | Klinefelter, sindrome di |
| **knee** *The joint at the distal femur and proximal tibia.* | ginocchio |
| **knee elbow position** *Knees and elbows are on the table and the chest is in the air.* | posizione genu-cubitale |
| **knee jerk reflex** *Contraction of the quadriceps, yielding leg extension when the quadriceps tendon is tapped.* | riflesso rotuleo |
| **kneecap** *Common term for patella.* | rotula |
| **kneeling** *Being on one's knees as in the prayer position.* | inginocchiarsi |
| **knock knees** *Common term for genu valgum.* | ginocchio valgo |
| **knot** *A fastening made by tying a suture, for instance.* | nodo chirurgico |
| **known** *Recognized or familiar.* | conosciuto |
| **knuckle** *A metacarpophalagngeal joint or a finger joint when the fist is closed.* | nocca |
| **koilonychia** *Thin and concave fingernails.* | coilonichia |
| **Koplik's spots** *Red buccal macules with a blue center; seen in measles.* | macchie di Koplik |
| **kopophobia** *A morbid fear of fatigue.* | kopofobia |
| **Köhler's disease** *A genetic disease characterized by osteonecrosis and subsequent collapse of the tarsal navicular bone.* | malattia di Köhler |
| **kraurosis vulvae** *Dryness and shrinkage of the vulva.* | craurosi vulvare |
| **Krebs cycle** *The process of aerobic respiration by which living cells generate energy.* | ciclo di Kreb |
| **kubisagari** *Vestibular neuronitis.* | vertigine paralizzante |
| **Kussmaul respiration** *The slow, deep breathing noted in patients with acidosis.* | respiro boccheggiante di Kussmaul |
| **Kyasanur Forest disease** *A viral fever noted in Mysore, India transmitted by Haemaphysalis spinigera. It is characterized by fever, headache, generalized pains, diarrhea, and intestinal bleeding.* | malattia di foresta Kyasanur |
| **kwashiorkor** *A form of malnutrition from inadequate protein intake.* | kwashiorkor |

| English | Italian |
|---|---|
| **kyphoscoliosis** *An abnormal outward and lateral curvature of the spine.* | cifoscoliosi |
| **kyphosis** *Abnormal outward curvature of the spine.* | cifosi |
| **lab result** *The data obtained from a laboratory test.* | risultato di laboratorio |
| **labial** *Referring to the lip.* | labiale |
| **labile** *Easily altered; emotionally unstable.* | labile |
| **labium majus (plural= labia majora)** *The folds of skin forming the lateral borders of the pudendal cleft.* | grande labbro della vulva |
| **labium minus (plural=labia minora)** *The folds of skin posterior to the labia majora.* | labbra meno |
| **labium** *Referring to any lip shaped structure.* | labbro |
| **labor onset** *The time when a pregnant woman begins uterine contractions in the process of childbirth.* | inizio di travaglio |
| **labor pains** *The intermittent pain associated with uterine contractions.* | travaglio |
| **labor room** *The hospital room used while a woman is in labor.* | sala parto |
| **laboratory** *A room equipped to run blood, tissue and fluid samples.* | laboratorio |
| **labyrinthitis** *Inflammation of the labyrinth.* | labirintite |
| **labrum** *An edge or lip. The labrum acetabular is the fibrocartilagous rim attached to the acetabulum.* | labbro dell'acetabolo |
| **labyrinth** *Inner ear structure concerned with balance.* | labirinto |
| **laceration** *An injury that produced a cut in the skin or tissue such as a tear during childbirth.* | lacerazione |
| **lacrimal** *Referring to the secretion of tears.* | lacrimale |
| **lacrimal fluid** *Fluid secreted by the lacrimal gland.* | fluido lacrimale |
| **lacrimation** *The secretion of tears.* | lacrimazione |
| **lactalbumin** *Proteins found in milk.* | lattalbumina |
| **lactase** *An enzyme that facilitates the breakdown of lactose to glucose and galactose.* | lattasi |
| **lactation** *The secretion of milk from mammary glands.* | lattazione |
| **lactic** *Referring to milk.* | lattico |
| **lactiferous duct** *A canal that carries milk.* | condotto lattifero |
| **lactose** *A disaccharide present in milk.* | lattosio |
| **lactose intolerance** *The inability of the small bowel to digest lactose.* | alattasia |
| **lacuna** *A small cavity or depression.* | lacuna |
| **lacunar infarction** *Small non-cortical cerebral infarcts.* | infarto lacunare |
| **lagophthalmos** *Characterized by the inability to close the eyelid completely over the eye.* | lagoftalmo |
| **laliophobia** *Abnormal fear of speaking or stuttering.* | lalofobia |
| **lalochezia** *Relief of stress by uttering obscenities.* | lalochezia |
| **lambdoid** *The suture connecting the parietal bones with the occipital bone.* | lambdoideo |
| **lamella** *A thin layer of bone.* | lamella |
| **laminectomy** *The surgical removal of part of a vertebrae.* | laminectomia |
| **lancet** *A small sharp instrument used to obtain a drop of blood for testing.* | lancetta; bisturi |
| **laparoscope** *A fiber-optic instrument used to visualize the peritoneal contents.* | laparoscopio |
| **laparoscopy** *A procedure utilizing a laparoscope.* | laparoscopia |
| **laparotomy** *A surgical incision of the abdomen.* | laparotomia |
| **laryngeal** *Referring to the larynx.* | laringeo |
| **laryngectomy** *Surgical removal of the larynx.* | laringectomia |
| **laryngismus stridulus** *Sudden, severe laryngeal spasm.* | laringismo stridulo |
| **laryngitis** *Inflammation of the larynx.* | laringite |

| English | Italian |
|---|---|
| **laryngology** *The study of the larynx and related diseases.* | laringologia |
| **laryngopharynx** *The pharyngeal space between the superior aspect of the glottis and the opening of the larynx.* | laringofaringe |
| **laryngospasm** *Sudden, involuntary muscle contraction of the larynx.* | laringospasmo |
| **laryngostenosis** *Abnormal narrowing of the larynx.* | laringostenosi |
| **laryngotomy** *Surgical creation of an opening in the larynx.* | laringotomia |
| **larynx** *A hollow muscular structure that contains the vocal cords.* | laringe |
| **last** *Final.* | finale |
| **late** *A time later than expected.* | tardivo |
| **lateral** *Referring to the side of the body.* | laterale |
| **laterodeviation** *Pushed to the lateral aspect.* | laterdeviazione |
| **lathyrism** *A disease characterized by tremors, spastic paralysis and paresthesias caused by Lathyrus sativus.* | latirismo |
| **laugh, to** | ridere |
| **laxity** *A description of a joint that is loose.* | mollezza |
| **layer** *A stratum or thickness.* | strato |
| **lead** *An element with an atomic number of 82.* | piombo |
| **lead poisoning** *The ingestion of lead, exhibited in severe cases by paralysis, encephalopathy, purple gingiva, and colic.* | avvelenamento da piombo |
| **leaflet** *Cusp.* | foglietto |
| **leakage** *Unintentional escape of gas or fluid.* | fuoriuscita |
| **learning** *The intentional acquisition of knowledge.* | apprendimento |
| **lecithin** *A compound widely used by tissues, derived from egg yolks and it consists of phospholipids linked to choline.* | lecitina |
| **leech** *An annelid used in some tropical regions for drawing out blood; they have an anticoagulant effect locally and have been attached to digits of persons with acute peripheral ischemia.* | sanguisuga |
| **left** | sinistro |
| **left-handed** *The preference of using the left hand for common tasks.* | mancino |
| **leg** *One of two lower extremities.* | gamba |
| **legionnaires' disease** *The name was derived after an outbreak at a convention of the American Legion; it is manifested by fever, chills, dyspnea, and cough.* | malattia del legionario |
| **leishmaniasis** *A condition caused by a flagellate protozoan parasite that is exhibited by visceral or dermatologic manifestations.* | leishmaniosi |
| **length** *The end to end measurement.* | lunghezza |
| **lengthening** *Becoming longer.* | allungamento |
| **lens** *The transparent chamber between the posterior chamber and the vitreous body.* | lente |
| **lenticular** *Referring to the lens of the eye.* | lenticolare |
| **lentigo** *A benign condition exhibited by flat brown patches on the skin.* | lentiggine |
| **leontiasis ossea** *Bilateral hypertrophy of the bones of the face and cranium.* | leontiasi ossea |
| **Leopold's maneuver** *Used to determine fetal position.* | manovra di Leopold |
| **leproma** *A superficial granulatomous papule that is seen in leprosy.* | leproma |
| **leprosy** *A contagious disease caused by Mycobacterium leprae that causes insensate papules and disfiguration.* | lebbra |
| **leptomeningitis** *A general term used to describe meningitis of the pia and arachnoid of the brain.* | leptomeningite |
| **leptospirosis** *A zoonosis caused by the spirochete Leptospira interrogans transmitted by rats and contaminated water.* | leptospirosi itteroemorragica |
| **lesbian** *A woman with same gender preference.* | lesbico |
| **less** *A smaller amount.* | minore |

| English | Italian |
|---|---|
| **lethal** *Deadly.* | letale |
| **lethal dose** *The amount of a drug required to cause death.* | dose letale |
| **lethargy** *Absence of energy.* | letargia |
| **leucinosis; maple syrup urine disease** *A condition characterized by an enzyme defect causing an increase in leucine in the urine.* | leucinosi |
| **leukemia** *A malignant disease causing an increase in the number of abnormal and immature leukocytes.* | leucemia |
| **leukine (or leucine)** *An amino acid obtained from hydrolysis of some proteins.* | leucina |
| **leukocyte** *A white blood cell.* | leucocito |
| **leukocythemia** *Synonym of leukemia.* | leucocitemia |
| **leukocytolysis** *Destruction of white blood cells.* | leucocitolisi |
| **leukocytosis** *An increase in the number of leukocytes.* | lecocitosi |
| **leukodermia** *A localized loss of skin pigment.* | leucoderma |
| **leukonychia** *A whitish discoloration of the fingernails and toenails.* | leuconichia |
| **leukopenia** *A decreased number of leukocytes in the blood.* | leucopenia |
| **leukopoiesis** *Production of white blood cells.* | leucopoiesi |
| **leukorrhea** *Thick white vaginal discharge.* | leucorrea |
| **levator** *A muscle that raises part of the body; the levator labii superioris raised the upper lip.* | sollevatore |
| **levulose** *Synonym for fructose.* | levulosio |
| **libido** *Sexual desire.* | libido |
| **Libman-Sachs syndrome** *A verrucous endocarditis associated with disseminated lupus erythematosus; also called nonbacterial verrucous endocarditis.* | sindrome di Libman-Sachs |
| **library** | biblioteca |
| **lice** *Plural for louse, a small parasite that lives on the skin. Pediculus humanus capitis is a head louse.* | pidocchio |
| **lichen** *A term used to describe a variety of papular skin diseases. Lichen planus is a shiny, flat, violaceous eruption of the mucous membranes, skin and genitalia.* | lichen |
| **life expectancy** *The length of time a person is anticipated to live.* | durata presumibile della vita |
| **life-threatening** *Potentially fatal.* | pericolo di vita |
| **lifetime** *Duration of a person's life.* | durata della vita |
| **lift, to** *Raise to a higher level.* | sollevare |
| **ligament** *A band of fibrous connective tissue that connects two bones or cartilage.* | legamento |
| **ligature** *A thread used to tie a vessel.* | legatura |
| **light** *Illumination, bright.* | luminoso |
| **light** *Not heavy.* | leggero |
| **light adaptation** *The pupillary adjustment after going from a dark environment to one of bright light.* | adattamento alla luc |
| **likelihood** *The probability or feasibility.* | probabilità |
| **limb** *An extremity or branch.* | membro |
| **limbus** *The margin of a structure, for example, of the cornea and sclera.* | lembo |
| **liminal stimulus** *Referring to a stimulus of threshold strength.* | stimolo liminale |
| **lincture** *A medicine mixed with a sweet substance.* | ellettuario |
| **linea alba** *The tendinous portion of the anterior abdomen between the two rectus muscles.* | linea alba |
| **lingua nigra** *A condition characterized by a dark fur-like covering on the dorsum of the tongue.* | lingua nigra |

| English | Italian |
|---|---|
| **lip, lower** *Labium inferius oris.* | labbro inferiore |
| **lip, upper** *Labium superius oris.* | labbro superiore |
| **lipase** *A pancreatic enzyme that facilitates the breakdown of fats.* | liipasi |
| **lipemia** *Abnormally high fat content in the blood.* | iperlipemia |
| **lipid** *A compound that is a fatty acid which is insoluble in water but soluble in organic solvents.* | lipide |
| **lipid-lowering agent** *A medication used to treat hyperlipidemia.* | lipidi abbassamento farmaco |
| **lipoatrophy** *Fatty tissue atrophy.* | lipoatrofia |
| **lipochondrodystrophy** *A congenital condition exhibited by short stature, kyphosis, mental deficiency and short fingers.* | lipocondrodistrofia |
| **lipocyte** *A fat cell.* | lipocito |
| **lipodystrophy** *Abnormal fat metabolism.* | lipodistrofia |
| **lipoid** *Referring to fat.* | lipoideo |
| **lipoidosis** *Abnormal lipid metabolism.* | lipoidosi |
| **lipoma** *A benign tumor consisting of fat cells.* | lipoma |
| **lipoprotein** *A soluble protein used to transport fat or lipids.* | lipoproteina |
| **lipotrophic substance** *A compound which causes an increase in body fat.* | sostanza lipotropo |
| **lisping** *A speech problem in which "s" and "z" are pronounced "th".* | essere bleso |
| **listeriosis** *A disease caused by Listeria monocytogenes that occurs in the pregnant and immunocompromised.* | listeriosi |
| **lithagogue** *A treatment of a calculus.* | litagogo |
| **litholapaxy** *The crushing and then removal of a calculus.* | litolapassi |
| **lithotomy** *Surgical removal of a calculus.* | litotomia |
| **lithotomy position** *Buttocks positioned at the end of the OR table, the hips and knees flexed and the feet strapped in. Dorsosacral position.* | posizione litotomia |
| **lithotriptor** *An instrument used to crush a calculus.* | litotribo |
| **litmus** *A dye that turns red with low pH and blue with high pH.* | tornasole |
| **liver** *A large glandular organ in the right upper quadrant that functions in digestive processes, as well as, neutralizing toxins.* | fegato |
| **liver abscess** *A localized collection of pus in the liver.* | ascesso fegato |
| **lobar** *Referring to a lobe.* | lobare |
| **lobe** *A body part divided by a fissure.* | lobo |
| **lobectomy** *Surgical removal of a lobe (generally lung or liver).* | lobectomia |
| **lobotomy** *Surgical incision into the prefrontal lobe; historically a treatment of mental illness.* | lobotomia |
| **Lobo's disease** *A condition exhibited by small, red, hard papules in the sacral region caused by Lacazia loboi.* | malattia di Lobo |
| **lobule** *A small lobe.* | lobulo |
| **localization** *Establishment of a site of a disease process.* | localizzazione |
| **localized** *Toward one point or area.* | localizzato |
| **lochia** *Vaginal secretions noted within two weeks of childbirth.* | lochiazione |
| **locked-in syndrome** *A neurologic condition characterized by a person being conscious of their surroundings but being unable to verbally communicate that understanding.* | sindrome del chiavistello |
| **loculated** *Divided into small cavities.* | loculato |
| **loiasis** *A disease caused by the filarial nematode Loa loa.* | Loa loa, infestazione de |
| **long-acting** *Referring to a drug with long lasting effects.* | lunga durata d'azione |
| **long-term care** *Generally referring to nursing home care.* | custodia a lungo termine |
| **long-standing** *Having existed for a long time.* | in atto da lungo tempo |
| **longevity** *Long life.* | longevità |
| **longsighted** *Synonym of hyperopia.* | ipermetrope |

| English | Italian |
|---|---|
| **loose** *Not tight.* | sciolto |
| **looseness** *Possessing a quality of not being tight.* | scioltezza |
| **lordosis** *An abnormal depth of the inward curvature of the spine.* | lordosi |
| **loss of consciousness** *Unresponsive to verbal and tactile stimuli.* | perdita di coscienza |
| **loss of function** *Inability to complete routine activities.* | perdita di funzione |
| **lost to follow-up** *This describes a situation in which a patient has a chronic medical problem but has not been seen regularly.* | perdita di successivo |
| **lots of** *An abundance of.* | molti |
| **low back pain** *Pain in the lumbar region.* | mal di schiena |
| **low nasal bridge** *A flattening of the top part of the nose.* | appiattimento del'aspetto superiore del naso |
| **low-fat foods** *Nutrients with lower than normal fat content.* | basso contenuto di grassi alimentari |
| **lower extremity edema** *Interstitial edema of the legs.* | edema dell'arto inferiore |
| **lubricant** *Emollient.* | lubrificante |
| **lumbago** *Pain in the region of the lumbar spine.* | lombaggine |
| **lumbar puncture** *Insertion of a needle into the spinal canal in the region of L3-4 to obtain a sample of CSF.* | puntura lombare |
| **lumbar** *Referring to the spinal region inferior to the thoracic spine.* | lombare |
| **lumen** *A hollow cavity.* | lume |
| **lump** *A protuberance.* | protuberanza |
| **lunate bone; os lunatum** *A carpal bone that articulates with the wrist.* | osso semilunare del carpo |
| **lung** *One of a pair of respiratory organs.* | polmone |
| **lung capacity, total** *The amount of air in the lungs after a maximal inhalation.* | capacità polmonare totale |
| **lunula** *The pale area at the base of a fingernail.* | lunula |
| **lupus erythematosous** *An autoimmune inflammatory disease exhibited by a butterfly shaped rash on the face along with visceral and connective tissue abnormalities.* | lupus eritematoso sistemico |
| **luteinizing hormone (LH)** *A pituitary hormone that stimulates ovulation in females and androgen in males.* | ormone luteinizzante |
| **luteotropic** *Synonym of prolactin.* | luteotropo |
| **Lyell's syndrome** *Also called toxic epidermal necrolysis, there are large portions of the skin that become erythematous with epidermal necrosis as seen with 2nd degree burns. This reaction can be seen with use of nevirapine or Bactrim.* | sindrome di Lyell |
| **lymph** *A transparent and sometimes opalescent fluid that flows in the lymph channels.* | linfa |
| **lymph node** *An area of organized lymphatic tissue.* | nodo linfa |
| **lymphadenitis** *Inflammation of a lymph node.* | linfadenite |
| **lymphangiectasis** *Distention of the lymph channels.* | linfangectasia |
| **lymphangioma** *A mass composed of newly formed lymph tissue.* | linfangioma |
| **lymphangitis** *Inflammation of the lymph vessels.* | linfangite |
| **lymphatic** *Referring to the lymph system.* | linfatico |
| **lymphocyte** *A white blood cell produced by the lymph tissue.* | linfocito |
| **lymphocythemia** *Abnormally high number of lymphocytes in the blood.* | linfocitosi |
| **lymphocytic leukemia** *Chronic accumulation of functionally incompetent lymphocytes.* | leucemia linfocito |
| **lymphocytopenia** *Decrease in the usual number of lymphocytes in the blood.* | linfocitopenia |
| **lymphocytosis** *The organization of cysts containing lymph.* | linfocitosi |
| **lymphoid** *Similar to lymph.* | linfoide |

| English | Italian |
|---|---|
| **lymphoma** *A malignant disease of the lymph system, Hodgkin's lymphoma for example.* | linfoma |
| **lymphosarcoma** *A malignant disease of the lymph system that does not include Hodgkin's lymphoma.* | linfosarcoma |
| **lysine** *An amino acid found in most proteins.* | lisina |
| **lysis** *The rupture of a cell wall or membrane.* | lisi |
| **lysosome** *An organelle contained in the cytoplasm of eukaryotic cells.* | lisosomi |
| **lysozyme** *An enzyme in tears that facilitates destruction of certain bacterial cell walls.* | lisozima |
| **lytic** *Referring to lysis.* | litico |
| **macrocheilia** *Abnormally large lips.* | macrocheilia |
| **macrocyte** *A large red blood cell.* | macrocito |
| **macrocytosis** *Referring to the status of an increased number of large erythrocytes as seen in Vitamin B12 deficiency.* | macrocitosi |
| **macrodactyly** *Abnormally large digits.* | macrodattilia |
| **macroencephaly** *Having an abnormally large head.* | macroencefalia |
| **macroglobulinemia** *A condition exhibited by an increase number of macroglobulins in the blood.* | macroglobulinemia |
| **macroglossia** *Abnormally large tongue.* | macroglossia |
| **macromastia** *Abnormally large breasts.* | macromastia |
| **macromelia** *Abnormally large head or extremity.* | macromelia |
| **macrophage** *A phagocytic cell that originates in the tissues.* | macrofago |
| **macrostomia** *Abnormal increase in the width of the mouth.* | macrostomia |
| **macula** *1. The area of the eye of greatest visual acuity that surrounds the fovea. 2. A small flat discoloration of the skin (synonym for macule).* | macchia; chiazza |
| **macula solaris** *Formal medical term describing a freckle.* | lentiggine |
| **maculopapule** *A skin lesion that is similar to both a macule and a papule.* | maculopapula |
| **mad cow disease** *Bovine spongiform encephalopathy, a disease that cause cerebral degeneration exhibited by ataxia.* | mucca pazza; encefalopatia spongiforme bovina |
| **madness** *Common term for insanity.* | alienazione mentale |
| **magnet** *A piece of iron with atoms ordered to make it magnetic.* | calamita |
| **magnetic** *Having the properties of a magnet.* | magnetico |
| **magnetic resonance imaging (MRI)** *Images are produced by evaluating the response of body tissue. nuclei to radio waves in a magnetic field.* | scanner della risonanza magnetica |
| **maiden name** *The surname a woman uses prior to being married.* | nome da ragazza |
| **maintenance therapy** *Continuing a form of treatment long-term.* | terapia di mantenimento |
| **Malabar itch.** *Pruritus associated with tinea imbricata which is characterized by overlapping rings of papulosquamous patches. It is also known as oriental ringworm.* | prurito di Malabar |
| **malacia** *The abnormal softening of a body part or tissue.* | malacia |
| **maladjustment** *Having the trait of being unable to cope normally.* | inadattabilità |
| **malaise** *A vague feeling of discomfort or unease.* | malessere |
| **malalignment (dental)** *Displacement of the teeth from their normal position.* | malallineamento |
| **malaria** *A condition caused by a protozoan of the genus Plasmodium. It is transmitted by mosquitos and is exhibited by fever, chills, headache. In the severe form it can lead to convulsions, increased ICP and death.* | malaria |
| **malignant** *Tendency of a tumor to invade normal tissue.* | maligno |
| **malignant hypertension** *Sudden, severe hypertension associated with neuroretinitis.* | ipertensione arteriosa maligno |
| **malingerer** *A person who feigns illness.* | simulazione di malattia |

| English | Italian |
|---|---|
| **malleolus** *A bony protrusion on medial and lateral aspect of each ankle.* | malleolo |
| **malleolus, lateral** *The lateral aspect of the distal fibula.* | malleolo esterno |
| **malleolus, medial** *The medial aspect of the distal portion of the tibia.* | malleolo tibiale interno |
| **mallet finger** *Flexion contracture of the distal phalanx.* | dito a martello di una mano |
| **malleus** *Small bone in the inner ear that articulates with the incus.* | martello |
| **Mallory-Weiss syndrome** *Upper GI bleeding related to a laceration at the gastroesophageal junction caused by vigorous vomiting.* | sindrome di Mallory-Weiss |
| **malnutrition** *Lack of appropriate nutrition.* | malnutrizione |
| **malpractice** *Negligent professional activity.* | scorrettezza professionale |
| **maltose** *A disaccharide hydrolyzed by amylase.* | maltosio |
| **malunion** *The union of a fracture in a faulty position.* | malunione |
| **mammaplasty** *Plastic surgery of the breast.* | mammoplastica |
| **mammary** *Referring to the breast.* | mammario |
| **mammary gland** *The mass of tissue posterior to the nipples which has the essential task of milk production.* | ghiandola mammaria |
| **mammillary** *Referring to a nipple.* | mammillare |
| **mammography** *Roentgenography of the breasts, used as a screening test for cancer.* | mammografia |
| **man** *Male human.* | uomo |
| **management** *The process of dealing with things or people.* | trattamento |
| **mandatory** *Obligatory.* | indispensabile |
| **mandible** *The lower jaw.* | mandibola |
| **mania** *A mental disorder exhibited by hyperexcitability, delusions and euphoria.* | mania |
| **manic-depressive psychosis** *A mental disorder exhibited by alternating periods of depression and mania.* | psicosi maniaco-depressiva |
| **manometer** *Device used for pressure monitoring.* | manometro |
| **manubrium sterni** *The superior segment of the sternum which articulates with the clavicle and first rib.* | manubrio dello sterno |
| **maple syrup urine disease** *A condition characterized by an enzyme defect causing an increase in leucine in the urine.* | malattia dell'urina a sciroppo diacero |
| **mapping** *A collection of data points showing spatial distribution.* | cartografia |
| **marasmus** *Progressive weight loss and emaciation.* | marasma |
| **Marfan syndrome** *A connective tissue disease exhibited by long limbs, joint laxity and cardiovascular defects.* | sindrome di Marfan |
| **marijuana** *Cannabis.* | marihuana |
| **marital counseling** *Therapy aimed at marriage reconciliation.* | consigliabile maritale |
| **marital status** *Single versus married status.* | stato coniugale |
| **marsupialization** *Creation of a surgical pouch.* | marsupializzazione |
| **mass** *Tumor.* | tumore, massa |
| **mast cell** *A cell containing basophilic granules that releases histamine and other substances during allergic reactions.* | mastzellen |
| **mastectomy** *Surgical resection of one or both breasts.* | mastectomia |
| **mastication** *Chewing.* | masticazione |
| **mastitis** *Inflammation of the breast.* | mastite |
| **mastodynia** *Breast pain.* | mastodinia |
| **mastoid** *Referring to the mastoid process.* | mastoide |
| **mastoid process** *The posterior part of the temporal bone bordered by the parietal bone superiorly and the occipital bone posteriorly.* | processo mastoideo |
| **mastoidectomy** *Surgical removal of the mastoid.* | mastoidectomia |
| **mastoiditis** *Inflammation of the mastoid process.* | mastoidite |

| English | Italian |
|---|---|
| **matching** *Corresponding in pattern or style.* | corrispondente in stile |
| **mattress** *A fabric case filled with material, used for sleeping.* | materasso |
| **mattress suture** *A double stitch that forms a loop and there is eversion of the edges when tied.* | sutura da materassaio |
| **maxilla** *The upper jaw that also forms the inferior portion of the orbit and part of the nose.* | mascella |
| **maxillofacial** *Referring to the maxilla and the face.* | maxillo-facciale |
| **mazamorra** *Dermatitis caused by hookworm larvae indigenous to Puerto Rico.* | mazamorra |
| **Mcdonald's maneuver** *A measurement of the uterus in centimeters that corresponds to gestational age in weeks.* | manovra di Mcdonald |
| **meaningless** *Having no significance.* | senza senso |
| **measles** *A childhood viral, infectious disease exhibited by rash and fever.* | morbillo |
| **meatus** *Opening to the body, such as urethral meatus.* | meato |
| **meconium** *The first newborn feces which are green.* | meconio |
| **meconium aspiration** *Presence of meconium on the newborn indicating there was fetal distress in-utero.* | aspirazione di meconio |
| **medial** *Situated toward the midline.* | mediale |
| **medianstinoscopy** *Visual inspection of the mediastinum with a scope.* | mediastinoscopia |
| **mediastinum** *The thoracic area between the lungs.* | mediastino |
| **medical record** *The electronic or paper report on a patient.* | cartella clinica |
| **medication** *A substance used for medical treatment.* | medicazione |
| **medicine** *A substance used for medical treatment or 2) the art and science of healing patients.* | medicina 2) medicamento |
| **medicosurgical** *Referring to medicine and surgery.* | medicochirurgico |
| **medulla oblongata** *The inferior portion of the brainstem.* | midollo allungato |
| **medullary** *1. The inner part of an organ. 2. Referring to the medulla oblongata.* | midollare |
| **medulloblastoma** *A malignant tumor of the cerebellum found mostly in children.* | medulloblastoma |
| **megacephaly** *Having a larger than normal cranial capacity.* | megalocefalia |
| **megacolon** *Abnormal enlargement and dilatation of the colon.* | megacolon |
| **megakaryocyte** *A cell found in the bone marrow that is a source of platelet production.* | megacariocito |
| **megaloblast** *A large red blood cell noted primarily in pernicious anemia.* | megaloblasto |
| **megalomania** *A mental disorder characterized by abnormal feelings of self-importance.* | megalomania |
| **meibomian cyst** *An enclosed fluid collection along a sebaceous gland of the eyelid.* | cisti di meibomio |
| **meiosis** *Cell division creating two daughter cells each with half the number of cells as the parent cell.* | meiosi |
| **melancholia** *Profound sadness.* | melancolia |
| **melanin** *A dark pigment found on the skin, hair or iris.* | melanina |
| **melanoma** *Malignant cancer, typically found in the skin.* | melanoma |
| **melena** *The passage of black, tarry stools indicative of upper gastrointestinal bleeding.* | melena |
| **melissophobia** *Also called apiphobia, a fear of bees.* | melissofobia |
| **melitis** *Inflammation of the cheek.* | melite |
| **member** *Referring to an extremity (arm or leg).* | membro |
| **memory** *Ability to remember.* | memoria |
| **menarche** *The time of the initial menstrual period.* | menarca |

| English | Italian |
|---|---|
| **meningeal** *Referring to the dura mater, arachnoid and the pia mater.* | meningeo |
| **meningioma** *A tumor of the meningeal tissue; generally benign.* | meningioma |
| **meningism** *Signs and symptoms of meningitis without infection of the meninges.* | meningismo |
| **meningitis** *Inflammation of the meninges exhibited by fever, photophobia, nuchal rigidity and in severe cases coma and convulsions.* | meningite |
| **meningocele** *A congenital defect exhibited by protrusion of the meninges through a defect in the spinal column.* | meningocele |
| **meningococcemia** *Presence of N. meningitidis in the blood.* | meningococcemia |
| **meniscectomy** *Surgical excision of a meniscus.* | menisectomia |
| **meniscus** *A thin cartilage between joint surfaces.* | menisco |
| **menopause** *The time when menstruation ceases.* | menopausa |
| **menorrhagia** *Abnormally large amount of menstrual blood.* | menorragia |
| **menses** *The blood and other material expelled from the uterus during menstruation.* | mestruazioni |
| **menstruation** *Synonym of menses.* | mestruazioni |
| **mental** *Cognitive or psychological.* | mentale |
| **mention, to** *Refer to or allude to.* | menzionare |
| **mesarteritis** *Inflammation of the middle layer of an artery.* | mesarterite |
| **mesencephalon** *Midbrain.* | mesencefalo |
| **mesenchyme** *Organized mesodermal cells that produce connective tissue, lymphatics and bone.* | mesenchima |
| **mesentery** *The fold of peritoneum that connects the small bowel, pancreas and spleen to the posterior portion of the abdominal wall.* | mesentere |
| **mesoappendix** *The portion of the mesentery vermiform appendix.* | mesoappendice |
| **mesocolon** *The mesentery connecting the colon to the posterior abdominal wall.* | mesocolon |
| **mesoderm** *The middle germ layer in an embryo that is the source of bone, muscle and skin.* | mesoderma |
| **mesonephroma** *Usually a tumor of the female genital tract that is thought to stem from the mesonephros.* | mesonefroma |
| **mesosalpinx** *A portion of the broad ligament supporting the fallopian tubes.* | mesosalpinge |
| **mesothelioma** *A tumor that stems from mesothelial tissue; a known cause is asbestos exposure.* | mesotelioma |
| **mesovarium** *The portion of the mesentery connecting the ovary with the abdominal wall.* | mesovario |
| **metabolic** *Referring to the physical and chemical reactions involved with keeping an organism functioning.* | metabolico |
| **metacarpal** *The name for any of the five hand bones.* | metacarpale |
| **metacarpophalangeal** *Referring to the metacarpus and the phalanges.* | metacarpofalangeo |
| **metaphysis** *The region between the diaphysis and the epiphysis.* | metafisi |
| **metaplasia** *Abnormal change in the nature or character of tissue.* | metaplasia |
| **metatarsal** *Any of the bones of the foot.* | metatarsale |
| **metatarsalgia** *Foot pain.* | metatarsalgia |
| **meter** *Unit if measurement. (instrument for measurement)* | metro |
| **methemoglobin** *A substance formed with the oxidation of hemoglobin.* | metaemoglobina |
| **methionine** *A sulfur-containing amino acid used in the biosynthesis of cysteine.* | metionina |
| **metric system** | sistema metrico |
| **metrorrhagia** *Uterine bleeding in normal amounts but at irregular intervals.* | metrorragia |
| **microbe** *A microorganism.* | microbo |

| English | Italian |
|---|---|
| **microbiology** *The study of microorganisms.* | microbiologia |
| **microcephalic** *A congenital deformity exhibited by an abnormally small head.* | microcefalico |
| **microcyte** *An unusually small erythrocyte associated with anemias, such as iron deficiency anemia.* | microcito |
| **micrognathia** *Abnormally small maxilla or mandible.* | micrognazia |
| **microgram** *One millionth of one gram.* | microgrammo |
| **micrometer** *One millionth of one meter.* | micrometro |
| **microorganism** *An organism only seen with a microscope.* | microorganismo |
| **microphthalmos** *A congenital condition characterized by smallness of the eyes.* | microftalmo |
| **microscope** *A instrument used to magnify and view small objects.* | microscopio |
| **micturition** *Synonym of urination.* | minzione |
| **midbrain** *The portion of the brainstem superior to the pons.* | mesencefalo |
| **middle ear** *The portion of the ear containing the stapes, incus and malleus.* | orecchio medio |
| **midline** *A median line of bilateral separation.* | linea mediana |
| **midstream urine** *A specimen of urine that is collected after the initial stream of urine is initiated and before one finishes urinating.* | urina centro della corrente |
| **midwife** *A person trained to assist in childbirth.* | ostetrica; levatrice |
| **midwifery** *The occupation of assisting in childbirth.* | ostetricia |
| **migraine** *An episodic, unilateral headache accompanied by nausea.* | emicrania |
| **mild** *Slight, nominal.* | mite |
| **milestone** *An event indicative of a certain stage of development.* | pietra miliare |
| **miliary** *Referring to a disease that is exhibited by small seed-like lesions (millet), such as miliary tuberculosis.* | miliare |
| **Milkman syndrome** *Osteomalacia with multiple pseudofractures.* | sindrome di Milkman |
| **milligram** *A unit of weight, 1/1000 of a gram.* | milligrammo |
| **milliliter** *A unit of volume, 1/1000 of a liter.* | millilitro |
| **millimeter** *A unit of measurement, 1/1000 of a meter.* | millimetro |
| **Milroy's disease** *Hereditary disease exhibited by leg edema.* | morbo di Milroy |
| **minute** *A unit of time.* | minuto |
| **minute** *Something very small.* | minuscolo |
| **mirror** *A device used for reflecting an image.* | specchio |
| **miryachit** *A disease of Siberia characterized by an exaggerated startle response; also referred to as jumping disease.* | miryachit |
| **misanthropy** *A severe dislike of homo sapiens.* | misantropia |
| **miscarriage** *Spontaneous abortion.* | aborto spontaneo |
| **misspelling** *Incorrect spelling of a word.* | sbagliare a scrivere |
| **mite fever** *Synonym of typhus fever.* | febbre da acaro |
| **mitochondria** *Organelle found in cells responsible for energy production.* | mitocondrio |
| **mitosis** *Cell division in which two daughter cells are formed that have the same number of chromosomes as the parent cell.* | mitosi |
| **mitral** *Referring to the mitral valve.* | mitrale |
| **mitral regurgitation** *Backflow of blood from the left ventricle to the left atrium because of dysfunctional valve.* | rigurgito mitrale |
| **mitral stenosis** *Narrowing of the left atrioventricular orifice.* | stenosi mitrale |
| **mitral valve** *The valve with two cusps between the left atrium and ventricle.* | valvola mitrale |
| **modiolus** *A column located in the cochlea.* | modiolo |
| **moist** *Damp or humid.* | madido |

| English | Italian |
|---|---|
| **molality** *The number of moles of a solution per kilogram of pure solvent.* | molalità |
| **molar tooth** *Any of the most posterior teeth bilaterally which includes 8 deciduous and usually 12 permanent teeth.* | dente molare |
| **molecule** *A combination of at least two atoms.* | molecola |
| **monitor** *A person that observes a process or a monitoring device.* | persona che controlla |
| **monkey-paw** *An appearance due to median nerve palsy causing atrophy of the thenar eminence with adduction and elevation of the thumb, resembling that of a simian.* | mano di scimmia |
| **monkeypox** *A viral disease that is similar to smallpox which occurs primarily in monkeys and rarely in humans.* | vaiolo delle scimmie |
| **monoamine oxidase inhibitor (MAOI)** *A drug used to treat depression that allows accumulation of serotonin and norepinephrine.* | inibitore monoamino-ossidasi |
| **monoclonal** *Asexual formation of a clone from a single cell.* | monoclonale |
| **monocyte** *A leukocyte with an oval nucleus and grey cytoplasm.* | monocito |
| **monocytosis** *An abnormal increase in the number of monocytes in the blood.* | monocitosi |
| **monodiplopia** *Double vision in only one eye.* | mondiplopia |
| **monomania** *A psychotic obsession about a single subject.* | monomania |
| **mononeuritis** *Inflammation of a single nerve.* | mononervite |
| **mononuclear** *A cell having only one nucleus.* | mononucleato |
| **mononucleosis** *An infectious disease exhibited by malaise and lymphadenopathy.* | mononucleosi |
| **monoplegia** *Paralysis of a single limb.* | monoplegia |
| **mons pubis** *The fleshy protuberance over the symphysis pubis.* | monte del pube |
| **mood** *A temporary state of mind or feeling.* | umore |
| **morbid** *Indicative of disease.* | morboso |
| **morbidity** *The state of disease.* | morbosità |
| **Morgagni's syndrome** *Also called metabolic craniopathy and Stewart-Morel syndrome, it is exhibited by hyperostosis frontalis interna, obesity and neuropsychiatric disorders.* | sindrome di Morgagni |
| **morgue** *A room where deceased patients are housed until sent to a funeral home.* | obitorio |
| **moribund** *Near death.* | moribondo |
| **morning sickness** *Nausea associated with pregnancy.* | nausea gravidica |
| **morphea** *A condition exhibited by an elevated or depressed patch of pink skin with a purple border.* | morfea |
| **morphine** *An opioid analgesic.* | morfina |
| **morphology** *The study of living organisms and the correlation between their structure.* | morfologia |
| **morula** *A solid mass created by the splitting of an ovum.* | morula |
| **mosquito net** *A fine mesh fabric hung over a bed as a mosquito repellent.* | zanzariera |
| **mossy fiber** *Nerve fibers that surround the nerve cells of the cerebellar cortex.* | fibre simili a muschio |
| **motion sickness** *Nausea associated with travel.* | chinetosi |
| **motor** *Referring to muscles.* | motore |
| **motor end plate** *The expansions on a motor nerve where the branches terminate on muscle fiber.* | placca neuromuscolare motore |
| **motor unit** *The complex of one motor cell and its attached muscle fibers.* | unità motore |
| **mottled** *An irregular arrangement of patches of color.* | screziato |
| **mourning** *A period of grieving.* | gemente |
| **mouth** *The orifice on the lower part of the face.* | bocca |

| English | Italian |
|---|---|
| **mouth to mouth resuscitation** *A form of emergency management of respiratory failure.* | rianimazione bocca a bocca |
| **mouthful** *A large quantity of something in one's mouth.* | boccata |
| **mucilage** *1. A viscous bodily fluid. 2. A polysaccharide used in medicines and glue.* | mucillagine |
| **mucin** *A glycoprotein that is the primary constituent in mucous.* | mucina |
| **mucocele** *An accumulation of mucous in a dilated cavity.* | mucocele |
| **mucoid** *Referring to mucous.* | mucoide |
| **mucolytic** *A substance that breaks down mucous.* | mucolitico |
| **mucopolysaccharidosis type I** *Also referred to as Hurler syndrome, persons cannot make lysosomal alpha-L-iduronidase which breaks down glycosaminoglycans.* | mucopolisaccaridosi tipo I |
| **mucopolysaccharidosis type II** *Also referred to as Hunter syndrome, persons with this inherited condition cannot produce iduronate sulfatase. There are mild to severe forms but all forms have deafness, coarse facial features, hypertrichosis and macrocephaly.* | mucopolisaccaridosi tipo II |
| **mucopolysaccharidosis type III** *Also referred to as Sanfilippo syndrome, persons cannot catabolize the heparan sulfate sugar chain. Symptoms include stiff joints, thick eyebrows, coarse facial features and developmental delays.* | mucopolisaccaridosi tipo III |
| **mucopolysaccharidosis type Is** *Also referred to as Scheie syndrome, persons cannot produce lysosomal alpha-L-iduronidase. Symptoms include cloudy cornea, hirsutism, prognathism and stiff joints.* | mucopolisaccaridosi tipo Is |
| **mucopolysaccharidosis type IV** *Also referred to as Morquio syndrome, persons do not produce galactosamine-6-sulfatase or in some cases beta-galactosidase. Symptoms include hypermobile joints, macrocephaly, short stature and wide spaced teeth.* | mucopolisaccaridosi tipo IV |
| **mucopolysaccharidosis type VI** *Also referred to as Maroteaux-Lamy syndrome. It is characterized by hydrocephalus, macroglossia and coarse facial features but normal intelligence.* | mucopolisaccaridosi tipo VI |
| **mucopurulent** *That which contains both mucous and pus.* | mucopurulento |
| **mucosa** *A mucous membrane like the buccal mucosa.* | mucosa |
| **Mucune-Albright syndrome** *Polyostotic fibrous dysplasia with cutaneous brown patches, endocrine dysfunction that exhibits in females as precocious puberty.* | sindrome di Mucune-Albright |
| **mucus** *A substance secreted by mucous membranes.* | muco |
| **multigravida** *A woman who has been pregnant more than once.* | multigravida |
| **multilocular** *The presence of more than one cell within a cavity.* | multiloculare |
| **multipara** *A woman with more than one live births.* | multipara |
| **multiple sclerosis** *A chronic neurologic disease exhibited by numbness, vision and speech problems, and motor incoordination.* | sclerosi multipla |
| **mumble, to** *To speak quietly and indistinctly.* | borbottare |
| **mumps** *A contagious viral disease that is exhibited by parotid swelling and puts males at risk for sterility. Also called epidemic parotitis.* | orecchioni |
| **mural thrombus** *A thrombus attached to a diseased portion of endocardium.* | trombo murale |
| **murmur** *An abnormal heart sound heard with a stethoscope.* | soffio |
| **muscle** *A band if fibrous tissue that can contract.* | muscolo |
| **muscle weakness** *Decreased muscular function.* | debolezza muscolare |
| **muscular** *Referring to muscles.* | muscolare |
| **muscular dystrophy** *A hereditary condition exhibited by progressive muscular weakness and muscle atrophy.* | distrofia muscolare |
| **mutation** *A gene alteration that can be passed to the next generation.* | mutazione |
| **mute** *Refraining from or being speechless.* | muto |
| **mutism** *Inability to speak.* | mutismo |

| English | Italian |
|---|---|
| **myalgia** *Muscle pain.* | mialgia |
| **myasthenia gravis** *An autoimmune disease characterized by fluctuating weakness of the ocular, limb and respiratory muscles.* | miastenia gravis |
| **mycetoma** *Persistent inflammation of the tissues caused by an infection.* | micetoma |
| **mycosis** *A disease caused by a fungal infection.* | micosi |
| **mycotoxin** *A substance toxic to fungus.* | micotossina |
| **mydriasis** *Pupillary dilation.* | midriasi |
| **myelin** *The substance that forms a sheath around some nerve fibers.* | mielina |
| **myelitis** *Inflammation of the spinal cord.* | mielite |
| **myelocele** *Protrusion of the spinal cord through a defect in the bony structure.* | mielocele |
| **myelogram** *CT scan or roentgenography of the spinal canal after injection of contrast media.* | mielogramma |
| **myeloid** *Referring to the bone marrow or spinal cord.* | mieloide |
| **myeloma** *Malignant tumor of the bone marrow.* | mieloma |
| **myelomatosis** *A leukemic disease in which there is an abnormally high amount of myeloblasts in the blood.* | mielomatosi |
| **myelomeningocele** *A protrusion of the spinal cord and its meninges through a defect in the vertebral canal.* | mielomeningocele |
| **myelopathy** *A condition of the spinal cord.* | mielopatia |

| English | Italian |
|---|---|
| **myocardial** *Referring to the muscular tissue of the heart.* | miocardico |
| **myocardial infarction** *The death of myocardial tissue as a result of an interruption in flow to the region supplied by a coronary vessel.* | infarto miocardico |
| **myocarditis** *An inflammation of the heart.* | miocardite |
| **myocardium** *The middle layer of the heart wall.* | miocardio |
| **myoclonus** *Contraction or spasm of a group of muscles.* | mioclonio |
| **myoglobin** *A protein within muscle that carries and stores oxygen.* | mioglobina |
| **myoma** *A benign neoplasm of muscular tissue.* | mioma |
| **myomectomy** *Surgical resection of a myoma.* | miomatectomia |
| **myometrium** *The smooth muscle layer of the uterus.* | miometrio |
| **myopathy** *Muscle disease.* | miopatia |
| **myopia** *Nearsightedness.* | miopia |
| **myosarcoma** *A mass with myoma and sarcoma characteristics.* | mioscaroma |
| **myosin** *A protein that when coupled with actin form the contractile complex of a muscle cells.* | miosina |
| **myositis** *Inflammation of muscle tissue.* | miosite |
| **myositis ossificans** *Inflammation of muscle tissue with presence of bony deposits.* | miosite ossificante |
| **myotomy** *The surgical removal of muscle tissue.* | miotomia |
| **myotonia dystrophica; Steinert's disease** *A condition exhibited initially by hypertonic muscles followed by atrophy of the facial and neck muscles.* | miotonia distrofica |
| **myringitis** *Inflammation of the tympanic membrane.* | miringite |
| **myringoplasty** *Surgical repair of tympanic membrane defects.* | miringoplastica |
| **myringotomy** *Surgical opening of the tympanic membrane.* | miringotomia |
| **mysophobia** *Severe fear of dirt or contamination from common objects.* | misofobia |
| **myxedema** *Diffuse edema with a wax-like appearance of the skin; this condition is associated with hypothyroidism.* | mixedema |
| **myxoma** *A tumor composed of mucous tissue.* | mixoma |
| **myxosarcoma** *A sarcoma that also has mucous tissue.* | mixosarcoma |
| **nail** *The hard surface on the dorsal surface of the toes or fingers.* | unghia |
| **nail bed** *The area just beneath a finger or toenail. Also called matrix unguis.* | letto ungueale |
| **nail biting** *A habit of chewing on one's fingernails.* | al cardiopalma |
| **nailing** *Referring to placement of an intramedullary rod in a long bone in order to treat a fracture.* | inchiodamento (di osso fratturato) |
| **name** *A word by which a person is known.* | nome |
| **nap** *A brief sleep or catnap.* | pisolino |
| **narcissism** *Abnormally excessive self-interest.* | narcisismo |
| **narcolepsy** *A condition exhibited by a strong desire to sleep and by sudden onset of sleep at increased intervals.* | narcolepsia |
| **narcosis** *A reversible medication-induced condition of excessive drowsiness or unconsciousness.* | narcosi |
| **narcotic** *A medication that produces narcosis.* | narcotico |
| **nasal** *Referring to the nose.* | nasale |
| **nasogastric tube** *A tube that is inserted into the nose with the distal tip in the stomach; it is used for irrigation or drainage of gastric contents.* | sonda nasogastrico |

| English | Italian |
|---|---|
| **nasogastric tube placement** *Insertion of a tube that is placed in the stomach via the nostril; it is used for administration of fluid or to suction gastric contents.* | sonda gastrico introdotta del naso |
| **nasolacrimal** *Referring to the nose and tear apparatus.* | nasolacrimale |
| **nasopharyngeal** *Referring to the nose and pharynx.* | nasofaringeo |
| **nasopharynx** *The part of the pharynx which lies superior to the soft palate.* | nasofaringe |
| **nausea** *A feeling that one wants to vomit.* | nausea |
| **navel** *Umbilicus.* | ombelico |
| **navicular** *1. boat shaped 2. Referring to the navicular bone of the hand or foot.* | navicolare |
| **navicular bone** *The most lateral bone in the proximal row of carpal bones.* | osso naviculare |
| **near** *In close proximity.* | vicino |
| **nebula** *An opaque spot on the cornea causing impaired vision.* | nebbiolina |
| **nebulizer** *A device used for transforming a liquid into a fine mist for inhalation as in nebulized albuterol for an acute exacerbation of asthma.* | nebulizzatore |
| **nebulizer treatment** *Administration of medication such as albuterol via a fine mist using a nebulizer.* | trattamento mediante nebulizzazione |
| **neck** *The part of the body that connects the body to the head.* | collo |
| **neck of the femur** *The portion of the femur between the shaft and head.* | collo del femore |
| **necropsy** *Synonym of autopsy.* | necropsia |
| **necrosis** *The death of most of the cells of the affected part.* | necrosi |
| **necrotic** *Referring to necrosis.* | necrotico |
| **need** *A want or obligation.* | bisogno |
| **needle** *The slender cylindrical device attached to a syringe.* | ago |
| **needle biopsy** *Use of a needle to aspirate body contents for microscopic or pathologic examination.* | ago biopsia |
| **needle for lumbar puncture** | ago per puntura lombare |
| **needle holder** *A surgical instrument used to grasp a needle during suturing.* | pinza per aghi; porta aghi |
| **needle-stick injury** *The inadvertent self-puncture with a needle that had been used previously to inject a patient.* | lesioni del ago-bastone |
| **negative** *Contrary or opposing.* | negativo |
| **nematode** *An endoparasite belonging to the class of the Nemathelminthes including roundworms and threadworms.* | nematode |
| **neonatal** *Referring to the first four weeks after birth.* | neonatale |
| **neonate** *The term for a newborn infant for the first four weeks.* | neonato |
| **neoplasm** *A new and abnormal growth.* | neoplasma |
| **nephrectomy** *Surgical removal of a kidney.* | nefrectomia |
| **nephritis** *A general term meaning inflammation of a kidney that is further categorized depending on the associated pathology.* | nefrite |
| **nephroblastoma** *Congenital tumor of the kidney, also called Wilms' tumor.* | nefroblastoma; tumore di Wilms |
| **nephrocalcinosis** *A condition exhibited by calcium phosphate deposition in the renal tubules; a cause of renal insufficiency.* | nefrocalcinosi |
| **nephrolithiasis** *A calculus in the kidney.* | nefrolitiasi |
| **nephrolithotomy** *Surgical removal of a renal calculus.* | nefrolitotomia |
| **nephroma** *A renal tumor.* | nefroma |
| **nephron** *A functional unit of the kidney that consists of the glomerulus, the proximal and distal convoluted tubules, the loop of Henle and the collecting tubule.* | nefrone |
| **nephropathy** *Renal disease.* | nefropatia |

| English | Italian |
|---|---|
| **nephropexy** *The surgical fixation of a kidney that was previously floating.* | nefropessi |
| **nephroptosis** *Inferior displacement of the kidney.* | nefroptosi |
| **nephrosclerosis** *Hardening of the kidney.* | nefrosclerosi |
| **nephrosis** *A kidney disease exhibited by edema and proteinuria; also called nephrotic syndrome.* | nefrosi |
| **nephrostomy** *Surgical creation of an opening between the renal pelvis and an opening in the skin.* | nefrostomia |
| **nephrotic** *Referring to nephrosis.* | nefrosico |
| **nephrotomy** *Surgical incision of the kidney.* | nefrotomia |
| **nerve** *A fibrous band made up of axons and dendrites that connects the nervous systems with other organs.* | nervo |
| **nerve impulse** *A signal transmitted along a nerve fiber.* | impulso nervo |
| **nerve block anesthesia** *Locally administered anesthesia.* | anestesia locale |
| **neural** *Referring to a nerve or nerve impulse.* | neurale |
| **neuralgia** *Severe pain along the course of a nerve.* | neuralgia |
| **neurapraxia** *Paralysis from nerve injury but no degeneration of the nerve.* | neuraprassia |
| **neurasthenia** *A psychoneurosis exhibited by severe fatigue.* | nervastenico |
| **neurectomy** *Excision of a section of a nerve.* | nervrectomia |
| **neurilemma** *The membrane covering a myelinated nerve fiber or the axon of an unmyelinated nerve fiber.* | neurilemma |
| **neuritis** *Inflammation of a nerve.* | nevrite |
| **neuroblastoma** *A nervous system malignant tumor composed of neuroblasts.* | neuroblastoma |
| **neurodermatitis** *A pruritic, thickened eruption in the axillary and inguinal thought to be exacerbated by emotions.* | neurodermatite |
| **neuroepithelium** *Cells specialized to serve as sensory cells such as cells of the cochlea and tongue.* | neuroepitelio |
| **neurofibroma** *A tumor formed by excessive growth of perineurium and endoneurium.* | neurofibroma |
| **neurofibromatosis** *A hereditary condition exhibited by formation of multiple soft tumors scattered throughout the skin surface. Also known as von Recklinghausen disease.* | neurofibromatosi |
| **neuroglia** *A type of connective tissue of the nervous system.* | nevroglia |
| **neuroleptic** *A drug that causes neurologic symptoms.* | neurolettico |
| **neuroleptic malignant syndrome** *A severe reaction to neuroleptic medications characterized by hyperthermia with autonomic and extrapyramidal symptoms.* | sindrome neurolettica maligna |
| **neurologist** *A physician who specializes in the study of the nervous system.* | neurolog |
| **neurology** *The study of the nervous system.* | neurologia |
| **neuroma** *A mass composed of nerve cells and fibers.* | neuroma |
| **neuron** *A nerve cell.* | neurone |
| **neuropathic** *Referring to neuropathy.* | neuropatico |
| **neuropathy** *Structural of pathologic changes of the peripheral nervous system.* | neuropatia |
| **neurosis** *A mental disorder.* | neurosi |
| **neurosurgery** *Surgery of the brain or spinal cord.* | neurochirurgia |
| **neurosyphilis** *Infection of the central nervous system with Treponema pallidum.* | neurosifilide |
| **neurotmesis** *The severing of a nerve.* | neurotmesi |
| **neurotomy** *Surgical incision into a nerve.* | neurotomia |

| English | Italian |
|---|---|
| **neurotransmitter** *A substance released at the end of a nerve fiber that facilitates transmission of an impulse.* | neurotrasmettitore |
| **neutropenia** *Diminished number of neutrophils in the blood.* | neutropenia |
| **neutrophil** *A polymorphonuclear leukocyte.* | neutrofilo |
| **nevus** *A benign, well-circumscribed growth of tissue of congenital origin.* | nevo |
| **next** *The following or upcoming.* | prossimo |
| **nick** *A small groove or notch.* | taglietto |
| **nicotinic acid** *A deficiency of this substance results in pellagra.* | acido nicotinico |
| **night blindness** *Common term for nyctalopia, it refers to low vision with reduced illumination, often seen with Vitamin A deficiency.* | nittalopia |
| **night shift** *The late shift, typically beginning at 19:00 or 23:00 hours.* | turno di notte |
| **night sweats** *Profuse sweating at night occurring with tuberculosis among other conditions.* | sudorazioni notturne |
| **night terror** *Sensation of profound fear upon wakening.* | pavor nocturnus |
| **nightmare** *An unpleasant or frightening dream.* | incubo |
| **nipple** *The small projection on the breast thru which milk is secreted.* | capezzolo |
| **nitrogen** *A colorless, odorless gas used as a coolant in the liquid form.* | azoto |
| **nitrous oxide** *An inhalant gas used as an anesthetic agent.* | ossido di azoto |
| **nocturia** *Urination at night.* | nocturia |
| **nocturnal emission** *Involuntary emission of semen at night.* | polluzione notturna |
| **nocturnal** *Referring to events that happen at night.* | notturna |
| **node** *A swelling or prominence.* | nodo |
| **nodule** *A small node in the skin of up to 1cm and in the lung up to 3cm.* | nodulo; nodo |
| **nonpitting edema** *Subcutaneous swelling that cannot be indented with compression.* | non conserva fossetta dopo compressione digitale |
| **non-rebreather mask** *A type of oxygen mask used to deliver a higher oxygen concentration.* | maschera a ossigeno a circuito aperto |
| **non-resorbable suture (nylon)** *Suture used to be permanent as it is not removed by normal body processes.* | sutura nailon |
| **noon** *The 12 o'clock mid-day hour.* | mezzogiorno |
| **norepinephrine** *A hormone secreted by the adrenal medulla and a synthetic drug used as a pressor agent.* | norepinefrina |
| **normoblast** *A precursor cell for erythrocytes.* | normoblasto |
| **normocyte** *A normal erythrocyte.* | normocito |
| **Norway itch** *A severe pruritus caused by scabies and is associated with immune disorders such as AIDS.* | prurito Norway |
| **nose** *The midface protuberance used for smelling and breathing.* | naso |
| **nosebleed** *Common term for epistaxis.* | epistassi |
| **nosocomial infection** *An infection occurring after admission to a hospital.* | infezione nosocomiale |
| **nosology** *The medical science of disease classification.* | nosologia |
| **nosophobia** *Unwarranted, excessive fear of any disease.* | nosofobia |
| **nostril** *One of two openings in the nose used for air passage.* | narice |
| **noxious** *Harmful or poisonous.* | nocivo |
| **nuclear magnetic resonance (NMR)** *A type a diagnostic body imaging utilizing electromagnetic radiation in a magnetic field.* | risonanza magnetica nucleare |
| **nuclear medicine** *The branch of medicine associated with the use of radioactive material in the evaluation and treatment of disease.* | medicina mucleare |
| **nuclear** *Referring to a nucleus.* | nucleare |
| **nucleic acid** *An organic compound found in living cells; its molecules contain nucleotides linked in long chains.* | acido nucleico |

| English | Italian |
|---|---|
| **nucleoprotein** A substance composed of a nucleic acid and a protein. | nucleoproteina |
| **nulligravida** A woman who has never been pregnant. | nulligravida |
| **nullipara** A woman who has never given birth. | nullipara |
| **numb chin syndrome.** Generally associated with metastatic breast or prostate cancer, it is characterized by unilateral sensory loss of the chin and lower lip. | sindrome intorpidita del mento |
| **numbness** Decreased sensation to tactile stimuli. | intorpidimento |
| **nummulation** Formed as round, flat discs. | nummulazione |
| **nurse** A person trained to care for the sick. | infermiera |
| **nurse practitioner** A person with advanced training capable of acting as a patient's primary care provider. | infermiera professionista |
| **nursing care** The assessment and treatment provided by nurses. | assistenza infermieristica |
| **nutation** Referring to nodding of the head. | nutazione |
| **nutrient** A substance that provides essential nourishment. | nutriente |
| **nutrient foramen** A conduit for passage of nutrient vessels in the marrow of bone. | forame nutrient |
| **nutrition** The process of supplying food needed for growth. | nutrizione |
| **nutritional status** The relative state of one's nutrition. | stato nutrizionale |
| **nystagmus** Rapid involuntary movement of the eyes; it can be horizontal, vertical or rotary. | nistagmo |
| **nyxis** Paracentesis or a puncture. | paracentesi |
| **obesity** Having a body mass index over 30kilograms/meters squared. | obesità |
| **obsession** A pathologic preoccupation. | ossessione |
| **obsolete** No longer in use; antiquated. | obsoleto |
| **obstetric** Referring to The management of pregnancy, labor and the peuperium. | ostetrico |
| **obstetrician** A physician who specializes in the management of pregnancy, labor and the peuperium. | ostetrico |
| **obstructed** To be blocked or halted. | fare ostruzionismo |
| **obturator** A device used to close an artificial or natural opening. | otturatore |
| **obtuse** Rather insensitive or hard to understand. | ottuso |
| **occipital** Referring to the back part of the head. | occipitale |
| **occipitofrontal muscle** Raises the eyebrows. | muscolo occipitofrontale |
| **occlusion** A pathway that is blocked or obstructed. | occlusione |
| **occlusive dressing** A synthetic covering for a wound that has a semipermeable membrane. | fasciatura occlusivo |
| **occult blood** Presence of blood from an unknown source. | sangue occulto |
| **occupational therapy** Rehabilitation focusing on activities of daily living. | terapia occupazionale |
| **ocular paralysis.** Paralysis of intraocular and extraocular muscles. | paralisi oculare |
| **ocular** Referring to the eye. | oculare |
| **oculogyric** Referring to movement of the eye around the anteroposterior axis. | oculogiro |
| **oculomotor nerve** Referring to cranial nerve III which is one of the nerves responsible for extraocular movements. | nervo oculomotore; III nervo cranico |
| **odiferous** Having an unpleasant or distinctive smell. | odorifero |
| **odontalgia** Tooth pain. | odontalgia |
| **odontoid** A prominence on the second cervical vertebra on which the first cervical vertebra pivots. | odontoide |
| **odontology** Synonym of dentistry. | odontologia |
| **odor** A smell that is given off someone or something. | odore |
| **odynophagia** Pain associated with swallowing. | odinofagia |
| **odynophonia** Pain associated with speaking. | odinofobia |

| English | Italian |
|---|---|
| **offspring** *One's children.* | progenie |
| **ointment** *A petroleum jelly based topical medication.* | unguento |
| **old age** *A relative term for the period of advanced years.* | vecchiaia |
| **older** *Being around more than compared with another.* | vecchio |
| **olecranon** *The bony protrusion at the proximal ulna at the elbow.* | olecrano |
| **olfactory** *Referring to the sense of smell.* | olfattivo |
| **oligodactyly** *Presence of fewer than 5 digits on a hand or foot.* | oligodattilia |
| **oligodendroglia** *The ectodermal cells forming part of the central nervous system.* | oligodendrociti |
| **oligohydramnios** *Inadequate amount of amniotic fluid.* | oligoidramnios |
| **oligomenorrhea** *Infrequent menstruation or low volume menstrual flow.* | oligomenorrea |
| **oligoptyalism** *Insufficient secretion of saliva; also oligosialia.* | oligoptialismo |
| **oligospermia** *Abnormally low sperm count.* | oligospermia |
| **oligotrophia or hypotrichosis** *Less than normal amount of head/body hair.* | oligotrofia |
| **oliguria** *Abnormally low urine output.* | oliguria |
| **ombrophobia** *An abnormal fear of rain.* | ombrofobia |
| **omentocele** *A herniated protrusion of omentum.* | omentocele |
| **omentopexy** *Surgically fastening the omentum to an adjacent tissue it was not previously attached to.* | omentopessia |
| **omentum** *A fold of peritoneum fastening the stomach to other organs in the viscera.* | omento |
| **omphalitis** *Inflammation of the umbilicus.* | onfalite |
| **omphalocele** *A large congenital, umbilical hernia with only a thin membranous covering.* | onfalocele |
| **on going** *Continuing.* | continuo |
| **oncologist** *A physician specializing in the treatment of cancer.* | oncologista |
| **oncology** *The study of cancer.* | oncologia |
| **onion bulb neuropathy** *Also known as hypertrophic interstitial neuropathy which is a sensorimotor polyneuropathy.* | neuropatia bulbo di cipolla; neuropatia ipertrofica interstiziale |
| **onset** *The beginning of an event.* | insorgenza |
| **onychia** *Inflammation of the toenail or fingernail matrix.* | onichia |
| **onychia sicca** *Brittle fingernails or toenails.* | onichia fragile |
| **onychocryptosis** *Ingrown toenail.* | onicocriptosi |
| **onychogryphosis** *A deformed nail that is incurved or hooked.* | onicogrifosi |
| **onychomycosis** *Fungal disease of the toenails or fingernails.* | onycomicosi |
| **onychophagia** *Habitually chewing on one's fingernails.* | onicofagia |
| **oocyte** *An ovarian cell that needs to undergo meiotic division to become an ovum.* | oocito |
| **oogenesis** *The initiation and development of an ovum.* | oogenesi |
| **oophorectomy** *Surgical removal of an ovary.* | ooforectomia |
| **oophoritis** *Inflammation of an ovary.* | ooforite |
| **oophoron** *Synonym for ovary.* | ovario |
| **oophorosalpingectomy** *Surgical removal of an ovary and fallopian tube.* | ooforosalpingectomia |
| **ooze, to** *To slowly leak.* | trasudare |
| **open reduction (of fractures)** *The realignment of a fractured bone using a surgical approach.* | riduzione aperta di una frattura |
| **operation** *A surgical procedure.* | operazione |
| **operative note** *A detailed description of a surgical procedure performed on a specific patient.* | sintesi operatorio |

| English | Italian |
|---|---|
| **ophthalmia** *Profound inflammation of the eye or its structures.* | oftalmia |
| **ophthalmic** *Referring to the eye.* | oftalmico |
| **ophthalmologist** *A physician specializing in diseases of the eye.* | oftalmologo |
| **ophthalmology** *The study of diseases of the eye.* | oftalmologia |
| **ophthalmoplegia** *Paralysis of the eye muscles.* | oftalmoplegia |
| **ophthalmoscope** *A device used to visually inspect the interior eye.* | oftalmoscopio |
| **opiate** *Referring to opium.* | oppiato |
| **opioid** *A substance similar to opium that binds to at least one of the opium receptors in the body.* | oppioide |
| **opisthotonos** *A profound spasm in which the head/neck is hyperextended, the feet are touching the bed and with the patient supine the body arched upward.* | opistotono |
| **opium** *An addictive drug derived from opium poppy; synthetic versions are used as analgesics.* | oppio |
| **Oppenheim reflex** *Extension of the toes elicited by scratching of the medial leg; present when the patient has cerebral irritation.* | segno di Oppenheim |
| **opponens** *Synonym for opponent muscle.* | opponente |
| **opsonin** *An antibody used to facilitate phagocytosis of a bacterium.* | opsonina |
| **optic** *Referring to the eye.* | ottico |
| **optic disk** *The area of the retina where the optic nerve enters.* | disco ottico |
| **optician** *A person who makes eyeglasses.* | ottico diplomato |
| **optometrist** *A person who practices optometry.* | optometrista |
| **optometry** *The profession of examination of the eyes for disease (not a medical doctor).* | optometria |
| **oral** *Relating to the mouth.* | orale |
| **oral contraceptive** *Tablet taken by mouth to prevent pregnancy.* | contraccettivo orale |
| **oral hygiene** *Cleansing of the mouth and associated structures.* | igiene orale |
| **orally** *By mouth.* | oralmente |
| **orbicular** *Rounded or circular.* | orbicolare; circolare |
| **orbit** *The bony structure enclosing the eyeball.* | orbita |
| **orbital** *Referring to the orbit.* | orbitario |
| **orchialgia** *Testicular pain.* | orchialgia |
| **orchidectomy** *Synonym of orchiectomy; removal of one or both testes.* | orchiectomia |
| **orchidopexy** *Surgical repair of an undescended testis.* | orchipessia |
| **orchiepididymitis** *Inflammation of the testis and epididymis.* | orchiepididimite |
| **orchitis** *Inflammation of one or both testes.* | orchite |
| **organ** *A part of the body that is self contained and serves a vital function.* | organo |
| **organomegaly** *Enlargement of an organ, typically referring to an intraabdominal organ.* | organomegalia |
| **oriental sore** *A stigmata of cutaneous leishmaniasis caused by a bite from a sand fly.* | piaga orientali |
| **orifice** *Synonym of foramen.* | orifizio |
| **ornithosis** *A viral infection transmitted by birds that is manifested by chills, headache, photophobia, fever, nausea and vomiting.* | ornitosi |
| **oropharynx** *The portion of the pharynx between the soft palate and the superior aspect of the epiglottis.* | orofaringe |
| **orthodontics** *A subspecialty of dentistry concerned with treatment of dental irregularities and malocclusion, including the use of braces.* | ortodonzia |
| **orthopedics** *A surgical specialty concerned with treatment of skeletal problems.* | ortopedia |
| **orthopnea** *The inability to breath comfortably except in the upright position.* | ortopnea |

| English | Italian |
|---|---|
| **orthosis** *Straightening of a malaligned part with the use of braces and other supportive devices.* | ortesi |
| **orthostatic** *Referring to the standing position. Orthostatic hypotension is low blood pressure in the standing position.* | ortostatico |
| **oscillating nystagmus** *Abnormal movement of the eyes in a wave-like pattern.* | nistagmo ondulatorio |
| **osmolality** *The concentration expressed in total number of solute particles per kilogram.* | osmolalità |
| **osmole** *The recognized unit of osmotic pressure.* | osmole |
| **osmosis** *The movement of a solvent from a solution of greater concentration to one of lower concentration through a semi-permeable membrane until the two solutions have equal concentration.* | osmosi |
| **osmotic** *Referring to osmosis.* | osmotico |
| **osseous** *Possessing the quality of bone.* | osseo |
| **ossicle** *A small bone. (auditory ossicle)* | ossicino |
| **ossification** *The formation of bone.* | ossificazione |
| **osteitis** *Inflammation of the bone.* | osteite |
| **ostensibly** *Synonym of apparently and seemingly.* | apparentemente |
| **osteoarthritis** *A long term, progressive degenerative joint disease.* | osteoartrite |
| **osteoarthrosis** *Arthritis without inflammation.* | osteoartrosi |
| **osteoblast** *A cell that matures from a fibroblast and produces bone.* | osteoblasto |
| **osteochondral** *Referring to bone and cartilage.* | osteocondrale |
| **osteochondritis** *Inflammation of bone and cartilage.* | osteocondrite |
| **osteochondroma** *A tumor with bony and cartilaginous characteristics.* | osteocondroma |
| **osteoclasis** *The surgical fracture of a bone usually in order to restore proper alignment.* | osteoclasia |
| **osteoclast** *A large bone cell that is associated with bone reabsorption and removal.* | osteoclasto |
| **osteoclastoma** *A tumor composed of giant cells or osteoclasts.* | osteoclastoma |
| **osteocyte** *An osteoblast within the bone matrix.* | osteocito |
| **osteodystrophy** *Abnormal bone formation.* | osteodistrofia |
| **osteogenesis** *Development of new bones.* | osteogenesi |
| **osteolytic** *Referring to the removal or loss of calcium from the bone.* | osteolitico |
| **osteomalacia** *Softening of the bones because of a deficiency of vitamin D, calcium or phosphorus.* | osteomalacia |
| **osteomyelitis** *Inflammation of the bone or bone marrow because of a microorganism.* | osteomielite |
| **osteopathy** *1. Any disease of the bone. 2. Medical practice concerning treatment of disease by manipulation and massage of bones, joints, and muscles.* | osteopatia |
| **osteopetrosis** *Increased bone density with no change in modeling.* | osteopetrosi |
| **osteophony** *The sound conduction of bone.* | osteofonia |
| **osteophyte** *Abnormal growth of a bone protuberance.* | osteofito |
| **osteoporosis** *Loss of bone substance because the osteoblasts fail to produce bone matrix.* | osteoporosi |
| **osteosarcoma** *A tumor composed of a sarcoma and osseous material.* | osteosarcoma |
| **osteosclerosis** *Abnormal hardening of bone.* | osteosclerosi |
| **osteotomy** *Creation of a surgical opening in bone.* | osteotomia |
| **ostium** *A vessel or body cavity opening.* | ostio |
| **osteogenesis imperfecta** *A connective tissue disorder characterized by bone fragility, skeletal deformity, blue sclerae, ligament laxity, and hearing loss.* | osteogenesi imperfetta |
| **otalgia** *Ear pain.* | otalgia |

| English | Italian |
|---|---|
| **otitis** *Inflammation of the ear. (otitis media or otitis externa)* | otite |
| **otolaryngologist** *Surgical specialist concerned with organs of the ears, nose and throat.* | otolaringologo |
| **otolith** *A calcium based calculus in the inner ear.* | otolito |
| **otology** *Study of conditions and anatomy of the ear.* | otologia |
| **otomycosis** *Fungal infection of the ear.* | otomicosi |
| **otosclerosis** *A hereditary condition exhibited by progressive hearing loss because of bone overgrowth in the inner ear.* | otosclerosi |
| **otoscope** *A device used for inspection of the tympanic membrane.* | otoscopio |
| **ototoxic** *A substance harmful to the ear or its nerve supply.* | ototossico |
| **outbreak (of a disease)** *A sudden start of a disease in a population.* | epidemia |
| **ouch-ouch disease** *Common term for Itai-Itai disease that is derived from "it hurts, it hurts" said by patients suffering from cadmium poisoning.* | morbo itai-itai |
| **outdated** *Something that has passed the expiration date.* | non più in uso |
| **ovarian cysts** *Generally used to describe benign tumors.* | ciste ovarico |
| **ovaritis** *Synonym for oophoritis.* | ovarite |
| **overdose** *An above normal dose of a medication.* | iperdosaggio |
| **overriding suture** *The overlapping of cranial sutures noted on vaginal exam when the head is descended.* | sutura sovrapporsi |
| **overt** *Not hidden.* | chiaro |
| **overweight** *Defined as BMI over 25kilograms per meters squared.* | sovrappeso |
| **oviduct** *The channel which an ovum passes from the ovary.* | ovidotto |
| **ovulation** *The release of an ova from the ovary.* | ovulazione |
| **ovule** *An immature ovum.* | ovulo |
| **owing to** *On account of.* | dovuto a |
| **oxaluria** *Existence of oxalates in the urine.* | ossaluria |
| **oxidation** *The process of a chemical combining with oxygen.* | ossidazione |
| **oximeter** *A medical device used to measure the percent of oxygen that is saturated in the blood (oxygen saturation).* | ossimetro |
| **oxycephaly** *The deformation of the skull so that it appears pointed.* | oxicefalia |
| **oxygen** *A colorless, odorless gas with atomic number 8.* | ossigeno |
| **oxygen consumption** *The body's utilization of oxygen per unit of time.* | utilizzo dell'ossigeno |
| **oxygen tent** *A manner of giving supplement oxygen to a neonate.* | tenda a ossigeno |
| **oxygen therapy** *Utilization of supplemental oxygen.* | terapia ossigeno |
| **oxygenation** *Saturated with oxygen.* | ossigenazione |
| **oxyhemoglobin** *The combination of oxygen and hemoglobin using a covalent bond.* | ossiemoglobina |
| **oxytocic** *Referring to rapid parturition.* | ossitocico |
| **oxytocin** *A natural hormone released by the pituitary or a synthetic hormone that facilitates uterine contraction.* | ossitocina |
| **ozena** *Various nasal conditions, all of which include fetid discharge.* | ozena |
| **ozone** *A toxic chemical that has profound oxidizing properties. It has three atoms in its molecule compared with oxygen which has two.* | ozono |
| **pace** *Consistent and continuous movement.* | passo |
| **pacemaker** *An electrical device used to stimulate the heart used for bradyarrhythmias.* | pacemaker |
| **pachydermia** *An abnormally thick skin.* | pachidermia |
| **pachymeningitis** *Inflammation of the dura mater.* | pachimeningite |
| **pad** *A thick piece of soft clothing.* | cuscinetto |
| **pagophagia** *Compulsive need to eat ice which is usually associated with iron deficiency anemia.* | pagofagia |
| **pain** *Physical suffering or discomfort.* | dolore |

| English | Italian |
|---|---|
| **painful** *Affected with pain.* | doloroso |
| **palatal myoclonus** *An involuntary, persistent, rapid regular tremor of the soft palate and face.* | clono del palato |
| **palate** *The roof of the mouth.* | palato |
| **palatoplegia** *Paralysis of the palate.* | palatoplegia |
| **palliative** *A treatment used to reduce pain when cure is not possible.* | palliativo |
| **pallidectomy** *Surgical resection of all or part of the palate.* | palliectomia |
| **pallor** *Unusually pale appearance.* | pallore |
| **palm** *The anterior aspect of the hand.* | palmo della mano |
| **palmar** *Referring to the palm.* | palmare |
| **palpation** *The assessment of the body with the use of one's hands.* | palpazione |
| **palpebra, palpebrae** *Eyelid, eyelids.* | palpebra |
| **palpitation** *Sensation of a forceful, rapid, irregular heartbeat present after exercise or with anxiety.* | palpitazioni |
| **palsy** *Paralysis that is usually associated with tremors.* | paralisi |
| **paludism** *Synonym of malaria.* | paludismo; malaria |
| **pamper, to** *Indulge with comfort and kindness.* | vezzeggiare |
| **panarthritis** *Inflammation of the joints.* | panartrite |
| **pancarditis** *Inflammation of pericardium, myocardium and endocardium.* | pancardite |
| **pancreas** *A gland that secretes digestive enzymes into the duodenum and insulin and glucagon into the blood.* | pancreas |
| **pancreatectomy** *Surgical excision of part or all of the pancreas.* | pancreatectomia |
| **pancreatitis** *Inflammation of the pancreas.* | pancreatite |
| **pancreozymin** *A duodenal mucosal enzyme that facilitates the secretion of amylase and other enzymes from the pancreas.* | pancreozimina |
| **pandemic** *When a disease is present over an entire region.* | pandemico |
| **panhypopituitarism** *Insufficiency of the anterior pituitary.* | panipopituitarismo |
| **panic attack** *Sudden, profound anxiety.* | attacco di panico |
| **panniculitis** *Inflammation of a section of subcutaneous tissue containing large amounts of fat.* | pannicolite |
| **panophthalmia** *Inflammation of the eye and all its structures.* | panoftalmite |
| **panotitis** *Inflammation of each part of a bone.* | panotite |
| **papilledema** *Swelling of the optic disc.* | papilledema |
| **papillitits** *Swelling of a papilla.* | papillite |
| **papilloma** *A benign, lobulated tumor coming from epithelium.* | papilloma |
| **papule** *A small, well-circumscribed elevation of the skin.* | papula |
| **para-aminobenzoic acid** *A natural product (not FDA approved) reportedly beneficial for Peyronie's disease and scleroderma. It is a component of folic acid.* | acido para-aminobenzoico |
| **para-aminohippuric acid (PAH)** *A chemical used for calculation of renal plasma flow.* | acido para-aminoippurico |
| **paracentesis** *A procedure involving aspiration of fluid from the abdominal cavity.* | paracentesi |
| **paracusia** *Any abnormality in the sense of hearing.* | paracusia |
| **paradoxical pupil** *Constriction of the pupil when exposed to darkness.* | pupilla paradossale |
| **paralysis agitans** *Synonym of Parkinson's disease (obsolete phrase).* | morbo di Parkinson |
| **paralytic** *1. Referring to paralysis. 2. A person who is paralyzed.* | paralitico |
| **paramedian** *Situated toward the middle of the body.* | paramediano |
| **paramedical** *Hospital support staff excluding physicians.* | paramedico |
| **parametritis** *Inflammation of the parametrium.* | parametrite |
| **parametrium** *The connective tissue and smooth muscle between the broad ligament serous layers.* | parametrio |

| English | Italian |
|---|---|
| **paramnesia** *A condition exhibited by a person's belief they have memory for an event that never happened.* | paramnesia |
| **paranasal sinuses** *Any of the sinuses (ethmoidal, frontal, maxillary or sphenoidal) that communicate with the nasal cavity.* | seni paranasali |
| **paranasal** *Situated adjacent to the nose.* | paranasali |
| **paranoia** *A mental condition exhibited by delusions of persecution.* | paranoia |
| **paranoid** *Having the symptom of paranoia.* | paranoideo |
| **paraphimosis** *A condition in which the foreskin is retracted but cannot be replace because of a restricted foreskin.* | parafimose |
| **paraplegia** *Paralysis of the lower extremities.* | paraplegia |
| **parapraxis** *1. Unable to perform purposeful movements. 1. Irrational behavior.* | paraprassia |
| **pararectal** *Adjacent to the rectum.* | pararettale |
| **parasite** *An organism that lives on or within another organism without benefit to the latter.* | parassita |
| **parasympathetic** *Part of the autonomic nervous system that opposes sympathetic stimulation.* | parasimpatico |
| **parathormone** *Synonym for parathyroid hormone.* | paratormone |
| **parathyroid** *Positioned adjacent to the thyroid.* | paratiroideo |
| **paravertebral** *Positioned adjacent to the vertebra.* | paravertebrale |
| **parenchyma** *The functional elements of an organ.* | parenchima |
| **parenteral** *Other than the alimentary canal.* | parenterale |
| **paresis** *Incomplete paralysis.* | paresi |
| **paresthesia** *An abnormal sensation usually described as pins and needles.* | parestesia |
| **parietal** *Referring to the wall of a part or cavity.* | parietale |
| **parietal cell** *Acid secreting cells of the stomach.* | cellula parietale |
| **Parkinson's disease** *A progressive neuromuscular disease exhibited by masklike facial expression, resting tremor, cogwheel rigidity and abnormal gait.* | morbo di Parkinson |
| **paronychia** *Inflammation of the tissue bordering a fingernail* | paronichia |
| **parosmia** *An alteration in the sense of smell.* | parosmia |
| **parotid** *A gland near the ear.* | parotico |
| **parotiditis** *Inflammation of the parotid gland.* | parotite |
| **paroxysmal** *Occurring in sudden attacks.* | parossistico |
| **parrot-beak nail** *A curved fingernail.* | unghia di becco di pappagallo |
| **parthenogenesis** *Reproduction that occurs without an egg being fertilized by sperm.* | partenogenesi |
| **parting** *Separating.* | separarsi |
| **parturition** *The process of giving birth.* | svolgimento del parto |
| **passive** *Not achieved through active effort.* | passivo |
| **past history** *Prior medical problems experienced by a patient.* | storia medica passata |
| **paste** *A thick, soft moist substance usually with medicine mixed in.* | pasta |
| **patch test** *A test used to determine which substances provoke an allergic response in a patient.* | cerottoreazione |
| **patella** *The bone situated in the anterior portion of the knee.* | patella , rotula |
| **patellectomy** *Surgical excision of the patella.* | patellectomia |
| **patellofemoral stress syndrome** *Overuse syndrome causing anterior knee pain from excessive lateral motion.* | sindrome femoro-rotulea da stress |
| **patent ductus arteriosus** *A condition exhibited by failure of the ductus arteriosus (communication between the aorta the the pulmonary artery normally noted in a fetus) to close.* | ductus arteriosus persistens |

| English | Italian |
|---|---|
| **patent foramen ovale** *A congenital anomaly in which there is a defect in the wall between the right and left atria; this can be a benign condition or result in cryptogenic strokes.* | forame ovale pervio |
| **pathogenesis** *The course of a disease.* | patogenesi |
| **pathogenic** *Referring to an organism that can cause disease.* | patogeno |
| **pathognomonic** *Characteristic of something.* | patognomonico |
| **pathological** *Referring to pathology.* | patologico |
| **pathology** *1. The branch of medicine dealing with the study of tissues and the forensic application. 2. Referring to a condition that is abnormal.* | patologia |
| **patient** *The client being treated for a medical or surgical condition.* | ammalato |
| **patient chart** *The file containing the client's medical record.* | scheda paziente |
| **peak flow** meter *A devic used to measure lung function in asthma.* | flussometro con indicatore limite di portata |
| **pectineal ligament** *A continuation of the lacunar ligament along the pectineal line in the pubis.* | legamento pettineo |
| **pectoral** *Referring to the pectoral muscle.* | pettorale |
| **pectoriloquy** *The examiner's voice is clearly audible when the patient speaks as when the examiner listens to an area of consolidation in the lungs of the speaker.* | pettoriloquia |
| **pediatrician** *Physician who is a specialist in pediatrics.* | pediatra |
| **pediatrics** *Medical specialty concerned with the treatment and prevention of childhood disease.* | pediatria |
| **pedicle** *Part of a skin/tissue graft temporarily left connected to the original site.* | innesto peduncolo |
| **pediculate** *Referring to pedicle.* | peduncolato |
| **pediculosis** *Lice infestation.* | pediculosi |
| **peduncle** *1. A stalk-like protrusion. 2. A bundle of nerve fibers connecting two parts of the brain.* | peduncolo |
| **pellagra** *A deficiency in nicotinic acid exhibited by diarrhea and dermatitis.* | pellagra |
| **pelvic inflammatory disease** *Generally a bacterial infection affecting a woman with potential involvement of the uterus, fallopian tubes, ovaries and cervix.* | malattia infiammatoria pelvica |
| **pelvic** *Referring to the pelvis.* | pelvico |
| **pelvimetry** *Measurement of the dimensions of the pelvis to determine whether a patient is capable of natural childbirth.* | pelvimetria |
| **pelvis** *The bony structure at the base of the spine.* | pelvi |
| **pemphigus** *A skin disorder with large bullous lesions.* | penfigo |
| **penetration** *The process of making a way through something.* | penetrazione |
| **penicillin** *A synthetic antibiotic originally produced from blue mold.* | penicillina |
| **penis** *Male genital organ used for the transfer of sperm and elimination of urine.* | pene |
| **pentosuria** *The presence of pentose in the urine (a monosaccharide with five carbon atoms in the molecule).* | pentosuria |
| **pepsin** *A proteolytic gastric enzyme.* | pepsina |
| **peptic** *Referring to pepsin or concerning digestion.* | peptico |
| **peptide** *A compound with low molecular weight and containing two or more amino acids.* | peptide |
| **percussion** *A manual procedure involving tapping a body part to determine the size or density (liquid or air) of a part.* | percussione |
| **perforation** *Presence of a hole.* | perforazione |
| **periaqueductal gray matter** *Refers to the brain gray matter adjacent to the periaqueductal.* | sostonaza grigia che circonda l'acquedotto |

| English | Italian |
|---|---|
| **periarthritis** *Inflammation of the tissues around a joint.* | periartrite |
| **pericardial** *Referring to around the heart.* | pericardico |
| **pericarditis** *Inflammation of the pericardium.* | pericardite |
| **pericardium** *The structure enclosing the heart which contains a fibrous outer layer and serous inner layer.* | pericardio |
| **perichondritis** *Inflammation of the perichondrium.* | pericondrite |
| **perichondrium** *The membrane that encloses a cartilage.* | pericondrio |
| **pericolitis** *Inflammation of the membrane covering the colon.* | pericolite |
| **pericorneal ring** *Also known as Kayser-Fleischer rings exhibited by presence of brown or grey-green rings on the cornea. This is from the deposition of copper and seen in Wilson's disease.* | anello pericorneale |
| **perilymph** *The fluid separating the membranous and osseous labyrinth.* | perilinfa |
| **perinatology** *The study of disease in the period just before and right after birth.* | perinataligo |
| **perineal** *Referring to the perineum.* | perineale |
| **perineal laceration** *Tearing of the tissue adjacent to the vaginal that can occur during childbirth.* | lacerazione perineale |
| **perineorrhaphy** *Surgical repair of the perineum.* | perineorrafia |
| **perinephric** *Around the kidney.* | perirenale |
| **perineum** *The area between the anus and scrotum or anus and vulva.* | perineo |
| **periodic paralysis** *A familial muscle disorder exhibited by recurrent episodes flaccid paralysis without change in level of consciousness.* | paralisi periodico |
| **periodontal disease** *Present around to a tooth.* | malattia periodontale |
| **periosteal** *Referring to the periosteum.* | periosteo |
| **periosteum** *A layer of connective tissue covering the bones.* | periosteo |
| **periostitis** *Inflammation of the periosteum.* | periostite |
| **peripheral** *Referring to an outward part or surface.* | periferico |
| **periproctitis** *Inflammation of the tissue encircling the anus and rectum.* | periproctite |
| **peristalsis** *The contraction of the longitudinal and circular muscle fibers of the alimentary canal so food is propelled.* | peristalsi |
| **peritomy** *Surgically creating an opening of the periosteum.* | peritomia |
| **peritoneal** *Referring to the peritoneum.* | peritoneale |
| **peritoneum** *The serous membrane covering the abdominal organs and lining the abdominal walls.* | peritoneo |
| **peritonitis** *Inflammation of the peritoneum.* | peritonite |
| **peritonsillar abscess** | ascesso peritonsillare |
| **peritonsillar** *Surrounding the tonsils.* | peritonsillare |
| **periurethral** *Surrounding the urethra.* | periuretrale |
| **permanent teeth** *Dentition that comes in after the primary teeth.* | denti permanenti |
| **pernicious** *1. Having a detrimental effect. 2. Pernicious anemia is a reduced red blood cell count due to Vitamin B12 deficiency.* | pernicioso, 2) anemia perniciosa |
| **peroneal** *Referring to the fibula or the outer part of the leg.* | peroneale |
| **peroneal atrophy** *Progressive muscle atrophy in the peroneal region.* | atrofia peroneale |
| **personality** *Qualities that form a person's unique character.* | personalità |
| **perspiration** *The process of sweating.* | traspirazione |
| **pertussis** *Synonym for whooping cough.* | pertosse |
| **pes cavus** *Excessive height of the longitudinal arch of the foot.* | piede cavo |
| **pes planus** *Medical term for flat foot.* | piede piatto |
| **pes valgus** *Abnormal longitudinal arch- it is flat.* | piede valgo |
| **pessary** *A supportive device placed in the rectum or vagina.* | pessario |
| **pet** *An animal kept for companionship.* | animale domestico |

| English | Italian |
|---|---|
| **PET scan Positron emission tomography.** *Production of tomographic images revealing biochemical tissue properties by analyzing positrons emitted when radioactively tagged substances are taken in tissues.* | tomografo a emissione di positroni |
| **petechia** *A small red or purple macule on the skin caused by bleeding.* | petecchia |
| **petrissage** *Massage using a kneading action.* | impastamento |
| **petrous** *Possessing a density of a stone.* | petroso |
| **Peyronie's disease** *Curvature of the penis during an erection to to plaque.* | morbo di Peyronie |
| **phagocyte** *A cell capable of surrounding and digesting microorganisms.* | fagocito |
| **phagocytosis** *The action of a phagocyte.* | fagocitosi |
| **phalanx** *One of the long bones of the fingers or toes.* | falange |
| **phantom limb pain** *Pain sensed in an area where one has had an amputation as though the limb is still present.* | dolore all'arto fantasma |
| **pharmacist** *A professional who prepares and sells medicine through various systems, including governmental organizations like the Veterans Administration.* | farmacista |
| **pharmacokinetics** *The study of the distribution, absorption and excretion of drugs within the body.* | farmacocinetica |
| **pharmacology** *The study of all aspects of medicines.* | farmacologia |
| **pharmacy** *A business that sells prescription medication.* | farmacia |
| **pharyngeal pouch** *A lateral diverticulum of the pharynx.* | diverticolo faringeo |
| **pharyngeal** *Referring to the pharynx.* | faringeo |
| **pharyngectomy** *Surgical excision of part of the pharynx.* | faringectomia |
| **pharyngitis** *Inflammation of the pharynx.* | faringite |
| **pharyngolaryngectomy** *Surgical removal of part of the pharynx and larynx.* | faringolaringectomia |
| **pharyngotympanic tube** *Synonym for eustachian tube.* | tromba faringoimpanico |
| **pharynx** *The membranous cavity from the mouth to esophagus.* | faringe |
| **phenotype** *The visual expression exhibited by a person from the association of the genotype with the environment.* | fenotipo |
| **phenylketonuria** *A hereditary condition in which a person cannot excrete phenylalanine; untreated it causes brain and spinal cord dysfunction.* | fenilchetonuria |
| **phimosis** *Stricture of the prepuce preventing it from being pulled back over the glans penis.* | fimosi |
| **phlebectomy** *Surgical excision of a vein.* | flebectomia |
| **phlebitis** *Inflammation of a vein.* | flebite |
| **phlebothrombosis** *Presence of a clot in a vein, without associated inflammation.* | flebotrombosi |
| **phlegmasia alba dolens** *Phlebitis of the femoral vein that can occur after pregnancy or typhoid fever.* | tromboflebite iliaco-femorale in puerperio |
| **phlegmasia** *Inflammation or fever.* | flegmasia |
| **phlyctenular** *Related to the formation of small vesicles on the cornea or conjunctiva.* | flittenulare |
| **phobia** *An profound fear of something.* | fobia |
| **phonation** *The vocalization of sounds.* | fonazione |
| **phoniatrics** *The treatment of speech abnormalities.* | foniatria |
| **phosphaturia** *Presence of phosphates in the urine.* | fosfaturia |
| **phospholipid** *A substance, such as lecithin, that when hydrolyzed produces fatty acids, glycerin, and a nitrogen compound.* | fosfolipide |
| **phosphonecrosis** *The breakdown of the mandible caused by excessive exposure to phosphorus.* | fosfonecrosi |
| **photophobia** *Abnormal sensitivity to light.* | fotofobia |

| English | Italian |
|---|---|
| **photosensitization** *The process of reacting to sunlight by developing edema and dermatitis.* | fotosensibilizzazione |
| **phrenic** *Referring to the diaphragm.* | frenico |
| **phrenicectomy** *Surgical excision of the phrenic nerve.* | frenicectomia |
| **phrenoplegia** *Paralysis of the diaphragm.* | frenoplegia |
| **physical exam** *Examination of a client to assess their medical status.* | esame fisico |
| **physical therapy** *Treatment of disease by heat, massage and exercise as opposed to medications.* | terapia fisica |
| **physician** *Medical practitioner.* | medico |
| **physiologic dead space** *The combination of anatomic and alveolar dead space.* | spazio morto fisiologico |
| **physiological saline** *0.9% normal saline.* | soluzione fisiologica |
| **physiology** *A subspecialty of biology that studies the normal functioning of the body.* | fisiologia |
| **physiotherapy** *Physical therapy.* | fisioterapia |
| **pia mater** *The first layer of three covering the brain and spinal cord.* | pia madre |
| **pica** *A desire for unusual substances as occurs in pregnancy and some psychological conditions.* | picacismo |
| **pill** *A medicated tablet or capsule.* | pillola |
| **pillow** *An encased fabric covering soft material used for a cushion.* | cuscino |
| **pilonidal cyst** *A small cone-shaped cluster of tissue situated posterior to the third ventricle of the brain.* | ciste pilonidale |
| **pin** *Hardware used in surgery.* | sottile chiodo metallico |
| **pin, intramedullary** *Hardware used for fracture management or during joint replacement.* | chiodo intramidollare |
| **pineal gland** *A small body posterior to the third ventricle of the brain.* | ghiandola pineale |
| **pinguecula** *The yellow tissue on the bulbar conjunctiva adjacent to the sclerocorneal junction.* | pinguecola |
| **pink eye** *Common term for acute contagious conjunctivitis.* | occhio rosa; congiuntivite acuta |
| **pinocytosis** *The absorption of fluid into a cell by the formation of vesicles on the cell membrane.* | pinocitosi |
| **pinworm** *Common term for Enterobius verminicularis; a nematode worm that is a parasite.* | verme sottilissimo |
| **pipet** *A slender tube with a bulb used for transferring liquids.* | pipetta |
| **pitting edema** *Edema of the lower extremities characterized by an indentation being left when the examiner applies pressure with their thumb.* | edema plastico |
| **pituitary gland** *A gland at the base of the hypothalamus.* | ipofisi |
| **pityriasis rosea** *A skin disease characterized by dry pink oval papulosquamous eruptions.* | pitiriasi rosea |
| **placebo controlled study** *When a study is placebo controlled it means part of the group received an inactive treatment while the other group received active therapy.* | studio controllato verso il placebo |
| **placenta** *The vascular tissue that nourishes a fetus through an umbilical cord.* | placenta |
| **placenta praevia** *A condition in which the placenta covers the cervical os.* | placenta previa |
| **placental** *Referring to the placenta.* | placentare |
| **plagiocephaly** *A condition characterized by an asymmetric skull because the cranial sutures do not close normally.* | plagiocefalia |
| **plantar** *Referring to the bottom of the foot.* | plantare |
| **plantar fibromatosis** *Deep fascia nodules on the plantar aspect of the feet.* | fibromatose plantare |

| English | Italian |
|---|---|
| **plantar wart** *A viral epidermal growth on the bottom of the foot.* | verruca plantare |
| **plasma cell** *A cell that produces only one type of antibody.* | cellula plasma |
| **plasmacytosis** *The existence of plasma cells in the blood.* | plasmacitosi |
| **plasmapheresis** *A method of removing blood and reinfusing it after the elimination of antibodies.* | plasmaferesi |
| **plaster cast** *Use of gypsum impregnated gauze to immobilize fractured extremities.* | modello in gesso |
| **plaster** *Dehydrated gypsum that has water added to it in order to immobilize fractured extremities.* | gesso |
| **platelet** *An oval cell without a nucleus used in coagulation; also called a thrombocyte.* | piastrina |
| **pledget** *A small plug of cotton or other synthetic material inserted into a wound.* | piccola compressa |
| **pleomorphism** *The ability of an organism or substance to attain distinct forms.* | pleomorfismo |
| **plethora** *An excess of something.* | pletora |
| **plethysmograph** *A device used to measure the amount of blood flowing through a body part; impedance plethysmography is used to check for deep venous thrombosis.* | pletismografo |
| **pleura** *The serous membrane lining each lung.* | pleura |
| **pleural effusion** *An abnormal collection of fluid between the internal chest wall and the pleura.* | effusione pleurico |
| **pleurisy** *Inflammation of the pleura.* | pleurite |
| **plica** *A fold, as in a fold in the peritoneum.* | plica |
| **Plummer-Vinson syndrome** *Also called sideropenic dysphagia. Exhibited by iron deficiency anemia, dysphagia, esophageal stenosis and atrophic glossitis. The cause is not known.* | sindrome di Plummer-Vinson |
| **pneumatocele** *1. A hernia-like protrusion of lung tissue. 2. A collection of gas in a sac such as the scrotum.* | pneumatocele |
| **pneumaturia** *Presence of air or gas in the urine.* | pneumaturia |
| **pneumococcus** *A bacterium causing pneumonia and meningitis. A common type is Streptococcus pneumoniae.* | pneumococco |
| **pneumoconiosis** *Fibrosis of the lung due to dust inhalation.* | pneumoconiosi |
| **pneumocystis jiroveci pneumonia**. *A pulmonary infection associated with AIDS. Formerly called pneumocystis carinii pneumonia* | polmonite pneumocisti jiroveci |
| **pneumonectomy** *Surgical excision of all or part of a lung.* | pneumonectomia |
| **pneumonia** *Inflammation of the lung due to an infection caused by a virus or bacterium.* | polmonite |
| **pneumoperitoneum** *Abnormal or induced presence of air or gas in the peritoneum.* | pneumoperitoneo |
| **pneumothorax** *Abnormal presence of air between the lung and chest wall.* | pneumotorace |
| **poikilocytosis** *The presence of abnormally shaped erythrocytes.* | piochilocitosi |
| **poikilothermy** *A condition of cold-blooded animals in which their temperature varies based on the ambient temperature.* | poichilotermia |
| **poison** *A substance that causes illness or death.* | veleno |
| **polioencephalitis** *Polio infection of the brain.* | polioencefalite |
| **poliomyelitis** *An infectious viral disease exhibited by constitutional symptoms that can lead to quadriplegia.* | poliomielite |
| **polyarteritis nodosa** *A systemic necrotizing vasculitis that effects medium sized arteries.* | periarterite nodosa |
| **polychondritis** *Inflammation of the cartilage at more than one site.* | policondrite |
| **polycystic** *Possessing more than one cyst.* | policistico |
| **polycythemia** *Excess in the number of erythrocytes in the blood.* | policitemia |

| English | Italian |
|---|---|
| **polycythemia vera** *Condition characterized by increase in erythrocytes, thrombocytes and leukocytes, as well as, splenomegaly.* | policitemia vera |
| **polydactyly** *Congenital anomaly exhibited by more than 5 digits on the hands and/or feet.* | polidattilia |
| **polydipsia** *Profound thirst.* | polidipsia |
| **polymenorrhea** *Increase in the frequency of menstruation.* | polimenorrea |
| **polymyositis** *Inflammation of several muscle groups at once.* | polimiosite |
| **polyneuritis** *Inflammation of more than one nerve.* | polinevrite |
| **polyneuropathy** *A condition involving more than one nerve.* | polineuropatia |
| **polyopia** *A condition in which one object is seen abnormally as two or more.* | poliopia |
| **polyposis** *The formation of multiple polyps.* | poliposi |
| **polypus** *Synonym of polyp (a prominent growth from a mucous membrane).* | poliposo |
| **polysaccharide** *A carbohydrate that upon hydrolysis forms more than ten monosaccharides.* | polisaccaride |
| **polysialia** *Abnormal increase in saliva.* | polisialia |
| **polytrauma** *A condition exhibited by multiple injuries from blunt or penetrating trauma.* | politraumatismo |
| **polyuria** *Abnormal increase in volume of urine excreted.* | poliuria |
| **pompholyx** *A condition exhibited by interdigital vesicles of the hands and feet.* | ponfolice |
| **pons** *The part of the brainstem that connects the medulla oblongata with the thalamus.* | ponte |
| **pontine** *Referring to the pons.* | pontino |
| **popliteal** *Referring to the posterior aspect of the knee.* | popliteo |
| **popliteal fossa** *The hollow in the posterior aspect of the knee joint.* | fossa popliteo |
| **porphyria** *A hereditary condition currently classified based on the specific enzyme deficiency. The most common form is porphyria cutanea tarda that causes blistering lesions.* | porfiria |
| **porphyrin** *A class of pigments that contain a flat ring of four heterocyclic groups.* | porfirina |
| **port-wine mark** *Also called nevus flammeus, it is a vascular anomaly characterized by purplish skin discoloration.* | nevo flammeus |
| **portal** *Referring to an entrance such as porta hepatis.* | portale |
| **portal hypertension** *Hypertension in the portal system of the liver as seen in conditions causing obstruction to the portal vein.* | ipertensione portale |
| **positive** *Indicating the presence of something.* | positivo |
| **post-mortem lividity** *The purplish discoloration occurring 30-120 minutes after death in dependent body parts.* | lividezza postmortem |
| **post-nasal drip** *The descent of sinus drainage.* | gocciolamento postnasal |
| **post-term birth** *An infant born after the normal length of pregnancy.* | post-termine nascita |
| **posterior** *Further back in position; opposite of anterior.* | posteriore |
| **posterior chamber of the eye** *An aqueous filled space between the cornea and the lens.* | camera posteriore |
| **posterior columns** *The dorsal portion of the gray matter of the spinal cord.* | colonna spinale posteriore |
| **postictal** *The period of time after a seizure.* | postaccessuale |
| **postmaturity** *Generally referring to a pregnancy that goes beyond the due date.* | postmaturità |
| **postpartum psychosis** *A episode of abnormal thought or hallucinations following delivery.* | psicosi postpartum |
| **postpone, to** *To delay.* | posporre |

| English | Italian |
|---|---|
| **postural hypotension** *A significant drop in blood pressure when going from the supine or sitting position to standing.* | ipotensione posturale |
| **postural** *Referring to position or posture.* | posturale |
| **potassium** *A chemical of the alkali metal group.* | potassio |
| **potency** *Strength or power.* | potenza |
| **Pott's disease** *Also referred to as tuberculous spondylitis it is caused by a spinal deformity caused by a tuberculosis infection of the spine.* | morbo di Pott; spondilite tubercolare |
| **Potter's syndrome** *A group of findings associated with oligohydramnios. Renal failure is the primary problem but the infant has abnormal limbs, broad nasal bridge, low set ears and receding chin. Death usually ensues due to renal and respiratory failure.* | sindrome di Potter |
| **poultryman's itch** *Pruritus associated with the mite Dermanyssus gallinae.* | prurito avicoltore |
| **powder** *Fine dry particles.* | polvere |
| **pox** *A general term for fluid filled papules that upon rupturing leave pockmarks.* | affezione erutiva o pustolosa |
| **preauricular** *Anterior to the ear.* | preauricolare |
| **precancerous** *Referring to an early stage in cancer development.* | precanceroso |
| **precipitin** *An antibody-antigen reaction producing a precipitate.* | preciptina |
| **precordialgia** *Pain in the precordium.* | precordialgia |
| **precordium** *The area occupying the epigastrium and lower sternum.* | precordio |
| **pre-eclampsia** *Hypertension with proteinuria and/or edema in the setting of pregnancy.* | pre-eclampsia |
| **pregnancy** *The period of being pregnant.* | gravidanza |
| **premature** *Occurring earlier than expected.* | prematuro |
| **premenstrual** *Occurring prior to the onset of menstruation.* | premesturale |
| **premenstrual syndrome** *A cluster of emotional, behavioral, and physical symptoms that occur in the premenstrual phase of the menstrual cycle and resolve with the onset of menstruation.* | sindrome premenstruale |
| **premolar** *The teeth anterior to the molars.* | premolare |
| **prenatal care** *Medical care received while one is pregnant.* | sorveglianza prenatale |
| **prenatal** *Referring to the time prior to birth.* | prenatale |
| **presbyacusia** *An age related, progressive hearing loss.* | presbiacusia |
| **presbyopia** *Farsightedness associated with aging.* | presbiopia |
| **prescription** *The action of prescribing a medication or treatment.* | ricetta |
| **presenting symptom** *The initial subjective complaint that initiated a visit.* | sintomi lamenti dal al momento della visita |
| **pressure dressing** *A dressing used for compression to reduce bleeding.* | medicazione compressiva |
| **pressure ulcer** *Loss in skin integrity due to a portion of the body being in the same position for too long and possibly other factors.* | piaga da decubito; ulcera da compressione |
| **presystolic** *The time just before systole.* | presistole |
| **prevent, to** *To stave off or hinder.* | prevenire |
| **priapism** *A painful and abnormally prolonged erection.* | priapismo |
| **prickly heat** *A rash with small vesicles that is pruritic and associated with a warm moist environment.* | miliaria rubra |
| **primipara** *A woman giving birth for the first time.* | primipara |
| **prior status** *Referring to a person's previous state of health.* | stato precedente |
| **probe** *A device used for exploration.* | specillo |
| **problem** *Difficulty or complaint.* | problema; difficoltà |
| **proctalgia** *A chronic high, dull rectal pain worse with sitting position.* | proctalgia |
| **proctectomy** *Surgical excision of the rectum.* | proctectomia |
| **proctitis** *Inflammation of the rectum.* | proctite |
| **proctocele** *A hernia-type protrusion of the rectum into the vagina.* | proctocele |

| English | Italian |
|---|---|
| **proctoscopy** *Inspection of the rectum with a scope.* | proctoscopia |
| **progeria** *A childhood disorder exhibited by signs of aging including gray hair, wrinkled skin and short height.* | progeria |
| **progesterone** *A steroid hormone that prepares the uterus for pregnancy.* | progestogeno |
| **proglottis** *Any segment of a tapeworm.* | apice della lingua |
| **prognathism** *Protrusion of the mandible which can cause malocclusion.* | prognatismo |
| **prognosis** *The likely course of a disease.* | prognosi |
| **progressive** *Developing gradually.* | progressivo |
| **prolactin** *A pituitary hormone that facilitates milk production.* | prolattina |
| **prolapse of the uterus** *Eversion of the uterus through the vagina.* | prolasso uterino |
| **prolapse of the umbilical cord** *Refers to the umbilical cord protruding from the cervix during active labor.* | epulsione prematura del cordone ombelicale durante il parto |
| **prolapse** *The slipping downward of a body part, such as rectal prolapse.* | prolasso |
| **prolonged rupture of the membranes** *Rupture of the membranes more than 24 hours before delivery.* | rottura delle membrane prolungata |
| **promonocyte** *An intermediate cell stage between monocyte and monoblast.* | promonocito |
| **promontory** *A protruding eminence.* | promontorio |
| **pronation** *Turning posteriorly. When the hand is pronated, it is turned medially until the palm is facing posteriorly (when the body was initially in the anatomic position).* | pronazione |
| **prone** *Lying with the abdomen and face downward.* | prono |
| **prophylaxis** *That which is done to prevent disease.* | profilassi |
| **proprioceptor** *A receptor that responds to sensory input including position sense.* | propriocettore |
| **proptosis oculi** *Synonym of exophthalmos; bulging of the eye.* | esoftalmo |
| **prostacyclin** *A prostaglandin that functions as an anticoagulant and vasodilator.* | prostaciclina |
| **prostaglandin** *A compound first found in semen (thus "prosta" in the name from prostate) with many effects including uterine contraction.* | prostaglandine |
| **prostate** *A gland found in men that surrounds the neck of the urethra and bladder.* | prostata |
| **prostatectomy** *Surgical excision of the prostate.* | prostatectomia |
| **prosthesis** *An artificial body part. (above the knee) [below the knee]* | protesi |
| **prostration** *Profound exhaustion.* | prostrazione |
| **protein** *A class of nitrogenous organic compound.* | proteina |
| **proteinuria** *The presence of protein in the urine.* | proteinuria |
| **proteolysis** *Enzyme action on proteins to form amino acids.* | proteolisi |
| **prothrombin** *A compound converted to thrombin during coagulation of blood.* | protrombina |
| **protoplasm** *The cytoplasm, organelles and nucleus of a living cell.* | protoplasma |
| **Protozoa** *A single celled microscopic organism including amoebas among others.* | Protozoi |
| **provoke, to** *To evoke or elicit.* | provocare |
| **proximal** *Situated closer to the center of the body (opposed to that which is farther away, as in distal).* | prossimale |
| **prurigo** *A chronic, pruritic papular skin eruption.* | prurigine |
| **pruritus** *A general term for conditions exhibited by itching.* | prurito |
| **pseudarthrosis** *Deossification of weight bearing long bones.* | pseudoartrite |

| English | Italian |
|---|---|
| **pseudobulbar palsy** *Sudden outbursts of laughter or tearfulness sometimes seen in amyotrophic lateral sclerosis.* | paralisi pseudobulbare |
| **pseudomnesia** *Sensing the memory of an event that has never happened.* | pseudomnesia |
| **psittacosis** *A chlamydial pneumonia that is transmitted by birds.* | psittacosi |
| **psoriasis** *A chronic papulosquamous dermatosis characterized by silver plaques.* | psoriasi |
| **psychasthenia** *Essentially any non-hysterical neuroses.* | psicastenia |
| **psychiatry** *A branch of medicine specializing in the treatment of mental disorders.* | psichiatria |
| **psychologist** *A professional specializing in psychology.* | psicologo |
| **psychology** *The study of the human mind and emotions.* | psicologia |
| **psychoneurosis** *A mental disorder that could include depression or anxiety but does not include hallucinations.* | psiconevrosi |
| **psychopathology** *Scientific examination of mental disease.* | psicopatologia |
| **psychosis** *A profound mental disorder that can include delusions and hallucinations.* | psicosi |
| **psychosomatic** *Physical ailments arising from mental disease.* | psicosomatico |
| **psychotherapy** *Treatment of mental disease with cognitive-behavioral approaches.* | psicoterapia |
| **pterygium** *A membrane in the interpalpebral fissure present from the conjunctiva to the cornea.* | pterigio |
| **ptosis** *Drooping of the upper eyelid usually due to paralysis of the third cranial nerve.* | ptosi (della palpebra superiore) |
| **ptyalin** *An enzyme found in saliva.* | ptialina |
| **puberty** *The time when adolescents become capable of sexual reproduction.* | pubertà |
| **pubic hair** *Hair present in the perineal area.* | peli del pube |
| **pubis** *The anterior inferior part of the hip bone on each side that articulates at the pubic symphysis.* | osso del pube |
| **pudendal** *Referring to the female genitalia* | pudendo |
| **pudendum** *The mons, pubis, labia majora, labia minora and the vagina.* | pudendo |
| **puerpera** *A woman who just gave birth.* | puerpera |
| **puerperium** *The six week period after childbirth.* | peurperio |
| **puffiness** *Having a soft, swollen area.* | tumidità |
| **pull, to** *To exert force on something.* | tirare |
| **pulmonary edema** *Characterized by abnormal fluid buildup in the lungs.* | edema polmonare |
| **pulmonary embolism** *A sudden blockage of a lung artery frequently emanating from a blood clot in one's leg.* | embolia polmonare |
| **pulmonary** *Referring to the lungs.* | polmonare |
| **pulmonary stenosis** *A stricture between the pulmonary artery and the right ventricle.* | stenosi polmonare |
| **pulp** *The tissue filling the root canals of a tooth.* | polpa |
| **pulpitis** *Dental pulp inflammation.* | pulpite |
| **pulsatile** *Relating to pulsation.* | pulsatile |
| **pulsation** *The action of expanding and contracting.* | pulsazione |
| **pulse** *The rhythmic throbbing of arteries felt at major vessels.* | polso |
| **pulsus alternans** *A regular alternation of weak and strong beats of the pulse.* | polso alternanza |
| **pupil** *The opening at the center of the iris.* | pupilla |
| **purpura** *The presence of patches of ecchymosis or petechiae.* | porpora |
| **purulent** *Referring to pus.* | purulento |

| English | Italian |
|---|---|
| **pus** *Thick yellow or green opaque liquid as seen with infection.* | pus |
| **putrefaction** *The rotting or decaying of organic matter.* | putrefazione |
| **pyelitis** *Renal pelvis inflammation.* | pielite |
| **pyelography** *Use of a contrast agent to radiologically study the kidney, ureters and bladder.* | pielografia |
| **pyelolithotomy** *Surgical excision of a calculus from the renal pelvis.* | pielolitotomia |
| **pyelonephritis** *Inflammation of the renal parenchyma usually due to bacterial infection.* | pielonefrite |
| **pyelonephrosis** *Term, rarely used anymore, used to describe disease of the renal pelvis.* | pielonefrosi |
| **pyemia** *Sepsis characterized by the presence of secondary abscesses.* | piemia |
| **pyknic** *Possessing a short, stocky physique.* | picnico |
| **pyknosis** *The degeneration of a cell with the nucleus shrinking.* | picnosi |
| **pyloric** *Referring to the pylorus.* | pilorico |
| **pyloroplasty** *Surgical enlargement of a pylorus that previously was stenotic.* | piloroplastica |
| **pylorus** *The opening at the distal stomach that opens into the duodenum.* | piloro |
| **pyoderma** *A purulent skin infection.* | piodermite |
| **pyogenic liver abscess** *A pus filled fluid collection in the liver.* | ascesso del fegato piogeno |
| **pyogenic** *Referring to the formation of pus.* | piogeno |
| **pyonephrosis** *Injury to the renal parenchyma due to pus.* | pionefrosi |
| **pyorrhea** *Emission of pus.* | piorrea |
| **pyosalpinx** *Purulent material in the oviduct.* | piosalpinge |
| **pyramidal** *A term that is used to describe various spinal tracts that originate in the cerebral cortex.* | piramidale |
| **pyrexia** *Fever.* | piressia |
| **pyridoxine** *Synonym for vitamin B6.* | piridossina; vitamina B6 |
| **pyrogen** *A fever producing substance released by bacteria.* | pirogeno |
| **pyrosis** *Synonym for heartburn.* | pirosi |
| **pyuria** *Presence of purulent material in the urine.* | piuria |
| **Q fever** *A disease caused by rickettsiae from the ingestion of unpasteurized milk.* | febbre Q |
| **quadranic hemianopia** *Loss of a quarter of the visual field in one or both eyes. If bilateral, it may be further described as homonymous, heteronymous, binasal, bitemporal, or crossed.* | emianopia a quadrante |
| **quadriceps jerk (reflex)** *Also referred to as the patellar reflex.* | riflesso rotulo; riflesso del tendine del quadricipite |
| **quadriceps** *The anterior thigh muscle composed of four muscles.* | quadricipite |
| **quadrigeminal bodies** *The cranial and caudal colliculi.* | corpi quadrigemino |
| **quadriplegia** *Paralysis of all four extremities.* | quadriplegia |
| **qualify** *To become eligible by fulfilling a necessary standard.* | qualificato |
| **quarantine** *A place of isolation for infectious persons until it can be certain it is safe to let them mingle.* | quarantena |
| **querulousness** *Whining or complaining.* | l'essere lamentoso |
| **quickening** *Signs of life noted by a mother as the fetus moves.* | primi movimento del feto nell'utero precepiti dalla madre |
| **quiescent** *A time of inactivity.* | quiescenza |
| **quiet** *Making little or no noise.* | quieto |
| **quinsy** *Peritonsillar inflammation or abscess.* | ascesso peritonsillare |

| English | Italian |
|---|---|
| **quintan fever** *Also known as trench fever as it was first noted during trench warfare in WW I. It is a rickettsial fever caused by Bartonella quintana and transmitted by a louse; signs and symptoms are myalgia, headache, malaise, fever and chills.* | morbo di Werner-His |
| **rabies** *An infectious viral disease transmitted through the bite of a mammal. Symptoms include hydrophobia, pharyngeal spasms and hyperactivity.* | rabbia |
| **racemose** *A gland having the form of a cluster.* | racemoso |
| **radial** *Referring to the radius.* | radiale |
| **radiation** *1. The emission of energy in the form of electromagnetic waves. 2. Divergence from a common point.* | radiazione |
| **radiculitis** *Inflammation of a spinal nerve root.* | radiocolite |
| **radioactive** *Referring to the emission of ionizing particles or radiation.* | radioattivo |
| **radioactive isotope** *An isotope with an unstable nucleus that is used in diagnostic imaging.* | isotopo radioattivo |
| **radiobiology** *The study of the effects of radiation on organisms.* | radiobiologia |
| **radioepithelitis** *The injury to epithelial cells due to effects of radiation.* | radiodermatite |
| **radiography** *The department where images are produced on sensitive film by x-rays.* | radiografia |
| **radiologist** *A physician specializing in radiology.* | radiologo |
| **radiology** *The branch of medicine concerned with roentgenography and other high-energy radiation.* | radiologia |
| **radionuclide** *A radioactive nuclide.* | radionuclide |
| **radiosensitivity** *The susceptibility of the skin to radiation.* | radiosensibilità |
| **radiotherapy** *Treatment of cancer with radiation.* | radioterapia |
| **rage** *Uncontrollable anger.* | rabbia |
| **raise, to** *To lift or bring up.* | sollevare |
| **rale** *An abnormal lung sound noted during auscultation.* | rantolo |
| **ramus** *A branch; a term used to describe a smaller vessel branching off from a larger one.* | ramo |
| **ranula** *A retention cyst formed because of obstruction of a salivary gland in the floor of the mouth.* | ranula |
| **rape** *Forced sexual relations.* | violenza carnale |
| **Rapid Eye Movement** *The movement of a person's eyes during this period of sleep.* | movimenti oculari rapidi |
| **rash** *Exanthema or urticaria.* | avventato; esantema |
| **rat bite fever** *As the name implies, it is a condition exhibited by fever, nausea and skin erythema after one is bitten by a rat.* | febbre da morso di ratto |
| **reaction** *A response to an action.* | reazione |
| **reactive** *A response to a stimulus.* | reattivo |
| **rebound** *A term used to describe a type of tenderness found with peritonitis.* | dolorabilità di rimbalzo |
| **receptor** *A cell or organ that accepts stimuli and transmits data to a sensory nerve.* | rrecettore |
| **recessive** *This refers to genetic controlled traits that are only inherited when code from both parents is the same.* | recessivo |
| **recollection** *Memory.* | memoria |
| **recovery room** *The immediate post-operative room where patients are stabilized prior to going to a general ward.* | sala postoperatoria |
| **rectal digital examination** *Use of a gloved finger to assess the rectal vault.* | esame rettale digitale |
| **rectal** *Referring to the rectum.* | rettale |
| **rectocele** *A herniation of the wall between the rectum and vagina.* | rettocele |

| English | Italian |
|---|---|
| **rectoscopy** *Visualization of the rectum with a scope.* | rettoscopia |
| **rectosigmoidectomy** *Surgical resection of the rectum and sigmoid colon.* | rettosigmoidectomia |
| **rectovesical septum** *The wall between the rectum and the urinary bladder.* | setto rettovescicale |
| **rectus abdominis muscle** *The pair of long, flat muscles that connect the sternum with the pubis.* | muscolo retto dell'addome |
| **recumbent** *Lying down.* | supino |
| **red nucleus** *A collection of gray matter near the subthalamus that receives data from the superior cerebellar peduncle.* | nucleo rosso |
| **reduction** *Return of a dislocated joint or fractured bone to its proper position.* | riduzione |
| **referred pain** *Pain felt in an area distinct from the original source.* | dolore eterotopico |
| **regardless of** *Without consideration of.* | nonostante tutto di |
| **regurgitation** *1. Backflow of blood in the heart. 2. Movement of gastric contents into the mouth.* | rigurgito |
| **relapse** *The return to a prior state of ill health.* | recidiva |
| **relapsing fever** *A recurrent bacterial infection, with fever, caused by Spirochetes.* | febbre recidivante |
| **related to** *Causally connected.* | associato; imparentato |
| **relation** *1. A person who has a blood or marriage connection.* | relazione |
| **relaxant** *Term generally used to refer to a muscle relaxant.* | rilassante |
| **relaxin** *A hormone secreted by the placenta which dilates the cervix.* | rilassina |
| **releasing hormone** *Hormones that come from one gland such as the thalamus that cause release of hormones from another gland such as the pituitary.* | ormoni liberatori |
| **reliable** *Trustworthy.* | attendibile |
| **relief** *Alleviation from pain or discomfort.* | attenuazione |
| **relieve, to (pain)** *To make less severe.* | alleviare |
| **REM (rapid eye movement) sleep** *This period of sleep is associated with irregular respirations and heart rate, involuntary movements and dreaming.* | movimenti oculari rapidi |
| **remission** *A decrease in severity or a temporary resolution.* | remissione |
| **removal** *The act of removing something.* | asportazione |
| **renal** *Referring to the kidney.* | renale |
| **renal colic** *Pain caused by passage of a calculus through the ureter.* | colica renale |
| **renal failure** *Diminution of kidney function.* | insufficienza renale |
| **renal pelvis** *The kidney collecting system.* | pelvi renale |
| **renin** *A renal enzyme that facilitates the production of angiotensin.* | renina |
| **resection** *The removal of tissue.* | resezione |
| **residual urine** *The amount of urine remaining in the bladder after a person voids.* | urina residuo |
| **residual volume (RV)** *The amount of air left in the lung after a maximal exhalation.* | volume residuo |
| **resin** *An organic substance that is insoluble in water. There are many types. Cholestyramine resin is used for hypercholesterolemia.* | resina |
| **resorbable suture (chromic)** *Suture that is not intended to be permanent as it is dissolved by normal body processes.* | sutura riassorbibile (cromico) |
| **respirator** *A device used to artificially ventilate a patient.* | ventilatore |
| **respiratory** *Referring to respiration or the organs of respiration.* | respiratorio |
| **respiratory distress syndrome** *A disease in infants that is caused by a surfactant deficiency.* | sindrome di ambascia respiratoria |
| **respiratory rate** *The number of breaths per minute.* | frequenza respiratoria |
| **rest** *Relaxation or respite.* | reposo |

| English | Italian |
|---|---|
| **restless legs** *Associated with a syndrome exhibited by continuous movement of the legs from uncertain etiology.* | gambe senza riposa |
| **retching** *Spasm of the stomach without presence of gastric material.* | conato di vomito |
| **reticular** *Referring to a matrix of membranous tubules inside the cytoplasm of a eukaryotic cells.* | reticolare |
| **reticulo-endothelial** *Referring to the system of phagocytes involved in the immune system.* | reticolo-endoteliale |
| **reticulocyte** *A red blood cell without a nucleus.* | reticulocito |
| **reticulocytosis** *An abnormal increase in circulating reticulocytes.* | reticolocitosi |
| **retina** *The innermost of three layers of the eyeball; it surrounds the vitreous body and is continuous with the optic nerve.* | retina |
| **retinal detachment** *A tear or hole in the retina caused by vitreous traction.* | distacco retinico |
| **retinitis** *Inflammation of the retina.* | retinite |
| **retinoblastoma** *A tumor consisting of retinal germ cells.* | retinoblastoma |
| **retinopathy** *Any one of a number of retinal inflammatory conditions.* | retinopatia |
| **retraction** *Being drawn back.* | retrazione |
| **retractor** *A device for pulling back tissue during surgery.* | divaricatore chirurgico |
| **retrobulbar optic neuritis** *An inflammatory, demyelinating condition in the retrobulbar region.* | neurite retrobulbare oculare |
| **retroflexed uterus** *Bending back of the uterus so that the top portion pushes against the rectum.* | utero retroflesso |
| **retrograde** *Referring to backward movement.* | retrogrado |
| **retroperitoneal** *Situated or referring to the area posterior to the peritoneum.* | retroperitoneale |
| **retropharyngeal abscess** *A collection of purulent material posterior to the pharynx.* | ascesso retrofaringeo |
| **retropharyngeal** *Referring to the area posterior to the pharynx.* | retrofaringeo |
| **Rett syndrome.** *A rare inherited disorder causing developmental delays and is seen mostly in girls.* | sindrome di Rett |
| **rhabdomyolysis** *A acute destruction of muscle documented by myoglobinemia and myoglobinuria.* | rabdomiolisi |
| **rhagade** *Fissures in the skin, particularly adjacent to body orifices.* | ragadi |
| **rheumatic** *Referring to rheumatism.* | reumatico |
| **rheumatic fever** *A febrile streptococcal disease causing pain and joint swelling.* | febbre reumatico |
| **rheumatic heart disease** *A manifestation of rheumatic fever, frequently causing valvular dysfunction.* | cardite reumatica |
| **rheumatism** *Any condition exhibited by inflammation and pain in the joints and muscles.* | reumatismo |
| **rheumatoid arthritis** *A symmetric peripheral polyarthritis.* | artrite reumatoide |
| **rhinitis** *A viral infection or allergic reaction exhibited by nasal mucosal inflammation.* | rinite |
| **rhinoplasty** *Plastic surgery performed on the nose.* | rinoplastica |
| **rhinorrhea** *Abundant nasal mucosal drainage.* | rinorrea |
| **rhinoscopy** *Examination of the nasal passages.* | rinoscopia |
| **rhizotomy** *Interruption of the spinal nerve roots within the spinal canal.* | rizotomia |
| **rhodopsin** *A reddish purple light sensitive pigment in the human retina.* | rodopsina |
| **rhomboid** *A back muscle that elevates, retracts and adducts the scapula.* | romboide |
| **rhonchus** *A coarse, dry sound heard on auscultation of the lungs.* | ronco |
| **rhythm** *The pattern or cadence.* | ritmo |
| **rib** *A series of curved paired boney articulations protecting the thorax.* | costole |

| English | Italian |
|---|---|
| **riboflavin** *Also called vitamin B2, this essential vitamin is present in food such as eggs and is synthesized in the small bowel.* | riboflavina; vitamina B2 |
| **ribonucleic acid** *An acid present in all living cells, it is a messenger for DNA.* | acido ribonucleico |
| **ribosomal RNA** *Four chains designated by their appropriate coefficients.* | acido ribonucleico ribosomiale |
| **rice-field fever** *An infection cause by a species of Leptospira, affecting rice workers in Italy and Sumatra.* | febbre di risaia |
| **rickets** *A condition exhibited by softening and bowing of the long bones; caused by Vitamin D deficiency.* | rachitismo |
| **Rickettsia** *A genus of bacteria transmitted by ticks or fleas; Rocky Mountain Spotted fever is one of many diseases caused by this bacterium.* | Rickettsia |
| **Rift valley fever** *A human febrile illness that is an endemic disease in sheep, transmitted by mosquitos and direct contact and caused by a virus of the family Bunyaviridae.* | febbre fossato tettonico |
| **right** *Opposite of left.* | destra |
| **right-handed** *Having a preference to use the right hand.* | destrimane |
| **rigor mortis** *The normal stiffening of the muscles and joints that occurs a few hours after death.* | rigidità cadaverica |
| **ring** *A small circular band.* | anello |
| **ringing in the ears** *Common term for tinnitus.* | ronzio nelle orecchie; tinnito |
| **ringworm** *A fungal skin infection exhibited by pruritic well circumscribed patches on the scalp or feet.* | epidermomicosi eritmatosquamosa |
| **risus sardonicus** *A spasm of the facial muscles causing what appears to be a smile on one's face.* | riso sardonico |
| **Ritgen's maneuver** *A procedure that controls the rate of delivery of the infant's head during childbirth.* | manovra di Ritgen |
| **rodent** *A gnawing mammal that includes rats and mice.* | animale roditore |
| **Roentgen** *One unit of ionizing radiation named after the German physicist Wilhelm Conrad Röntgen.* | roentgen |
| **room** *A division in a building surrounded by walls.* | sala; camera |
| **root** *An embedded part of an organ or structure.* | radice |
| **rosacea** *Erythema of the cheeks and nose caused by chronic vascular and follicular dilation.* | acne rosacea |
| **Rossolimo reflex** *Flexion of the toes when the tips of the toes are flicked. This abnormal response is present in pyramidal tract lesions.* | riflesso Rossolimo |
| **rotation** *Movement around an axis.* | rotazione |
| **rotator cuff** *The structure around the capsule of the shoulder joint formed by the infraspinatus, supraspinatus, teres minor and subscapularis muscles.* | cuffia dei muscoli rotatori |
| **round ligament of the uterus** *The supporting structure of the uterus.* | ligamentum teres uteri |
| **rub** *A sound heard at times with pericarditis called more specifically a pericardial friction sound.* | sfregamento |
| **rubefacient** *A substance that reddens the skin.* | rubefacente |
| **rubella** *Also called German measles, it is characterized by a rash, fever, headache.* | rosolia |
| **Rubeola** *Another term for measles, an acute exanthematous disease.* | morbillo |
| **rude** *Ill-mannered.* | maleducato |
| **rugine** *A surgical instrument that resembles a rasp.* | raschiaperiostio |
| **rule out, to** *To perform a test or exam to exclude an illness or disease.* | squalificare |
| **running suture** *A method of sewing a wound in which there is a knot at each end and continuous otherwise.* | sutura continua |

| English | Italian |
|---|---|
| **rupia** *A sign of tertiary syphilis in which there are bullae or vesicles formed on the skin that erupt and form crusts.* | rupia |
| **rupture** *An instance of bursting suddenly.* | rottura |
| **sacral** *Referring to the sacrum.* | sacrale |
| **sacral canal** *The portion of the vertebral canal that progresses into the sacrum.* | canale sacrale |
| **sacralization** *The fusion of the fifth lumbar vertebra to the sacrum.* | sacralizzazione |
| **sacrum** *The bone formed by five fused vertebrae that is situated between the two hip bones.* | osso sacro |
| **saddle joint** *A joint that exhibits two saddle type surfaces at a 90 degree angle to each other, such as the carpometacarpal joint.* | articolazione sella |
| **sadness** *The state of being sad.* | tristezza |
| **sagittal suture** *The line where the two parietal bones meet.* | sutura sagittale del cranico |
| **Saint Ignatius' itch** *Pruritus noted with a cluster of symptoms related to niacin deficiency. Generally referred to as pellagra.* | prurito di Saint Ignatius; pellagra |
| **Saint Vitus' dance** *Historic name for chorea minor characterized by hypotonia and emotional lability months after a streptococcal infection.* | corea minor |
| **saline** *A solution of sodium chloride.* | salino |
| **saliva** *The watery liquid secreted by the salivary glands.* | saliva |
| **salivary gland** *The parotid, submandibular and sublingual glands that secrete saliva.* | ghiandole salivari |
| **salivation** *The process of secreting saliva.* | salivazione |
| **salpingectomy** *Surgical resection of the fallopian tubes.* | salpingectomia |
| **salpingitis** *Inflammation of the fallopian tubes.* | salpingite |
| **salpingography** *Roentgenography of the fallopian tubes after administration of contrast media.* | salpingografia |

| English | Italian |
|---|---|
| **salpingostomy** *A surgical procedure involving cutting the fallopian tube.* | salpingostomia |
| **salt** *Typically referring to sodium chloride.* | salato |
| **saluretic** *An agent that promotes excretion of sodium and chloride in the urine.* | saluretico |
| **sampling** *The taking of samples.* | campionatura |
| **sandfly fever** *A febrile illness transmitted by a sandfly, from the genus Phlebotomus, and found in the Mediterranean.* | febbre di mosca della sabbia |
| **sanitary napkin** *Cloth or synthetic material used to absorb menstrual blood.* | assorbente |
| **saphena** *Referring to either of the two superficial saphenous veins.* | safena |
| **saponify,to** *The creation of soap from oil using an alkali.* | saponificare |
| **saprophyte** *Any organism living on dead organic material.* | saprofita |
| **sarcoid** *Referring to sarcoidosis.* | sarcoide |
| **sarcoidosis** *A chronic disease characterized by lymphadenopathy and widespread granulomas.* | sarcoidosi |
| **sarcolemme** *The sheath that covers skeletal muscle fibers.* | sarcolemma |
| **sarcoma** *A non-epithelial malignant tumor.* | sarcoma |
| **sartorius muscle** *The thigh muscle that runs from the pelvis to the proximal, medial aspect of the tibia.* | muscolo sartorio |
| **saturation** *An amount, expressed in a percentage, that expresses the degree something is absorbed versus the maximal absorption possible.* | saturazione |
| **saw** *A hand or power-driven tool used for cutting.* | sega |
| **scabies** *A skin condition exhibited by intense pruritus and a macular rash commonly in the perineal and interdigital spaces.* | scabbia |
| **scald** *A burn injury from extremely hot water.* | scottatura |
| **scale** *A device to check a person's weight.* | scala |
| **scalp** *The skin covering the head except for the face.* | cuoio capelluto |
| **scalp avulsion** *An injury causing the skin along with some subcutaneous tissue to be pulled from the skull.* | ripugnanza del cuoio capelluto |
| **scalpel** *A knife used during surgery for incision of skin and tissue.* | scalpello |
| **scaphocephaly** *A condition exhibited by a long narrow skull because of early closure of the sagittal sutures.* | scafocefalia |
| **scaphoid bone** *The most lateral of the carpal bones; it articulates with the radius.* | osso scafoide |
| **scapula** *Medical term for the shoulder blade.* | scapola |
| **scarification** *Multiple small scratches of the skin, as is sometimes used for vaccine administration.* | scarificazione |
| **scarlet fever** *A condition caused by streptococci that is exhibited by fever and a bright red (scarlet) rash.* | scarlattina |
| **scatter** *The degree to which repeated measurements differ.* | dispersione |
| **scheme** *A program or plan.* | schema |
| **schistocyte** *Part of a red blood cell seen in hemolytic anemia.* | schistocito |
| **schistosomiasis** *A condition, sometimes known as bilharzia, which involves infestation with flukes of the genus Schistosoma.* | schistosomiasi |
| **schizophrenia** *A chronic mental condition exhibited by delusions, hallucinations, and faulty perception.* | schizofrenia |
| **Schmorl's nodule** *Protrusion of the nucleus pulposus through the vertebral body endplate into the adjacent vertebra.* | nodulo di Schmorl |

| English | Italian |
|---|---|
| **sciatica** *Pain radiating from the buttock down the back of the leg; it is caused by a compressed spinal nerve root.* | sciatica |
| **scimitar sign** *An abnormal radiologic finding associated with anomalous pulmonary venous drainage.* | segno di scimitar |
| **scirrhus** *A cancer that is hard to palpation.* | scirro |
| **scissors** *A cutting instrument with two blades, joined at the middle.* | forbici |
| **sclera** *The white outer covering of the eyeball.* | sclera |
| **scleritis** *Inflammation of the eyeball.* | sclerite |
| **sclerodactylia** *Scleroderma of the digits.* | sclerodattilia |
| **scleroderma** *A systemic disease of the connective tissues.* | sclerodermia |
| **sclerotomy** *Surgical incision of the sclera.* | sclerotomia |
| **scolex** *The front end of a tapeworm.* | scolice |
| **scoliosis** *A lateral curvature of the spine.* | scoliosi |
| **scopophilia** *Sexual pleasure attained by viewing sexual organs.* | scopofilia |
| **scotoma** *A blind spot within an otherwise normal visual field.* | scotoma |
| **scrape** *An injury caused by having a body part rubbed against a rough surface.* | raschiatura |
| **scratch** *A long, narrow superficial wound.* | scalfittura |
| **screening** *An evaluation as part of a methodical study.* | indagine di massa |
| **scrofula** *Cervical tuberculous lymphadenitis.* | scrofola |
| **scrotal** *Referring to the scrotum.* | scrotale |
| **scrotal hydrocele** *A benign collection of fluid in the scrotum.* | idrocele scrotale |
| **scrotum** *The sac which contains the testes.* | scroto |
| **scurvy** *A disease of vitamin C deficiency exhibited by bleeding gums.* | scorbuto |
| **scutulum** *A crust of tinea capitis.* | scutulo |
| **scybalum** *A hard, dry formation of stool in the bowel.* | scibale |
| **seal** *A device or substance used to bind two things together.* | sigillo |
| **sebaceous** *Referring to a sebaceous gland or what it secretes.* | sebaceo |
| **sebaceous gland** *A gland in the skin that secretes sebum.* | ghiandola sebaceo |
| **seborrhea** *Abnormal amount of sebum production.* | seborrea |
| **secretin** *A hormone that increases secretion from the pancreas and liver.* | secretina |
| **secretion** *The discharge of substances from cells or glands.* | secrezione |
| **sedative** *A medication used to facilitate sleep or calm a person.* | sedativo |
| **seizure** *An episode of tonic/clonic movement noted in epilepsy.* | attaco; crisi epilettica |
| **semen analysis** *Evaluation of semen used as part of a fertility workup.* | analisi del seme |
| **semicircular canal** *The anterior, posterior and lateral canals in the inner ear that assist in balance control.* | canale semicircolare |
| **seminiferous tubules** *Used for transport of semen.* | tubuli seminifero |
| **seminoma** *A malignant tumor of the testis.* | seminoma |
| **senescence** *The normal process of deterioration with age.* | senescenza |
| **senile** *Generally referring to mental deterioration associated with aging.* | senile |
| **senility** *The process of being senile.* | senilità |
| **sensation** *A perception when one is touched.* | sensazione |
| **sensibility** *Ability to feel or perceive.* | sensibilità |
| **sensible** *When referring to a choice, chosen with wisdom.* | sensibile |
| **sensitization** *The change in an organ by a hormone so it will respond to another stimulus.* | sensibilizzazione |
| **sensitized** *Being abnormally sensitive to a substance.* | sensibilizzato |
| **sensory nerve** *A nerve that receives input from various receptors.* | nervo sensitivo |

| English | Italian |
|---|---|
| **sepsis** *A condition exhibited by overwhelming inflammation due to infection.* | sepsi |
| **septic** *Referring to a state of sepsis.* | settico |
| **septicemia** *A systemic disease in which microorganisms or their toxins are in the blood stream.* | setticemia |
| **septum** *A wall separating two chambers, the nasal septum for example.* | setto |
| **sequela** *A medical problem related to an initial injury or disease.(late sequelae)* | sequela |
| **sequestrum** *Necrotic bone present in an injured or diseased bone.* | sequestro osseo |
| **serial** *In a series.* | seriato |
| **serotonin** *A neurotransmitter that constricts blood vessels.* | serotonina |
| **serous** *Referring to serum or similar to serum.* | sieroso |
| **serpiginous** *A skin lesion having wavy margin.* | serpiginoso |
| **serum** *The fluid that isolates out when blood coagulates.* | siero |
| **sessile** *Having a broad base with no stalk.* | sessile |
| **severe** *Intense or very great.* | severo |
| **sex** *Gender.* | sesso |
| **sexual intercourse** *The act of copulation.* | rapporto sessuale |
| **sexually transmitted disease (STD)** *A condition one obtains from another during sexual relations.* | malattia trasmessa sessualmente |
| **Sézary syndrome** *Symptoms are exfoliative dermatitis with intense itching caused by cutaneous infiltration by mononuclear cells,* | sindrome di Sézary |
| **shake, to** *To tremble uncontrollably.* | scuotere |
| **sharp (pain)** *When describing pain, a piercing sensation.* | tagliente |
| **sheath** *A covering.* | guaina |
| **sheet (bed)** *A rectangular fabric covering a bed.* | traversa |
| **shellfish** *An aquatic shelled crustacean or mollusk.* | mollusco |
| **shield** *A protective device, as in eye shield.* | schermo |
| **shin** *Refers to the anterior tibial region.* | cresta tibiale |
| **shingles** *A reactivation of herpes zoster.* | zona |
| **shiver** *A trembling.* | brivido non intenso |
| **shock** *A condition characterized by systemic hypoperfusion.* | shock cardiaco |
| **shoe** *Article of clothing worn on each foot.* | scarpa |
| **shortening** *Notable for having a shorter length.* | accorciamento |
| **shoulder** *The joint were the scapula joins the clavicle and humerus. (right shoulder, left shoulder)* | spalla |
| **shunt** *An alternate path for blood or fluid.* | cortocircuito |
| **sialadenitis** *Inflammation of a salivary gland.* | sialadenitis |
| **sialogogue** *A substance that increase salivary flow.* | agente sialagogo |
| **sialolith** *A calculus in a salivary duct.* | sialolito |
| **sibling** *A brother or sister.* | fratello (m); sorella (f) |
| **sickle-cell anemia** *A hereditary type of anemia characterized by crescent shaped red blood cells.* | anemia drepanocitica |
| **sickness** *Illness or a state of disease.* | infermità; malattia |
| **side** *A position medial or lateral to center.* | laterale |
| **side effect** *An expected but unwanted effect of a medication.* | effetto collaterale |
| **siderosis** *Discoloration of a part due to iron deposition.* | siderosi |
| **sigh** *A long deep exhalation that expresses an emotion, as in relief.* | sospiro |
| **sigmoid flexure** *The S shaped curve located between the descending colon and rectum.* | flessura iliaca del colon |
| **sigmoid** *Referring to the portion of the colon that leads into the rectum.* | sigmoide |
| **sigmoidoscopy** *Visualization of the sigmoid colon with a scope.* | sigmoidoscopia |

| English | Italian |
|---|---|
| **sigmoidostomy** *Formation of an opening in the sigmoid colon that communicates with the outside of the body.* | sigmoidostomia |
| **silent** *Absence of noise or no indication of something.* | silente |
| **silicosis** *Grinders's disease; fibrotic lung disease caused by inhalation of silica.* | silicosi |
| **silver** *A precious metal with atomic number 47.* | argento |
| **silver nitrate stick** *A medical device used to treat hypergranulation tissue.* | bastoncino di nitrato d'argento |
| **simultaneous** *Occurring at the same time.* | simultaneo |
| **single** *Only one.* | solo |
| **single** *Not married.* | single |
| **sinistrocardia** *Location of the heart toward the left (more than normally seen).* | sinistrocardia |
| **sinistrotorsion** *Distorsion toward the left; in reference to the eye generally.* | sinistrotorsione |
| **sinoatrial** *Referring to the cardiac node of the same name.* | senoatriale |
| **sinoatrial node** *A mass of cardiac tissue that acts as the pacemaker.* | nodo senoatriale |
| **sinus arrhythmia** *Cardiac dysrhythmias related to sinoatrial nodal dysfunction.* | aritmia sinusale |
| **sinusitis** *Inflammation of the sinuses.* | sinusite |
| **sinusoid** *An irregular vessel having almost no adventitia that is found in the liver, heart, parathyroid, spleen and pancreas.* | sinusoide |
| **sip, to** *To slowly take small drinks of a fluid.* | sorseggiare |
| **Sister Mary Joseph nodule** *A nodule at the umbilicus associated with metastatic abdominal cancer.* | nodulo di Suor Maria Giuseppa |
| **site** *Location.* | sito |
| **size** *The dimensions of something.* | dimensioni |
| **Sjogren's syndrome.** *Characterized by dryness of the mouth and eyes, it is sometimes linked to rheumatoid arthritis.* | Sjogren, sindrome di |
| **skeletal traction** *Use of a pulley system to reduce a fracture.* | trazione scheletrica |
| **skeleton** *Internal bony framework.* | scheletro |
| **skin** *Flesh.* | pelle |
| **skin fold** *An overlapping of skin formed by subcutaneous tissue.* | piega della pelle |
| **skin lesion** *An abnormal but not necessarily cancerous lesion.* | lesione cutanea |
| **skin rash** *Dermal exanthema.* | eurzione cutanea |
| **sleep** *A nap or a snooze.* | sonno |
| **sleep apnea** *Episodic apnea during sleep that is exhibited by daytime symptoms of fatigue, difficulty concentrating and sleepiness.* | apnea del sonno |
| **sleeping sickness** *Also called Trypanosomiasis, this disease is caused by a parasitic protozoa and transmitted by the tsetse fly.* | malattia del sonno; tripanosomiasi |
| **slice** *A sliver or shaving.* | fettina |
| **slide** *A thin, rectangular piece of glass used for viewing specimen under a microscope.* | vetrino portaoggetti per microscopio |
| **slight** *Minor or small.* | lieve |
| **sling** *A device used to give support to an injured extremity.* | bendaggio a fionda o a triangolo |
| **slow** *Unhurried.* | lento |
| **sludge** *A viscous fluid.* | deposito |
| **slurring** *Indistinct yet comprehensible speech.* | strascicato |
| **smallpox** *Variola.* | vaiolo |
| **smear** *Used to refer to a specimen smeared on a slide.* | effettuare uno striscio |
| **smegma** *A thick curdled secretion found around the clitoris and the prepuce.* | smegma |

| English | Italian |
|---|---|
| **smoke, to** *To inhale on a cigarette.* | fumare |
| **sneeze, to** *To suddenly expel air from the nose and mouth because of nasal irritation.* | starnutire |
| **sniffing** *Short, rapid nasal inhalation.* | atto dell'annusare |
| **snore, to** *To snore or grunt while breathing during sleep.* | russare |
| **soap** *A compound made with fats/oils and an alkali; it is used for washing.* | sapone |
| **sob, to** *To cry uncontrollably.* | singhiozzare |
| **socket** *An anatomical hollow that is part of an articulation. (eyeball socket)* | incavo |
| **socks** *Worn on the feet before one puts on shoes.* | calzino |
| **sodium chloride** *A colorless, crystalline compound; also table salt.* | sodio cloruro |
| **soft** *Easy to mold or compress.* | soffice, dolce |
| **solar plexus** *A cluster of ganglia and nerves, located at the base of the sternum, that surround the celiac trunk.* | plesso solare |
| **sole of foot** *Common term for plantar aspect of the foot.* | pianta del piede |
| **soleus muscle** *Assists with ankle plantar flexion.* | soleo |
| **solvent** *Able to dissolve with other chemicals.* | solvente |
| **somatic** *Referring to the body.* | somatico |
| **somnambulism** *Sleepwalking.* | sonnambulisomo |
| **somnolence** *Drowsiness.* | sonnolenza |
| **soporific** *Promoting drowsiness or sleep.* | soporifero |
| **sore throat** *Common term for pharyngitis.* | mal di gola |
| **sorrow** *A feeling of deep despair.* | pena |
| **sound** *Vibrations that travel through air and are heard when reaching the ears.* | sano |
| **sour** *An acid or bitter taste.* | agro |
| **span** *A distance between two objects.* | spanna |
| **sparing** *Economical.* | frugale |
| **spasm** *An involuntary contraction of muscles.* | spasmo |
| **spasmolytic** *A substance that diminishes spasms.* | spasmolitico |
| **spastic** *Stiff, awkward movement of the muscles.* | spastico |
| **spasticity** *Refers to continuous spastic movement.* | spasticità |
| **specific** *Clearly defined.* | specifico |
| **specimen** *A sample for medical testing.* | campione |
| **spectrometry** *The use of a device to measure spectra.* | spettrometria |
| **spectroscope** *A device for producing and recording spectra.* | spettroscopio |
| **speculum** *A device used to open a canal for inspection. (vaginal speculum)* | speculo |
| **speech** *Oral articulation.* | linguaggio |
| **speech therapist** *A person trained to assist people with speech and language disorders.* | logopedista |
| **sperm** *Short term for spermatozoon.* | sperma |
| **spermatic cord** *The structure containing the ductus deferens, testicular artery, and nerves that goes from the inguinal ring to the testis.* | funicolo spermatico |
| **spermatocele** *A cyst in the epididymis containing spermatozoa.* | spermatocele |
| **spermatogenesis** *The production of spermatozoa.* | spermatogenesi |
| **spermatozoon** *A mature male germ cell that is capable of fertilizing an ovum.* | spermatozoo |
| **spermicide** *A substance capable of killing sperm.* | spermicida |
| **sphenoidal sinus** *Part of the sphenoid bone; it communicates with the most superior aspect of the nasal meatus.* | seno sfenoidale |

| English | Italian |
|---|---|
| **spherocyte** *An erythrocyte without the usual central pallor; it is noted in spherocytosis and some hemolytic anemias.* | sferocito |
| **spherocytosis** *The presence of spherocytes in the blood.* | sferocitosi |
| **sphincter** *A muscle the surrounds an orifice or duct so it closes when the muscle contracts.* | sfintere |
| **sphincterotomy** *Surgical incision of the anal sphincter.* | sfinterotomia |
| **sphygmomanometer** *Device for measuring blood pressure.* | sfigmomanometro |
| **spica** *A figure of eight bandage.* | bendaggio a spiga |
| **spicule** *A sharp, slender part.* | spicola |
| **spider nevus** *A papule with telangiectases radiating from the center.* | nevo ragno |
| **spinal** *Referring to the spine.* | spinale |
| **spinal cord abscess** *A localized collection of purulent material in or adjacent to the spinal cord.* | ascesso del midollo spinale |
| **spinal cord** *The bundle of nerves that with the brain comprise the central nervous system.* | midollo spinale |
| **spinal ganglion** *The ganglion located on the dorsal root of each spinal nerve.* | ganglio spinale |
| **spinal nerve** *The term for each of the thirty pairs of nerves that originate in the spine and traverse between the vertebrae. There are eight cervical, twelve thoracic, five lumbar, five sacral and one coccygeal nerve pairs.* | nervo spinale |
| **spinal reflex** *A reflex that has an arc passing through the spine.* | riflesso spinale |
| **spinal shock** *Hypotension related to injury or intervention of the spine.* | shock spinale |
| **spine** *The spinal column or a thorny protrusion.* | spina dorsale |
| **spirograph** *A device used to record respiratory movements.* | spirografo |
| **spirometer** *A device used to measure pulmonary capacity.* | spirometro |
| **spit** *A term used to describe saliva that is ejected from the mouth.* | saliva |
| **splanchnic nerves** *The nerves supplying the abdominal viscera and blood vessels.* | nervi splancnico |
| **spleen** *The visceral organ that is involved with production and removal of blood cells.* | milza |
| **splenectomy** *Surgical excision of the spleen.* | splenectomia |
| **splenic flexure of the colon** *The portion of the colon that turns from the transverse to the descending colon.* | flessura splenico del colon |
| **splenic** *Referring to the spleen.* | splenico |
| **splenomegaly** *An abnormally enlarged spleen.* | splenomegalia |
| **splint** *A rigid support used to immobilize and extremity.* | stecca di immobilizzazione |
| **splinter** *A small, thin object; usually refers to the object being imbedded in the body.* | scheggia |
| **spondylitis** *Inflammation of the vertebrae.* | spondilite |
| **spondylolisthesis** *The overlapping of one vertebra over another.* | spondilolistesi |
| **spondylolysis** *Dissolution of the vertebra.* | spondilolisi |
| **sponge** *Sterile fabric used to soak up fluid during surgery.* | spugna |
| **spongiosis** *Edema of the spongy layer of the skin.* | spongiosi |
| **spontaneous** *Occurring without provocation.* | spontaneo |
| **spoon nail** *Also referred to as koilonychia, the nail is concave and is generally associated with anemia.* | unghia a cucchiaio |
| **spoonful** *A measurement that does not specify teaspoon or tablespoon.* | cucchiaiata |
| **sporotrichosis** *A Sporotrichum schenckii infection manifested by formation of lymphatic and subcutaneous nodules.* | sporotricosi |
| **sprain** *A joint injury without fracture.* | distorsione |
| **spray** *Liquid blown through the air in the form of fine droplets.* | spruzzo |

| English | Italian |
|---|---|
| **sputum** *A mixture of respiratory tract secretions and saliva.* | muco |
| **squama** *A scale or platelike body.* | squama |
| **squamous** *Scaly.* | squamoso |
| **square root** *The result noted when a number is multiplied by itself.* | radice quadrata |
| **squeeze, to** *To apply pressure.* | passare appena |
| **squint, to** *To look at something with the eyes partially closed.* | essere strabico |
| **squirt, to** *To eject a liquid from a small opening.* | spremere |
| **stab wound** *An injury occurring with a sharp object.* | ferita da arma bianca |
| **stabbing pain** *A sharp piercing quality to pain.* | dolore trafittura |
| **stagger, to** *To walk in an unsteady fashion.* | vacillare |
| **staging** *Refers to a stratification of cancer for example.* | stadiazione |
| **stamina** *Ability to maintain physical or mental exertion for a long period.* | capacità di resistenza |
| **stammering** *The impulse to repeat the first letter of words and involuntary pauses while speaking.* | balbuzie |
| **standing** *Position or status.* | stato |
| **stapedectomy** *Surgical excision of the stapes.* | stapediectomia |
| **stapedius muscle** *Located in the tympanic interior, it reduces stapedial movement.* | muscolo stapedio |
| **stapes** *This auditory ossicle is the innermost of three ossicles and is shaped like a stirrup.* | stapedio |
| **staphyloma** *Protrusion of the cornea due to inflammation.* | stafiloma |
| **staphylorrhaphy** *Surgical repair of a defect between the soft palate and uvula.* | stafilorrafia |
| **starvation** *Death related to starvation.* | inanizione |
| **stasis** *Lack of movement.* | stasi |
| **state** *Status.* | stato; condizione |
| **statement** *A written or oral commentary.* | dichiarazione |
| **static** *Not changing.* | statico |
| **status** *Position or condition* | stato, condizione |
| **steady state** *In equilibrium.* | equilibrio dinamico |
| **steatoma** *A sebaceous cyst or lipoma.* | steatoma |
| **steatorrhea** *Excrement with an abnormally high fat content.* | steatorrea |
| **steatosis** *Fatty degeneration; when referring to the liver it involves invasion of fat into hepatocytes.* | steatosi |
| **stellate ganglion** *Formed by the seventh cervical, eighth cervical and first thoracic ganglia.* | ganglio stellato |
| **stenosis** *Narrowing of an orifice.* | stenosi |
| **stercobilin** *A substance created by the reduction of bilirubin and gives excrement the brown hue.* | stercobilina |
| **stereognosis** *The ability to identify an object by touch.* | sterognosia |
| **sterile** *1. Infertile 2. Refers to equipment that is free of contamination.* | infecundo 2) asettico |
| **sterilization** *A procedure done to prevent production of offspring.* | sterilizzazione |
| **sternal** *Referring to the sternum.* | sternale |
| **sternocleidomastoid** *The pair of muscles that connect the sternum, clavicle and mastoid process.* | sternocleidomastoideo |
| **sternum** *Commonly called the breast bone, it consists of the corpus, manubrium and xiphoid process.* | sterno |
| **sterol** *Unsaturated steroid alcohols such as cholesterol.* | sterolo |
| **stethoscope** *Device used to auscultate the heart, lungs and over arteries to assess for abnormalities.* | stetoscopio |
| **stiff** *Not easily bent.* | duro; rigido |
| **stiff-neck** *Cervical sprain with reduced range of motion.* | rigidità nucale |

| English | Italian |
|---|---|
| **stillborn** *Refers to a newborn that died in utero.* | nato morto |
| **sting** *A small puncture as in a bee sting.* | pungiglione |
| **stippling** *Having numerous small specks or spots.* | punteggiatura |
| **stirrup** *An attachment to an exam table where a woman puts her legs to assist examination of the genitalia.* | staffa (utilizzata durante l'esame pelvico) |
| **stomach** *Organ of digestion between the esophagus and small bowel.* | stomaco |
| **stomach cramps** *Sensation of muscle contraction in the epigastric area.* | campi allo stomaco |
| **strabismus** *An anomaly of ocular movement.* | strabismo |
| **strain** *As in a muscle strain.* | tensione o distensione eccessiva |
| **strait-jacket** *A device used to temporarily restrain the arms of patients who are psychotic and violent.* | camicia di forza |
| **strange** *Unusual in an unsettling way.* | strano |
| **straw itch** *Pruritus associated with exposure to straw that is infested with the mite Pyemotes ventricosus. Also referred to as dermatitis pediculoides ventricosus.* | dermatosi da Pediculoides ventricosus della paglia |
| **strawberry tongue** *A characteristic discoloration of the tongue seen in an early phase of scarlet fever.* | lingua fragola |
| **stream** *The flow of a liquid.* | corrente |
| **strength** *Force, might or vigor.* | forza |
| **stress** *Strain or pressure.* | pressione, tensione |
| **stress fracture** *A long bone fracture caused by repetitive mechanical stress.* | frattura da sforza |
| **stretcher** *A device used to carry a patient in the supine position.* | lettiga |
| **stria** *A narrow bandlike body.* | stria |
| **stricture** *A narrowing of a canal or duct.* | restringimento |
| **stride** *Walk with long definitive steps.* | falcata |
| **stridor** *An abnormal, high-pitched, musical sound caused by an obstruction in the larynx or stenosis of the vocal cords.* | stridore |
| **stroke** *Common term for cerebrovascular accident.* | colpo apoplettico |
| **stroke volume** *The amount of blood ejected from the ventricle with each contraction.* | gittata ventricolare sistolica |
| **stroma** *A term used to describe the framework of an organ.* | stroma |
| **strong** *Having the power to move heavy objects.* | forte |
| **stump** *Term used to designate what remains of an amputated extremity.* | moncone di arto amputato |
| **Strümpell's disease** *Also known as spondylitis deformans, it is characterized by arthritis and osteitis deformans of the spinal cord with a rounded kyphosis and rigidity.* | malattia di Strümpell |
| **Strümpell reflex** *Flexion of the leg and adduction of the foot elicited by stroking of the thigh or abdomen.* | riflesso di Strümpell |
| **stupor** *A reduced level of consciousness.* | stupore |
| **stuttering** *Involuntary repetition of the first consonant.* | balbuziente |
| **sty** *Also called hordeolum externum, it is inflammation of the sebaceous gland of an eyelash.* | orzaiolo |
| **stylet** *A thin wire within a catheter that is removed after the catheter is in place.* | stiletto |
| **subacute** *A stage between acute and chronic.* | subacuto |
| **subarachnoid** *The layer of the brain covering between the arachnoid and pia mater.* | subaracnoideo |
| **subareolar abscess** *A purulent fluid collection in the areolar gland.* | ascesso subareolare |
| **subclavian** *Refers to the area under the clavicle; the subclavian vein runs below the clavicle.* | sottoclaveare |

| English | Italian |
|---|---|
| **subclavian steal syndrome** *Retrograde vertebral artery flow due to ipsilateral subclavian artery stenosis.* | sindrome del furto della succlavia |
| **subdural** *The area between the dura mater and the arachnoid membrane.* | subdurale |
| **subdural hematoma** *Formation of a blood clot between the dura mater and the arachnoid membrane.* | ematoma subdurale |
| **suberosis** *A type of hypersensitivity pneumonitis related to inhalation of moldy cork dust.* | suberosi |
| **sublingual** *Situated under the tongue.* | sublinguale |
| **submaxillary** *Situated below the maxilla.* | submaxillare |
| **subphrenic** *Referring to below the diaphragm.* | subfrenico |
| **succussion** *The presence of a splashing sound when a body cavity is moved indicating presence of both air and fluid.* | succussione |
| **suck, to** *As in, to suction fluid.* | succhiare |
| **suckle, to** *An infant taking to his mother's nipple.* | allattare al seno |
| **sudamina** *White vesicles noted because of retained sweat in the layers of the epidermis.* | sudamen |
| **sudden infant death syndrome** *A leading cause of death of infants from one month to one year; the etiology is unknown.* | sindrome di morte infantile improvvisa |
| **suffer, to** *To be affected by an illness or sickness.* | soffrire |
| **suffocation** *To die from a lack of air or inability to breathe.* | soffocamento |
| **sugar** *A sweet crystalline substance made from a plant such as sugar cane.* | zucchero |
| **suicide** *To kill oneself intentionally.* | suicidio |
| **sulcus** *A groove, like in the brain.* | solco |
| **sulfonamide** *A class of drugs derived from sulfanilamide that are antibacterial.* | solfonamidi |
| **sulfur** *A chemical element with atomic number of 16.* | zolfo |
| **summer itch** *Pruritus noted upon exposure to hot weather, also known as pruritus aestivalis.* | prurito aestivalis |
| **superciliary arch** *The area superior to the upper border of each orbit.* | arco sopracciliare |
| **superfecundation** *The fertilization of two different ova by spermatozoa of two different males.* | superfecondazione |
| **superficial inguinal ring** *The opening of the aponeurosis of the external oblique muscle for the round ligament or spermatic cord.* | canale inguinale superficiale |
| **superior** *In a position above something else.* | superiore |
| **supination** *Turning the sole of the foot or the palm of the hand upward..* | supinazione |
| **supine** *Flat on one's back.* | supino |
| **supplies** *Stock or reserves.* | provviste |
| **suppository** *A delivery system for medication placed in an orifice.* | suppositorio |
| **suppuration** *Formation of purulent material.* | suppurazione |
| **supranuclear ophthalmoplegia** *A disorder that effects the extraocular movements especially limiting the upward movement of the eyes.* | oftalmoplegia sovranucleare |
| **supraorbital** *Situated above the orbit.* | sovraorbitario |
| **suprapubic** *Situated above the pubis.* | sovrapubico |
| **sural** *Referring to the calf of the leg.* | surale |
| **surfactant** *A substance that reduces surface tension in the lungs.* | surfattante |
| **surgeon** *A physician who performs surgery.* | chirurgo |
| **surgery** *The incision of a body part using sterile technique in order to treat disease or injury.* | operazione chirurgica |
| **surgical** *Referring to surgery.* | chirurgico |
| **surname** *One's given "last" name that generally changes for women upon marriage to that of the man's surname.* | cognome |

| English | Italian |
|---|---|
| **sustain, to** *To keep or maintain.* | sostenere |
| **sustained release tablet** *Describes a medicine that is slowly dispersed so it has a lasting effect.* | compressa preparati ritardo |
| **suture** *Thread used for sewing together a wound.* | sutura |
| **swab** *An absorbent material used for cleaning wounds or applying ointment.* | tampone |
| **swallow, to** *To cause something to pass down the esophagus.* | inghiottire |
| **sweat** *Moisture exuded through the pores of the skin.* | sudorazione |
| **sweat, to** *The action of releasing moisture through pores of the skin.* | sudare; traspirare |
| **swelling** *An abnormal enlarged from fluid collection.* | tumefazione; rigonfiamento |
| **swimmer's itch** *Pruritus caused by exposure to schistosomes.* | prurito del nuotatore |
| **swollen (distended) abdomen** | addome gonfio |
| **sycosis** *A bacterial infection affecting the hair follicles on a person's face.* | sicosi |
| **Sydenham chorea** *Historically known as Saint Vitus' dance, it is a childhood chorea associated with rheumatic fever.* | corea di Sydenham |
| **symbiosis** *The living together of two organisms.* | simbiosi |
| **symmetry** *Being equally bilaterally.* | simmetria |
| **sympathectomy** *The surgical resection of a sympathetic nerve to reduce undesired effects.* | simpatectomia |
| **sympathetic nervous system** *The nerves responsible for the flight or fight response.* | sistema nervoso simpatico |
| **symptom** *A physical feature that is characteristic of disease.* | sintomo |
| **synapse** *The intersection of two nerve cells.* | sinapsi |
| **synarthrosis** *Adjacent bones connected by a joint but the joint is fixed.* | sinartrosi |
| **synchondrosis** *A joint with little motion that uses cartilage such as the vertebral bodies.* | sincondrosi |
| **syncope** *Sudden loss of consciousness.* | sincope |
| **syncytial knot** *Aggregation of syncytiotrophoblastic nuclei in the villi of the placenta during early pregnancy.* | nodo sinciziale |
| **synechia** *The adhesion of two body parts, such as synechia vulvae in which the labia minora are congenitally adherent.* | sinechia |
| **synovectomy** *Surgical resection of a synovial membrane.* | sinoviectomia |
| **synovial fluid** *The fluid that surrounds, for example, the knee within a capsule.* | liquido sinoviale |
| **synovitis** *Inflammation of the synovium.* | sinovite |
| **syphilis** *A infectious disease caused by Treponema pallidum that causes a painless penile ulcer in the primary stage but can lead to irreversible brain damage in the untreated tertiary stage.* | sifilide |
| **syringe** *A device used for administering medication through various routes.* | siringa |
| **syringomelia** *A condition exhibited by fluid-filled cavities in the spinal cord.* | siringomielia |
| **syrup** *A thick sweet liquid.* | sciroppo |
| **systole** *The phase of the cardiac cycle in which the ventricles contract.* | sistole |
| **systolic** *Referring to systole or that which occurs during systole.* | sistolico |
| **tablespoon** *An eating utensil that holds 15milliliters of fluid.* | cucchiaio da tavola |
| **tablet** *A small disk of a compressed solid substance.* | tavoletta, compressa |
| **tachycardia** *Heart rate higher than physiologic normal.* | tachicardia |
| **tachypnea** *Breathing faster than normal.* | tachipnea |
| **tactile** *Able to be felt.* | tattile |
| **talipes calcaneus** *A foot deformity exhibited by abnormal dorsiflexion.* | talipo calcaneare |

| English | Italian |
|---|---|
| **talipes equinovaro** *Medical term for what is commonly known as club foot.* | talipo equinovaro |
| **talipes equinus** *A foot deformity exhibited by abnormal plantar flexion.* | talipo equino |
| **talus** *The most superior tarsal bone that articulates with the tibia.* | talo; astragalo |
| **tampon** *Disposable intravaginal product used to collect blood from menstruation.* | batuffolo di cotone (utilizzato per raccogliere le mestruazioni |
| **tamponade** *1. Stopping bleeding during surgery with a cotton pledget. 2. When referring to cardiac tamponade, it is the limitation of cardiac contraction because of blood or fluid accumulation in the pericardial sac.* | tamponamento 2) tamponamento cardiaco |
| **tap** *A puncture with the intent of draining fluid as in spinal tap.* | percuotere leggermente |
| **tape measure** *A long length of tape, marked at intervals for measuring.* | metro a nastro |
| **tapeworm** *A parasitic, intestinal flatworm.* | verme solitario |
| **tarantula** *A large hairy spider found mainly in the tropics.* | tarantola |
| **target** *An objective towards which efforts are directed.* | targa |
| **target cell** *An abnormal cell that is present in liver disease and certain hemoglobinopathies.* | cellule a bersaglio |
| **tarsal** *Referring to any bone in the tarsus.* | tarsale |
| **tarsal tunnel syndrome** *Characterized by impingement of various nerves of the ankle.* | sindrome del tunnel tarsale |
| **tarsalgia** *Pain in any of the tarsal bones.* | tarsalgia |
| **tarsectomy** *Surgical excision of all or part of the tarsus.* | tarsectomia |
| **tarsorrhaphy** *Suturing the eyelids in order to tighten the palpebral fissure.* | tarsorrafia |
| **tarsus** *The group of seven bones of the ankle or foot (three cuneiform bones, talus, calcaneus, navicular, cuboid bones).* | tarso |
| **taste** *Sensation of flavor perceived in one's mouth.* | gusto |
| **tattoo** *A design made by inserting indelible ink into the skin.* | tatuaggio |
| **taurocholic acid** *A bile acid composed of cholic acid and taurine.* | acido taurocolico |
| **tear** *As in, to shed a tear.* | lacrima |
| **tear, vaginal** *Referring to a vaginal tear after childbirth.* | strapparsi vaginale |
| **teaspoon** *A measure instrument that holds 5 milliliters of fluid.* | cucchiaino da tè |
| **tectum** *A roof-like body.* | tetto |
| **tectum mesencephali** *The posterior portion of the mesencephalon including the sup. and inf. colliculi and tectal lamina.* | mesencefali tetto |
| **telangiectasis** *A condition exhibited by red, dilated capillaries on the skin.* | telangettasia |
| **telemetry** *Use of radio signals to transmit patient data. The most common form is for electrocardiography in a patient who is ambulatory.* | telemetria |
| **temperature** *The degree of internal heat in a person's body.* | temperatura |
| **temporomandibular joint** *The hinged joint of the temporal bone and mandible.* | articulazione temporomandibolare |
| **tendinitis** *Inflammation of a tendon.* | inflammazione delle guaine tendinee |
| **tendon** *Fibrous tissue that connects muscle to bone.* | tendine |
| **tendon reflex** *A deep reflex elicited by gently tapping the tendon.* | riflesso tendine |
| **tenesmus** *The attempt to defecate but attempts elicit pain and are ineffective.* | tenesmo |
| **tennis elbow** *Inflammation at the lateral aspect of the epicondyle where the muscle and tendon join; lateral epicondylitis.* | gomito del tennista; epicondilalgia omerale |
| **tenoplasty** *Surgical repair of a tendon.* | tenoplastica |
| **tenorrhaphy** *The surgical repair with suture of a separated tendon.* | tenorrafia |

| English | Italian |
|---|---|
| **tenosynovitis** *Inflammation and swelling of an articulation.* | tenosinovite |
| **tenotomy** *Incision of a tendon as is done for strabismus.* | tenotomia |
| **tepid** *Lukewarm.* | tiepido |
| **teratogen** *A substance that induces fetal anomalies.* | teratogene |
| **teratoma** *A tumor made up of tissue not usually at the location (a mass of hair, teeth and gingival tissue in a leg tumor for instance).* | teratoma |
| **terebrant** *Having a piercing quality.* | terebrante |
| **terminal illness** *A disease with no viable treatment with death being inevitable.* | morbo terminale |
| **tertian fever** *A febrile syndrome caused by Plasmodium vivax which produces a fever spike every 48 hours.* | febbre terzana |
| **tertiary** *Third in order or designating medical care at a specialized hospital.* | terziario |
| **test tube** *A glass or plastic tube used to hold a medical specimen.* | provetta |
| **testicle** *One of a pair of organs in the male scrotum that produces sperm.* | testicolo |
| **testicular torsion** *Rotation of the spermatic cord resulting in testicular ischemia.* | torsione testicolare |
| **testosterone** *This steroid hormone produces secondary male sexual characteristics.* | testosterone |
| **tetanus** *A condition caused by Clostridium tetani which produces spasm and rigidity of voluntary muscles.* | tetano |
| **tetany** *A condition caused by the hypocalcemic effect of hypoparathyroidism, exhibited by periodic muscle spasms, convulsions, and peri-oral numbness.* | tetania |
| **tetracycline** *An antibiotic used for gram positive and gram negative infections.* | tetraciclina |
| **tetradactylous** *Referring to a condition of having only four digits on a hand or foot.* | tetradattilo |
| **thalamic syndrome** *Caused by an infarct of the posteroinferior thalamus, there is transient hemiparesis, severe sensory loss with preserved crude pain in the hypalgic limbs.* | sindrome talamico |
| **thalamus** *A paired structure located adjacent to the third ventricle.* | talamo |
| **thalassemia** *A hereditary hemolytic anemia first observed in people from the Mediterranean area.* | talassemia |
| **thalidomide** *A drug used originally as a sedative, after it was found to cause congenital anomalies, its use was restricted. Now it is used for a few conditions such as multiple myeloma.* | talidomide |
| **theca** *A tendon or ovarian follicle sheath.* | teca |
| **thecoma** *A tumor composed of theca cells.* | tecoma |
| **thenar eminence** *Formed by the bellies of the abductor pollicis brevis, flexor pollicis brevis and opponens pollicis.* | eminenza tenar |
| **therapeutic range** *The highest to lowest value that will produce a desired effect.* | finestra terapeutica |
| **thermometer** *A device used to measure temperature.* | termometro |
| **thiamine** *Also called vitamin B1; a deficiency causes beriberi.* | tiamina |
| **thigh** *The body region between the inguinal crease and knee.* | coscia |
| **thin** *Lean or slender.* | magro |
| **thirst** *The desire to drink.* | sete |
| **thoracentesis** *Insertion of a needle into the pleural space to drain and or obtain a specimen for analysis.* | toracentesi |
| **thoracic** *Referring to the thorax.* | toracico |
| **thoracoplasty** *Surgical removal of ribs.* | toracoplastica |
| **thoracoscopy** *Visualization of the thoracic cavity with a scope.* | toracoscopia |

| English | Italian |
|---|---|
| **thoracotomy** *Surgical incision of the thorax.* | toracotomia |
| **thorax** *The part of the body between the neck and abdomen.* | torace |
| **three way foley** *A urinary tube used for irrigation of the bladder.* | caterere urinario a tre vie |
| **threonine** *An amino acid needed for the growth in infants.* | treonina |
| **throat** *The anterior aspect of the neck.* | gola |
| **throb, to** *The beat with strong regular rhythm.* | battere |
| **thrombectomy** *Excision of a thrombus from a vein or artery.* | trombectomia |
| **thrombin** *An enzyme that is a catalyst for the conversion of fibrinogen to fibrin in the formation of a clot.* | trombina |
| **thromboangiitis** *Inflammation and thrombosis in a blood vessel.* | tromboangioite |
| **thromboarteritis** *Thrombosis of an inflamed artery.* | tromboarterite |
| **thrombocytopenia** *Abnormal decrease in the number of blood platelets.* | trombocitopenia |
| **thrombophlebitis** *Inflammation of a venous wall associated with a thrombus.* | tromboflebite |
| **thrombosis** *Formation of a clot in a vein or artery.* | trombosi |
| **thrush** *Candida albicans* | mughetto |
| **thumb** *The first digit of each hand.* | pollice |
| **thymectomy** *Surgical excision of the thymus.* | timectomia |
| **thymine** *A chemical with a pyrimidine base found in DNA.* | timina |
| **thymocyte** *A lymphocyte located in the thymus.* | timocito |
| **thymoma** *A tumor composed of thymic tissue and is sometimes associated with myasthenia gravis.* | timoma |
| **thymus** *A body organ located in the neck and it produces T cells to improve immune function.* | timo |
| **thyroglossal cyst** *A common congenital growth in the thyroglossal duct.* | cisto tireoglosso |
| **thyroid** *A gland in the neck that secretes hormones regulating metabolism.* | tiroideo |
| **thyroid stimulating hormone (TSH)** *A thyroid secreted by the pituitary that regulates the thyroid.* | ormone tireotropo |
| **thyroidectomy** *Surgical resection of all or part of the thyroid.* | tiroidectomia |
| **thyrotoxicosis** *Abnormal increase in thyroid activity exhibited by thinning hair, hypertension, tachycardia and at times atrial fibrillation.* | tireotossicosi |
| **thyroxine** *An iodine containing hormone, referred to T4.* | tiroxina |
| **tibia** *The larger of two long bones in the lower leg.* | tibia |
| **tic** *Periodic spasmodic facial muscle contractions.* | tic |
| **tic douloureux** *Also referred to as trigeminal neuralgia.* | nevralgia del trigemino |
| **tick bite** | puntura di zecca |
| **tick-borne fever** *A relapsing fever caused by a spirochete of the genus Borrelia.* | febbre di zecche |
| **tickle, to** *To lightly touch a person to cause one to laugh.* | fare il solletico |
| **tidal volume** *The amount of air inspired with each breath. One can set a ventilator to deliver a preset number of milliliters of oxygenated air with each breath.* | volume corrente |
| **tight junction** *An intercellular junction with an impermeable membrane.* | giunzione stretto |
| **tincture** *1. A very small amount of something. 2. A medicine dissolved in alcohol.* | tintura |
| **tinea barbae** *Ringworm on the face in the region a man shaves.* | tigna della barba |
| **tinea capitis** *Ringworm of the scalp, a fungal infection.* | tigna del capo |
| **tinea corporis** *Ringworm of the body, a fungal infection.* | tigna del corpo |
| **tinea cruris** *Ringworm in the inguinal region, a fungal infection.* | tinea cruris |

| English | Italian |
|---|---|
| **tinea** *Medical term for ringworm.* | tigna |
| **tinea pedis** *Ringworm of the feet, a fungal infection.* | tigna piede |
| **tingling** *Prickling or stinging sensation.* | formicolio |
| **tinnitus** *Medical term for ringing in the ears. It is associated with Meniere's syndrome among other conditions.* | tinnito |
| **tired** *Fatigued.* | affaticato |
| **tissue** *Any of the distinct materials people are made of.* | tessuto |
| **tocopherol** *Vitamin E.* | tocoferolo |
| **toe** *Any of the digits of of the feet.* | dito del piede |
| **toenail** *The nail at the tip/dorsal aspect of each toe.* | unghia delle dita dei piedi |
| **tongs** *A medical device used for holding or grasping.* | tenaglie |
| **tongue** *The fleshy muscular organ of the mouth.* | lingua |
| **tongue depressor; tongue blade** *As the name implies, the stick pushes the tongue down so the posterior aspect of the mouth can be viewed more readily.* | abbassalingua |
| **tonometer** *A device used to measure ocular pressure in glaucoma.* | tonometro |
| **tonsil** *A rounded mass of lymphoid tissue, most commonly referring to the pharyngeal tonsil.* | tonsilla |
| **tonsillectomy** *Excision of the tonsils.* | tonsillectomia |
| **tonsillitis** *Inflammation of the tonsils.* | tonsillite |
| **tooth** *One of a set of hard, bony enamel coated structure in the jaw.* | dente |
| **toothache** *Dental pain.* | odontalgia; mal di dente |
| **toothless** *Edentulous.* | senza denti; edentato |
| **torpor** *Unresponsiveness to normal stimuli.* | torpore |
| **torsade de pointe** *Ventricular cardiac rhythm disturbance.* | tachicardia ventricolare multiforme |
| **torsion** *Refers to twisting. Testicular torsion is the twisting of the spermatic cord that can lead to ischemia and gangrene of the testicle.* | torsione |
| **torsion spasm** *Also called dystonia musculorum deformans, a genetic condition exhibited by twisting contortions sideways and forward while walking.* | distonia muscolare deformante progressiva |
| **torso** *The trunk of the body.* | tronco |
| **torticollis** *A condition exhibited by the head being turned to one side continuously.* | trocicollo |
| **touch** *Tactile stimulation.* | senso del tatto |
| **tourniquet** *A device tied tightly around an extremity to diminish blood flow or blood loss.* | tourniquet |
| **toxemia** *The release of toxic substances into the blood stream from a local infection. Toxemia of pregnancy is a synonym for preeclampsia.* | tossiemia |
| **toxic** *Relating to or caused by poison.* | tossico |
| **toxicology** *The study of the nature, effects and detection of poisons.* | tossicologia |
| **toxin** *A poison of plant or animal origin.* | tossina |
| **toxoid** *A chemically modified toxin that can be used as a vaccine.* | tossoide |
| **toxoplasmosis** *A disease caused by an organism from the genus Toxoplasma. One can have simple malaise to central nervous system involvement.* | toxoplasmosi |
| **trabecule** *A connective tissue strand that goes from a capsule to the enclosed organ.* | trabecola |
| **trabeculotomy** *A surgery for open angle glaucoma.* | trabecolotomia |
| **trachea** *The ringed canal between the pharynx and bronchi.* | trachea |
| **tracheitis** *Inflammation of the trachea.* | tracheite |
| **trachelorrhaphy** *Surgical repair of a lacerated cervix.* | trachelorrafia |

| English | Italian |
|---|---|
| **tracheobronchitis** *Inflammation of the trachea and bronchi.* | tracheobronchite |
| **tracheostomy** *Creation of a surgical opening in the trachea so a tube could be placed in the trachea.* | tracheostomia |
| **tracheotomy** *Surgical incision of the trachea.* | tracheotomia |
| **trachoma** *An infection of the cornea and conjunctiva caused by Chlamydia.* | tracoma |
| **tract** *A large bundle of fibers or a major passage in the body.* | tratto |
| **traction** *Sustained pull on a muscle or bone to correct alignment.* | trazione |
| **tragus** *The fleshy prominence anterior to the opening of the ear.* | trago |
| **tranquilizer** *A medication used to diminish anxiety.* | tranquillante |
| **transabdominal** *Through the abdominal wall.* | transaddominale |
| **transaminase** *An enzyme that facilitates the transfer of an amino group to an amino acid.* | transaminasi |
| **transdermal** *Through the skin.* | transdermico |
| **transfusion** *Administration of blood products intravenously.* | transfusione |
| **transient ischemic attack** *Cerebral ischemic changes resulting from transitory hypoperfusion.* | infarto bianco o ischemia |
| **transpire, to** *To release vapor from the skin or respiratory mucosa. 2) to come about* | sudare 2) accadere |
| **transplant,to** *To move a body part from one location to another.* | trapiantare |
| **transplantation** *The grafting of tissues.* | trapianto |
| **transrectal ultrasound** *Insertion of an ultrasound probe into the rectum to view adjacent structures.* | ultrasuono transrettale |
| **transudation** *The movement of body tissue through a membrane that is usually the result of inflammation.* | trasudazione |
| **transvaginal ultrasound** *Insertion of an ultrasound probe in the vagina to view adjacent structures.* | ecografia transvaginale |
| **trapezium** *The lateral bone in the distal row of carpal bones.* | ossa dell carpo |
| **trapezius muscle** *The muscle with an origin of occipital bone and seventh cervical vertebra, insertion of clavicle and scapula, and it draws the scapula backward.* | muscolo trapezio |
| **trapezoid bone** *A bone that articulates with the second metacarpal, trapezium, capitate and scaphoid.* | osso del carpo (situato fra trapezio e capitato) |
| **trauma** *A physical injury or emotional shock.* | ferita fisica o psichica |
| **treadmill** *An exercise machine on a continuous belt used for walking.* | tapis roulant |
| **treat, to** *Medical care one receives for illness or injury.* | fare un trattamento |
| **trematoda** *A parasitic fluke such as Schistosoma.* | Trematoda |
| **tremor** *Involuntary contraction and relaxation of small muscle groups.* | tremore |
| **trench mouth** *Inflammation and ulceration of the gingivae.* | stomatite di Vincent |
| **trephination** *Cutting away a circular disc of bone or the cornea.* | trapanazione |
| **triceps** *Referring to something having three heads like the triceps muscle.* | muscolo tricipite |
| **triceps reflex** *A tendon reflex causing extension of the arm when the triceps tendon is gently tapped.* | riflesso tricipite |
| **trichiasis** *Inversion of the eyelashes.* | trichiasi |
| **trichinosis** *A disease caused by meat infected by Trichinella spiralis causing fever and gastrointestinal effects.* | trichinosi |
| **trichomoniasis vaginitis** *Infection related to a species of Trichomonas.* | Trichomonas vaginite |
| **trichophytosis** *A skin or nail fungal infection caused by Trichophyton.* | tricofitosi |
| **tricuspid valve** *The cardiac valve located between the right atrium and right ventricle.* | valvola tricuspide del cuore |
| **trigeminal** *Generally refers to the fifth cranial nerve.* | trigeminale |

| English | Italian |
|---|---|
| **trigeminal nerve** *The fifth cranial nerve which supplies the motor function of mastication and has three sensory branches, the ophthalmic, maxillary and mandibular.* | nervo trigemino |
| **trigeminal neuralgia** *Pain in the region of one or more branches of the fifth cranial nerve sensory branches.* | neuralgia trigeminale |
| **trigger finger** *A condition in which one's finger gets stuck in the flexed position and when extended it snaps like a trigger. Also called stenosing tenosynovitis.* | dito a grilletto |
| **trigone of bladder** *Refers to the area at the base of the bladder between the openings of the ureters and the urethra.* | trigono vescicale |
| **triplegia** *Paralysis of three extremities.* | triplegia |
| **triplets** *Three infants born during one birth.* | tre gemelli |
| **triploid** *Referring to a cell with three homologous sets of chromosomes.* | triploide |
| **trismus** *Commonly called lockjaw, it is a spasm of the muscles supplied by the trigeminal nerve and is an early symptom of tetanus.* | trisma |
| **trisomy 21** *A congenital anomaly in which chromosome 21 is effected and results in Down's syndrome.* | sindorme di trisomia 21 |
| **trisomy** *A general category of congenital anomalies in which there is an extra set of chromosomes in the cell nucleus.* | trisomia |
| **trivial** *Of little importance or value.* | insignificante |
| **trocar** *A device enclosed in a catheter that is used to withdraw fluid from a body cavity.* | trequarti |
| **trochanter** *Refers to the greater or lesser trochanter; the prominences on the femoral neck.* | trocantere |
| **trochlea** *A pulley-shaped structure such as the groove at the distal humerus.* | troclea |
| **trochlear** *Referring to a trochlea.* | trocleare |
| **trochlear nerve** *The fourth cranial nerve that supplies the superior oblique muscle of the eyeball.* | nervo trocleare |
| **trophoblast** *A layer of endodermal tissue that helps attach an ovum to the uterine wall.* | trofoblasto |
| **truncal** *Referring to the trunk of a body or a nerve.* | tronco |
| **truss** *A synthetic device for containing a hernia within the abdomen.* | cinto erniario |
| **trypanosomiasis** *A disease caused by a protozoa of the genus Trypanosoma that can cause sleeping sickness and Chagas' disease.* | tripanosomiasi |
| **trypsin** *An enzyme whose precursor is secreted by the pancreas that breaks down proteins in the intestine.* | tripsina |
| **trypsinogen** *The precursor to trypsin that is secreted by the pancreas.* | tripsinogeno |
| **tryptophan** *An amino acid that is a precursor of serotonin. If present in the body in appropriate levels it can prevent pellagra even if niacin levels are low.* | triptofano |
| **tsetse fly** *An insect that transmits the protozoa trypanosoma and can cause sleeping sickness.* | mosca tse-tse |
| **tsutsugamushi disease** *An acute febrile infectious disease caused by Rickettsia tsutsugamushi. It is characterized by fever, pain lymphadenopathy, small black lesions on the genitals, neck or axilla.* | morbo tsutsugamushi |
| **tubal** *Referring to a tube, as in fallopian tube.* | tubale |
| **tubercle** *1. A granulomatous nodule produced by Mycobacterium tuberculosis. 2. A small prominence on a bone.* | tubercolo |
| **tuberculin** *A solution containing M. tuberculosis or M. bovis that is used to test for tuberculosis by injecting the solution intradermally and looking for a reaction.* | tubercolina |
| **tuberculoma** *1. A tuberculous growth in the brain. 2. A mass that is produced from enlargement of a caseous tubercle.* | tuberuloma |
| **tuberculosis** *Any infectious disease caused by Mycobacterium.* | tubercolosi |

| English | Italian |
|---|---|
| **tuberculous** *Referring to tuberculosis.* | tubercoloso |
| **tuberosity** *A protuberance. For instance the iliac tuberosity is a prominence on the surface of the ilium.* | tuberosità |
| **tuberous sclerosis** *An inherited neurocutaneous disorder exhibited by benign hamartomas of the brain, lung, kidney, skin and other organs.* | sindrome di Bourneville |
| **tubo-ovarian** *Referring to the fallopian tube or ovary.* | tubo-ovarico |
| **tubular** *Referring to a hollow, round-shaped organ.* | tubulare |
| **tularemia** *An infectious disease caused by Francisella tularensis. The symptoms range from mild constitutional complaints to septic shock.* | tularemia |
| **tumefaction** *An area of swelling.* | tumefazione |
| **tumor** *A benign or malignant overgrowth of tissue.* | tumore |
| **tunica** *Generally a covering of a body part or organ. The tunica mucosa nasi is the mucous membrane lining the nasal cavity.* | tunica |
| **tuning fork** *A device used to distinguish between perceptive and conductive hearing loss.* | diapason |
| **tunnel vision** *Constriction in the visual field as though looking through a tube or hollow cylinder. Also called tubular vision.* | visione a galleria |
| **turbinate bones** *The three curved shelves in the nasal cavity.* | osso turbinato |
| **turbinectomy** *Surgical excision of a turbinate bone.* | turbinectomia |
| **turgid** *Congested and swollen.* | turgido |
| **turgor** *Referring to the elasticity of skin. If one pinches skin and it remains in place the patient is dehydrated.* | turgore |
| **twins** *Two infants born at the same birthing.* | gemelli |
| **twitch** *A sudden jerking movement.* | angoscia lancinante |
| **two times** *One action being done on two occasions.* | due volte |
| **tympanic** *Referring to the tympanic membrane or having a resonant quality to percussion.* | timpanico |
| **tympanic cavity** *The air chamber medial to the tympanic membrane in the temporal bone, between the external acoustic meatus and the inner ear.* | timpanoeustachiano |
| **tympanic membrane** *The membrane between the external and middle ear.* | membrana timpanica |
| **tympanoplasty** *Restoration of the tympanic membrane's continuity.* | timpanoplastica |
| **typhoid fever** *A condition caused by ingestion of food or water containing salmonella typhi that is exhibited by fever and abdominal signs and symptoms.* | tifo |
| **typhus fever** *A rickettsiae infection exhibited by rash, fever, headache and myalgia.* | febbre tifo |
| **tyrosine** *An amino acid important in the synthesis of hormones.* | tirosina |
| **ulcer** *A concave wound caused by a break in the integrity of skin or mucous membrane. (duodenal ulcer)* | ulcera |
| **ulcerative** *Referring to ulceration.* | ulcerativo |
| **ulcerative colitis** *Recurrent episode of inflammation of the membranous layer of the colon.* | colite ulcerativo |
| **ulnar nerve** *Arises from the C8-T1 nerves and supplies the hand. (Injury to the ulnar nerve causes loss of flexion of the metacarpophalangeal joints and extension at the interphalangeal joints, thus the common term, claw hand.)* | nervo ulnare |
| **ultrasonography** *Visualization of body structures with the echoes of ultrasound pulses.* | ultrasonografia |
| **ultrasound** *A sound or vibration of ultrasonic frequency.* | ultrasuono |
| **ultraviolet rays** *Electromagnetic radiation with wavelength longer than x rays.* | raggi ultravioletti |
| **umbilical cord** *The stalk between the placenta and the unborn infant.* | cordone umbelicale |
| **umbilicated** *Referring to depressed areas that resemble the umbilicus.* | ombelicato |

| English | Italian |
|---|---|
| **umbilicus** *The scar that denotes the end of the umbilical cord.* | ombelico |
| **unciform** *Another term for hamate bone in the wrist.* | unciforme |
| **uncinariasis** *Hookworm infestation of genus Uncinaria.* | uncinariasi |
| **unciforme bone** *Hamate bone. The bone on the ulnar side of the distal row of the carpus. It articulates withe the 4th and 5th metacarpal, triquetral, lunate and capitate.* | osso uncinato del carpo |
| **unconsciousness** *Unable to respond to sensory stimuli.* | incoscienza |
| **under; infra** *Sometimes used when indicating a patient is "under treatment" for a condition (active treatment).* | sotto |
| **underlying** *Causative, unexposed, or fundamental.* | che sta sotto |
| **undulant fever** *Wave-like variations in the fever, going from very high to normal and back again, as seen in Brucellosis.* | febbre ondulante |
| **unexpected** *Unforeseen.* | imprevisto |
| **unicellular** *A term describing organisms like protozoans that only have cell.* | unicellulare |
| **unilateral** *One side only.* | monolaterale |
| **uniovolar** *Referring to one fertilized ovum.* | mono-ovulare |
| **unknown** *Uncertain or undisclosed.* | sconosciuto |
| **unstable knee** *A condition with giving way of the knee due to ligamentous or cartilaginous dysfunction.* | ginocchio instabile |
| **unsteady** *Unstable or wobbly.* | incerto |
| **upper limb** *Referring to either arm.* | dell'arto superiore |
| **upper respiratory tract** *Generally considered the part of the respiratory tract superior to the vocal cords.* | tratto respiratorio superiore |
| **upright** *Vertical or standing.* | dritto |
| **urachus** *A connection between the bladder and the allantois in the fetus.* | uraco |
| **urate** *The salt of uric acid.* | urato |
| **urea** *A nitrogenous product of protein metabolism; excreted in urine.* | urea |
| **uremia** *An excess of urea and creatinine in the blood.* | uremia |
| **ureter** *The conduit between each kidney and the urinary bladder.* | uretere |
| **ureteral** *Referring to one of two tubes from the kidneys to the bladder that carry urine.* | ureterale |
| **ureterectomy** *Surgical resection of one or both ureters.* | ureterectomia |
| **ureteritis** *Inflammation of the ureter.* | ureterite |
| **ureterocele** *Protrusion of the distal portion of the ureter into the bladder.* | ureterocele |
| **ureterolith** *Presence of a stone in the ureter.* | ureterolito |
| **ureterolithotomy** *Removal of a ureteral stone.* | ureterolitotomia |
| **ureterovaginal** *Referring to the ureter and vagina.* | ureterovaginale |
| **ureterovesical** *Referring to the ureter and urinary bladder.* | ureterovescicale |
| **urethra** *The canal connecting the urinary bladder with the outside of the body.* | uretra |
| **urethral** *Referring to the urethra.* | uretrale |
| **urethritis** *Inflammation of the urethra.* | uretrite |
| **urethrocele** *A prolapse of the urethra through the meatus.* | uretrocele |
| **urethrography** *Imaging of the urethra after instillation of contrast media.* | uretrografia |
| **urethroplasty** *Surgical repair of the urethra.* | uretroplasica |
| **urethroscope** *A scope used to visualize the inside of the urethra.* | uretroscopio |
| **urethrotomy** *A surgical opening of the urethra.* | uretrotomia |
| **urgency** *Emergency or priority.* | urgenza |

| English | Italian |
|---|---|
| **uric acid** *Uric acid is a purine-derived product of nitrogen metabolism that can increase the risk of gout and calculi.* | acido urico |
| **urinal** *Device used by men to void while in bed or sitting.* | orinale |
| **urinalysis** *Chemical and microscopic examination of the urine.* | esame delle urine |
| **urinary** *Referring to the urine.* | urinario |
| **urinary bladder** *The organ collecting urine from the ureters prior to discharge via the urethra.* | vescica urinaria |
| **urinary casts** *A protein precipitated from renal tubules and excreted in the urine.* | cilindro urinario |
| **urinary incontinence** *Involuntary micturition.* | incontinenza urinaria |
| **urinary sediments** *The debris that settles in a urine sample when left undisturbed.* | sedimento urinario |
| **urinary tract** *The organs and canals associated with urine secretion including the kidneys, ureters, bladder and urethra.* | tratto urinario |
| **urine** *The fluid concentrated by the kidneys and expelled via the urethra.* | urina |
| **urinometer** *A device for measuring urine specific gravity.* | urometro |
| **urobilin** *A brownish pigment that is an oxidized form of urobilinogen.* | urobiline |
| **urobilinogen** *A colorless substance produced in the intestines when bilirubin is reduced.* | urobilinogeno |
| **urochrome** *A yellow pigment in the urine that gives urine its color.* | urocromo |
| **urodynamics** *A study done to determine whether a person has the contractile capacity in the bladder to void spontaneously.* | indagine urodinamica |
| **urogenital** *Referring to the urinary and genital systems.* | urogenitale |
| **urography** *Roentgenography of the urinary tract after administration of contrast media.* | urografia |
| **urolith** *Urinary calculi.* | urolito |
| **urology** *Surgical specialty involving medical and surgical treatment of the urogenital system.* | urologia |
| **urticaria** *A diffuse pruritic macular rash, caused by an allergy.* | orticaria |
| **usual** *Typical or normal.* | usuale |
| **uterine** *Referring to the uterus.* | uterino |
| **uterine bleeding** *Bleeding that emanates from the uterus.* | sanguinamento uterino |
| **uterine fibroids** *Benign tumors made up of muscular and fibrous tissue in the uterus. This is an older term for what is now known as leiomyoma.* | fibroma uterino |
| **uterine prolapse** *Protrusion of the uterus out the vagina.* | prolasso uterino |
| **uterovesical** *Referring to the uterus and urinary bladder.* | uterovescicale |
| **uterus** *The hollow organ in the female pelvis where a fertilized ovum embeds and grows.* | utero |
| **utricle** *A small sac. It can refer to a division of the membranous labyrinth.* | utricolo |
| **uveitis** *Inflammation of the uvea.* | uveite |
| **uvula** *A fleshy pendent at the back of the soft palate.* | uvula |
| **uvulectomy** *Excision of the uvula.* | uvulectomia |
| **uvulitis** *Inflammation of the uvula.* | stafilite |
| **vaccination** *The act of receiving a vaccine.* | vaccinazione |
| **vaccine** *A solution of attenuated microorganisms given to prevent or treat a disease.* | vaccino |
| **vaccine certificate** *A document that denotes what vaccines have been received by the holder.* | certificato di vaccinazione |
| **vacuole** *A cavity that develops in a cell.* | vacuolo |
| **vagal** *Referring to the vagus nerve.* | vagale |
| **vagina** *The canal in a female that extends from the vulva to the cervix.* | vagina |

| English | Italian |
|---|---|
| **vaginal** *Referring to the vagina.* | vaginale |
| **vaginismus** *Involuntary contraction of the vagina muscles that causes a painful spasm.* | vaginismo |
| **vagitus** *An infant cry that can be further defined as vagitus vaginalis in which the infant cries while its head is in the vaginal canal.* | vagito |
| **vagotomy** *Incision of the vagus nerve.* | vagotomia |
| **vagus nerve** *The tenth cranial nerve that supplies the heart, lungs visceral organs; its function is tested by assessment of elevation of the uvula.* | nervo vago |
| **valgus** *Refers to a joint being abnormally angulated away from the midline of the body.* | valgo |
| **valine** *An essential amino acid that assists with nitrogen equilibrium.* | valina |
| **Valsalva's maneuver** *A technique in which one attempts to exhale with the mouth and nose closed; this equalizes pressure in the ears.* | manovra di Valsalva |
| **valvulotomy** *Surgical incision of a valve.* | valvulotomia |
| **varicella** *A virus that causes chickenpox and shingles. Also called herpes zoster.* | varicelle |
| **varicocele** *A cluster of varicose veins in the scrotum.* | varicocele |
| **varicose** *Referring to an abnormally distended, irregular vein.* | varicose |
| **varix** *A twisted, distended vein, artery or lymph vessel.* | varice |
| **varus position** *Refers to a joint being abnormally angulated toward the midline of the body.* | posizione varo |
| **vascular** *Referring to a blood vessel.* | vascolare |
| **vasculitis** *Inflammation of a blood vessel.* | vasculite |
| **vasectomy** *The surgical separation of each vas deferens with the intent of producing a sterile person.* | vasectomia; deferentectomia |
| **vasoconstriction** *The process of making the blood vessels smaller which increases blood pressure.* | vasocostrizione |
| **vasodilatation** *The process of making the blood vessels larger which decreases blood pressure.* | vasodilatazione |
| **vasomotor** *Referring to the constriction or dilation of vessels.* | vasomotore |
| **vasopressin** *A hormone secreted by the pituitary that facilitates the retention of sodium and water and also increases blood pressure.* | vasopressina |
| **vasospasm** *The abrupt constriction of a blood vessel.* | vasospasmo |
| **vasovagal** *Referring to overstimulation of the vagus nerve, exhibited by hypotension, pallor, nausea and diaphoresis.* | vasovagale |
| **vector** *An organism that transmits disease.* | vettore |
| **vegetation** *Abnormal growth, such as cardiac valve vegetations as found in endocarditis.* | vegetazione |
| **vein** *A vessel carrying blood back toward the heart.* | vena |
| **velum** *A veil-like part or covering of the palate; soft palate; Velum palatinum.* | velo |
| **vena cava** *The large vein that carries deoxygenated blood to the right atrium.* | vena cava |
| **vena cava filter** *A screen placed in the inferior vena cava to prevent blood clots from causing a pulmonary embolism.* | filtro vena cava inferiore |
| **venereal disease** *A condition transmitted via sexual intercourse.* | morbo venereo |
| **venereal wart** *Common term for condyloma acuminatum.* | verruca venereo |
| **venography** *Roentgenography of a vein after administration of contrast media.* | venografia |
| **venom** *A term used to describe the toxin injected via a bite or sting.* | veleno di serpente |
| **venous** *Referring to the veins.* | venoso |
| **ventilation** *The movement of air into the lungs; generally meant to suggest by an artificial process.* | ventilazione |

| English | Italian |
|---|---|
| **ventral** *Referring to the underside but in humans, a ventral hernia, for example, refers to an abdominal hernia.* | ventrale |
| **ventricle** *1. One of two chambers of the heart. 2. The four interconnected cavities in the center of the brain.* | ventricolo |
| **ventricular septal defect** *An abnormal communication between the right and left ventricles via a hole in the septum.* | difetto del setto ventricolare |
| **ventriculography** *Roentgenography of the ventricles after administration of contrast media.* | ventricolografia |
| **ventriculostomy** *A tube placed into the third ventricle to relieve increased intracranial pressure.* | ventricolostomia |
| **venula** *The vessels that connect the capillary plexuses to veins.* | venula |
| **verminous** *Referring to presence of worms.* | elmintico |
| **verminous ileus** *Obstruction due to masses of intestinal parasites.* | ileo elmintico |
| **verruca** *A hyperplastic epidermal lesion, sometimes referred to as plantar wart.* | verruca |
| **vertebra** *A term for each bone surrounding the spine.* | vertebra |
| **vertebral column** *The cervical, thoracic and lumbar vertebrae.* | colonna vertebrale |
| **vertebrobasilar insufficiency** *Diminished flow to the vertebral and basilar arteries causing posterior fossa symptoms.* | sindrome dell'arteria basilare |
| **vertex** *The crown of the head.* | vertice |
| **vertigo** *A sensation of imbalance with many possible causes.* | vertigini |
| **vesical** *Referring to the urinary bladder.* | vescicale |
| **vesicovaginal** *Referring to the urinary bladder and vagina.* | vescicovaginale |
| **vesiculitis** *Inflammation of the urinary bladder.* | vescicolite |
| **vestibular** *Referring to a vestibule.* | vestibolare |
| **vestigial** *Rudimentary.* | vestigiale |
| **viable** *Referring to a fetus that can survive childbirth.* | vitale |
| **vial** *A small cylindrical container typically used to hold liquid medicine.* | fiala |
| **vibration** *An instance of oscillation of parts.* | vibrazione |
| **villous** *Covered with many villi.* | villoso |
| **villus** *A small vascular prominence from a membrane surface.* | villo |
| **virilization** *The result of androgen; a process of development of masculine characteristics.* | virilizzazione |
| **virology** *The study of viruses.* | virologia |
| **virulence** *The potential severity of a disease or poison.* | virulenza |
| **visceral** *Referring to the organs in the abdominal or thoracic cavity.* | viscerale |
| **viscometer** *A device used to measure viscosity.* | viscosimetro |
| **viscous** *Having a thick, sticky consistency.* | viscoso |
| **vision** *State of being able to see.* | visione |
| **vision, blurred** *Haziness of the visual field.* | visione offuscata |
| **visual field** *The complete area a person can see with their eyes in a fixed position.* | campo visivo |
| **vital capacity (VC)** *The maximal amount of air exhaled after a maximal inhalation.* | capacità vitale |
| **vital signs** *The designation for blood pressure, pulse, respirations and temperature.* | segni vitali |
| **vitamin B12 neuropathy** *Abnormal sensation related to a chronic deficiency of cyanocobalamin;also called subacute combined degeneration of the spinal cord or Putnam-Dana syndrome.* | neuropatia di carenz di vitamina B12 |
| **vitelline** *Referring to the yolk of an egg or ovum.* | vitellino |
| **vitiligo** *The appearance of non-pigmented white patches on otherwise normal skin; hair is usually white in the affected areas.* | vitiligine |

| English | Italian |
|---|---|
| **vitreous** *Glass appearance; used to describe the vitreous body of the eye.* | vitreo |
| **vivisection** *Animal surgery done for purposes of research.* | vivisezione |
| **vocal** *Referring to that which emanates from the vocal cords.* | vocale |
| **vocal cords** *Paired folds of mucous membranes stretched across the larynx.* | corde vocali |
| **voice** *The sound produced through the larynx and out the mouth.* | voce |
| **voiding** *The act of urinating.* | svuotamento |
| **voiding cystography** *Roentgenography of the bladder and urethra after administration of contrast media.* | cistografia svuotamento |
| **volunteer** *A person who performs work without expecting compensation.* | volontario |
| **volvulus** *Twisting of the bowel leading to obstruction and sometimes perforation.* | volvolo |
| **vomit** *The gastric contents that are expelled through the mouth.* | vomito |
| **vomit, to** *To expel gastric contents out the mouth.* | vomitare |
| **vulval cleft** *The area between the labia majora where the vagina and urethra rest.* | fessura vulvare; rima pudendi |
| **vulvectomy** *Surgical resection of the vulva.* | vulvectomia |
| **vulvitis** *Inflammation of the vulva.* | vulvite |
| **vulvovaginitis** *Inflammation of the vulva and vagina.* | vaginite |
| **waddling gait** *Walking in short steps in a swaying fashion.* | andatura ondeggiante |
| **walker** *A metal frame used to facilitate walking.* | camminatore |
| **walking cast** *A cast used for simple fractures of the lower leg.* | camminando ingessatura |
| **ward** *A section of a hospital where patients reside.* | reparto osedaliero |
| **wart** *A flesh colored growth that is also called verruca.* | verruca |
| **wasp** *Any one of a winged hymenopterous insects.* | vespa |
| **water** *A colorless, odorless liquid.* | acqua |
| **wax** *Cerumen.* | cera |
| **weak** *Feeble or deconditioned.* | debole |
| **weakness** *Feebleness.* | debolezza |
| **weekly** *That which occurs every seven days.* | settimanale |
| **weep, to** *To ooze fluid, such as from a wound.* | colare |
| **weep, to** *To shed tears.* | lacrimare |
| **wet** *Covered in moisture.* | acquoso |
| **wheal** *A circumscribed urticarial lesion.* | stria |
| **wheelchair** *A wheeled device used for propulsion.* | sedia a rotelle |
| **wheezing** *A whistling or musical sound made by air passing through a narrowed airway.* | ansimante |
| **whiplash** *Common term for cervical strain following a sudden deceleration.* | colpo di frusta |
| **whipworm** *A parasitic, intestinal nematode worm of the genus Trichuris.* | Trichinella spiralis |
| **whisper** *Speech in a volume that is barely discernible.* | sussurro |
| **whispered pectoriloquy** *The sound heard through the stethoscope when listening to a person's lungs. The sound resonates as it would when listening over a bronchus if there is an area of consolidation.* | pettoriloquia bisbigliata |
| **whisper test** *The examiner whispers into one ear while blocking the other ear to see if the patient can hear in the ear whispered into.* | prova sussurro |
| **whisper, to** *To speak in a volume that is barely discernible.* | bisbigliare; sussurrare |
| **whistle, to** *To make a high pitch noise by forcing air through the lips.* | fischiare |
| **white** *Of the color of snow.* | bianco |

| English | Italian |
|---|---|
| **white matter** *The brain tissue consisting of myelin sheaths and nerve fibers.* | sostanza bianca |
| **whitlow** *An abscess occurring on the palmar surface of the fingertips.* | paronichia |
| **whooping cough** *Pertussis* | pertosse |
| **wick** *A drain using a thin piece of cloth or tubing.* | stoppino |
| **widespread** *Encompassing or spanning.* | disseminato |
| **width** *Side to side measurement.* | larghezza |
| **wisdom tooth** *Third molar.* | dente del giudizio |
| **wise** *Possessing much knowledge.* | profondo |
| **withdrawal** *The action of being without drugs or alcohol.* | ritrattazione |
| **withhold, to** *To refuse to give something.* | trattenere |
| **World Health Organization (WHO)** | Organizzazione Mondiale della Sanità |
| **worm** *Any of long, slender, legless, soft-bodied invertebrates.* | verme |
| **worry, to** *To fret or have unease.* | preoccupare |
| **worsen, to** *To deteriorate.* | deteriorare |
| **wound** *A tissue injury of varying severity.* | ferita |
| **wound care** *The treatment applied to a tissue injury.* | cura della ferita |
| **wrist** *The articulation of the hand and radius/ulna.* | polso |
| **wrist drop** *The inability to hyperextend the wrist due to radial nerve injury.* | carpoptosi |
| **x-ray** | raggi x |
| **xanthine** *A purine derivative that is found in the blood and urine after the metabolism of nucleic acids to uric acid.* | xantina |
| **xanthochromia** *A yellow tone to the skin or spinal fluid.* | xantocromia |
| **xanthoma** *A lipid deposition on the skin exhibited by an irregular yellow patch.* | xantoma |
| **xerodermia** *A mild form of ichthyosis.* | xeroderma |
| **xerophthalmia** *A manifestation of Vitamin A deficiency exhibited by dryness of the cornea and conjunctiva.* | xerooftalmia |
| **xeroradiography** *A form of radiography using photoelectric cells.* | xeroradiografia |
| **xerosis** *Pathological dryness of the skin or mucous membranes.* | xerosi |
| **xerostomia** *A dry mouth from salivary gland hypofunction.* | xerostomia |
| **xiphoid process** *The inferior segment of the sternum.* | processo xifoideo dello sterno |
| **yawn** *Opening one's mouth and inhaling deeply due to sleepiness/boredom* | sbadiglio |
| **yaws** *A tropical disease characterized by ulcers on the extremities, caused by Treponema pertenue.* | framboesia |
| **year** *A time period that covers 365 days.* | anno |
| **yearly** *Occurring once each year.* | annualmente |
| **yeast** *A unicellular fungus.* | lievito |
| **yell, to** *To speak in a loud tone.* | chiamare |
| **yellow** *A color between green and orange in the spectrum* | giallo |
| **yellow fever** *A viral, hemorrhagic fever transmitted by mosquitos.* | febbre gialla |
| **young** *Having lived for a short period.* | giovane |
| **youth** *The time between childhood and being an adult.* | giovinezza |
| **zero** *No quantity.* | zero; nulla |
| **Ziehl-Neelsen carbolfuchsin stain** *A stain used to detect acid-fast bacilli that appear red on the methylene blue background.* | colorante di Ziehl-Neelsen |
| **zinc** *A chemical with atomic number 30.* | zinco |
| **zonula** *A small zone or junction.* | zonula |

| English | Italian |
|---|---|
| **zoology** *The study of animals.* | zoologia |
| **zoonosis** *An animal-born disease that can be transmitted to humans, such as rabies.* | zoonosi |
| **zygomatic bone** *The triangular cheek bone.* | osso zigomatico |
| **zygote** *A fertilized ovum.* | zigote |
| **zymogen** *An inactive compound that is metabolized to an active state.* | zimogeno |

| Italian | English |
|---|---|
| a caso | **at random** *Occurring by chance alone.* |
| a dire il vero | **indeed** *As a matter of fact.* |
| abasia | **abasia** *Inability to walk due to impaired coordination.* |
| abbassalingua | **tongue depressor; tongue blade** *As the name implies, the stick pushes the tongue down so the posterior aspect of the mouth can be viewed more readily.* |
| abducente | **abducent** *Abducting or to separate.* |
| abduttore pollicis brevi | **abductor pollicis brevis** *Abducts the thumb.* |
| abduttore pollicis lungo | **abductor pollicis longus** *Abducts and flexes the thumb.* |
| abito sterile | **gown** *A sterile gown used during surgical procedures.* |
| abitudine | **habit** *A custom or inclination.* |
| abitudine alla droga e disturbo di salute mentale | **dual diagnosis** *Term used to describe the presence of alcohol/drug addiction associated with a psychiatric diagnosis such as depression.* |
| ablazione | **ablation** *Surgical removal or amputation.* |
| aborto | **abortion** *Premature expulsion of the fetus from the uterus.* |
| aborto indotto | **induced abortion** *Surgical or medical evacuation of the fetus.* |
| aborto spontaneo | **miscarriage** *Spontaneous abortion.* |
| abruptio placentae | **abruptio placentae** *The premature detachment of a normally implanted placenta resulting in maternal decompensation.* |
| abusi | **abuse (sexual abuse)** |
| acalasia | **achalasia** *Inability to relax the smooth muscle fibers of the gastrointestinal tract. In the case of esophageal achalasia one has dilatation and hypertrophy of the esophagus.* |
| acalcolia | **acalculia** *The inability to perform mathematical calculations.* |
| acantoma | **acanthoma** *An adult cornifying squamous carcinoma.* |
| acantosi | **acanthosis** *Hypertrophy of the prickle cell layer of the skin.* |
| acantosi nigricans | **acanthosis nigricans** *A skin disorder characterized by dark, thick, velvety skin in the body folds and creases.* |
| acapnia | **acapnia** *A condition of lower than normal carbon dioxide level in the blood.* |
| acariasi | **acariasis** *Mite infestation.* |
| acaricide | **acaricide** *A treatment for mite infestation.* |
| acaro | **acarus** *A mite.* |
| acaro dei Thrombiculidae | **chigger** *A parasitic mite of the genus Trombicula.* |
| acatalasia | **acatalasia** *A condition characterized by the congenital absence of the enzyme catalase.* |
| acatisia | **acathisia** *The inability to sit quietly or to have motor restlessness.* |
| acatisia | **akathisia** *A condition exhibited by motor restlessness and inability to sit quietly.* |
| accelerare | **accelerate** *(To accelerate the healing process).* |
| accesso | **access** *Means of entry.* |
| accesso anorettale | **anorrectal abscess** *A localized collection of pus in the anorrectal region.* |
| accessorio | **accessory** *Complimentary or concomitant.* |
| accidente | **accident** |
| accomodazione | **accommodation** *A term used to describe the ability of the eye to adjust to various distances.* |
| accomodazione consensuale | **consensual light reflex** *Constriction of the pupil of one eye in sync with the other pupil upon exposure to light.* |

| Italian | English |
|---|---|
| accorciamento | **shortening** *Notable for having a shorter length.* |
| accordo | **agreement** *Accordance in opinion or feeling.* |
| acefalo | **acephalous** *A absence of a head.* |
| acetabulo | **acetabulum** *The cup-shaped cavity with which the head of the femur articulates.* |
| acetaminofene | **acetaminophen** *Mild analgesic drug used for pain relief.* |
| acetilcolina | **acetylcholine** *A reversible acetic acid ester of choline.* |
| acetonemia | **acetonemia** *The presence of acetone in the blood.* |
| acetonuria | **acetonuria** *The presence of acetone in the urine.* |
| achilia | **achylia** *The absence of chyle.* |
| achillodinia | **achilliodynia** *Pain around the calcaneal tendon.* |
| acida | **acid** *Substance with a pH less than 7.* |
| acidemia | **acidemia** *A lower than normal pH in the blood.* |
| acidità | **acidity** *Referring to an acid state.* |
| acido acetilsalicilico | **acetylsalicylic acid** *The chemical name for common aspirin.* |
| acido ascorbico | **ascorbic acid** *Commonly known as vitamin C; a deficiency of this vitamin causes scurvy.* |
| acido cloridrico | **hydrochloric acid** *A solution with a low pH formed by dissolving hydrogen chloride in water.* |
| acido desossiribonucleico | **deoxyribonucleic acid (DNA)** *The carrier of genetic information.* |
| acido desossiribonucleico | **DNA Deoxyribonucleic acid.** *The hereditary material in humans and almost all other organisms.* |
| acido folico | **folic acid** *Also called pteroylglutamic acid; a deficiency can cause megaloblastic anemia.* |
| acido grasso | **fatty acid** *A carboxylic acid occurring as a an ester in fats and oils.* |
| acido nicotinico | **nicotinic acid** *A deficiency of this substance results in pellagra.* |
| acido nucleico | **nucleic acid** *An organic compound found in living cells; its molecules contain nucleotides linked in long chains.* |
| acido para-aminobenzoico | **para-aminobenzoic acid** *A natural product (not FDA approved) reportedly beneficial for Peyronie's disease and scleroderma. It is a component of folic acid.* |
| acido para-aminoippurico | **para-aminohippuric acid (PAH)** *A chemical used for calculation of renal plasma flow.* |
| acido ribonucleico | **ribonucleic acid** *An acid present in all living cells, it is a messenger for DNA.* |
| acido ribonucleico ribosomiale | **ribosomal RNA** *Four chains designated by their appropriate coefficients.* |
| acido taurocolico | **taurocholic acid** *A bile acid composed of cholic acid and taurine.* |
| acido urico | **uric acid** *Uric acid is a purine-derived product of nitrogen metabolism that can increase the risk of gout and calculi.* |
| acinesia | **akinesia** *An absence of movement or sparsity of movement.* |
| acinestesia | **akinesthesia** *Lack of perception of movement.* |
| acino | **acinus** *A very small grape shaped portion of an acinous gland.* |
| acloridria | **achlorhydria** *The absence of hydrochloric acid in gastric secretions.* |
| acne | **acne** *Inflamed or infected sebaceous glands.* |
| acne congestiva | **acne rosacea** *A chronic disease characterized by the presence of flushing of the skin of the nose, forehead and cheeks.* |
| acne rosacea | **rosacea** *Erythema of the cheeks and nose caused by chronic vascular and follicular dilation.* |
| acne volgare | **acne vulgaris** *Chronic acne occurring on the face, chest and back of youth.* |
| acolia | **acholia** *The lack of bile.* |
| acondroplasia | **achondroplasia** *A congenital inadequacy of enchondral bone formation resulting in a type of dwarfism.* |

| Italian | English |
|---|---|
| acorea | **acorea** *The absence of the pupil of the eye.* |
| acqua | **water** *A colorless, odorless liquid.* |
| acqua potabile | **drinking water** *Water clean enough to ingest orally.* |
| acqueo | **aqueous** *Use of water as a solvent or medium.* |
| acquoso | **wet** *Covered in moisture.* |
| acrocefalia | **acrocephaly** *A condition characterized by a pointed head.* |
| acrocianosi | **acrocyanosis, Raynaud's disease** *A benign condition in which the feet and hands are cyanotic, cold and sweating.* |
| acrodermatite | **acrodermatitis** *Inflammation of the skin of the hands and/or feet.* |
| acrodinia | **acrodynia** *An infantile condition exhibited by swollen bluish-red extremities and later polyarthritis..* |
| acrofobia | **acrophobia** *The morbid fear of heights.* |
| acromatopsia | **achromatopsia** *Inability to differentiate yellow, blue, red or their intermediates.* |
| acromegalia | **acromegaly** *Hyperplasia of the nose, jaw, fingers and toes.* |
| acromion | **acromion** *The flattened process extending laterally from the spine of the scapula which forms the most prominent point of the shoulder.* |
| acrosarcomatosi di Kaposi | **Kaposi sarcoma** *Typically seen in AIDS patients, it is characterized by cutaneous reddish-purple macules and plaques.Also called multiple idiopathic hemorrhagic sarcoma.* |
| acrotico | **acrotic** *Referring to great weakness or absence of a pulse.* |
| actina | **actin** *A protein in the muscle that, along with myosin, facilitates muscle contraction and relaxation.* |
| actinic dermatitis | **actinic dermatosis** *A skin disease caused by exposure to radiation from the sun, ultraviolet waves or gamma radiation.* |
| actinomicina | **actomyosin** *Myosin and actin complex present in muscles.* |
| actinomicosi | **actinomycosis** *A chronic bacterial infection that effects the face and neck and is caused by Actinomyces israelii. In rare cases it can cause a pulmonary infection.* |
| acustico | **acoustic** *Referring to the auditory system.* |
| acustico | **auditory** *Referring to hearing.* |
| acutezza | **acuity** *1. Relating to accuracy of hearing, as in hearing acuity. 2. Severity of illness as in, "What is the patient's acuity?"* |
| acuto | **acute** *Abrupt onset.* |
| adattamento alla luc | **light adaptation** *The pupillary adjustment after going from a dark environment to one of bright light.* |
| adattamento scotopico | **dark adaptation** *Adjustment to low light by reflex dilation of the pupil.* |
| adattarsi | **adjust, to** *To modify a plan.* |
| adattilo | **adactylia** *A congenital condition exhibited by the absence of toes and fingers.* |
| addome | **abdomen** *The portion of the body bordered by the diaphragm and the pelvis.* |
| addome gonfio | **swollen (distended) abdomen** |
| addominale riflesso | **abdominal reflexes** *Elicited by stroking the abdomen lightly from mid-axillary line to umbilicus. A normal response is contraction of the umbilicus toward the stimulated side.* |
| addominocentesi | **abdominocentesis** *Puncturing of the abdominal wall for drainage purposes.* |
| addormentato | **asleep** *To be in a dormant or inactive state.* |
| adduttore | **adductor** *A muscle that brings a part to the midline.* |
| adduzione | **adduction** *To bring toward the midline.* |
| adenectomia | **adenectomy** *The removal of a gland.* |
| adenite | **adenitis** *The inflammation of a gland.* |
| adenoacatoma | **adenocanthoma** *Malignant tumor comprised of glandular tissue.* |

| Italian | English |
|---|---|
| adenocarcinoma | **adenocarcinoma** *Cancer from glandular tissue.* |
| adenofibroma | **adenofibroma** *Connective tissue with glands that form a tumor.* |
| adenoide | **adenoid** *Referring to a gland.* |
| adenoidectomia | **adenoidectomy** *Removal of the adenoids.* |
| adenoidi | **adenoids** *Pharyngeal tonsils.* |
| adenoidite | **adenoiditis** *Inflammation of the adenoids.* |
| adenoipofisi | **adenohypophysis** *The anterior portion of the pituitary gland.* |
| adenolinfoma | **adenolymphoma** *A salivary gland tumor, also called Warthin's tumor.* |
| adenoma cistico | **cystadenoma** *Adenoma associated with cysts of neoplastic origin.* |
| adenomioma | **adenomyoma** *A tumor characterized by the overgrowth of endometrial and uterine muscle tissue.* |
| adenomiosi | **adenomyosis** *A condition characterized by the overgrowth of endometrial and uterine muscle tissue.* |
| adenopatia | **adenopathy** *Generally referring to a condition of the lymphatic glands.* |
| adenosindifosfato | **adenosine triphosphate (ATP)** *A chemical that represents the energy reserve of the muscle.* |
| adenosindifosfato | **adenosine diphosphate** *A product of hydrolysis of ATP.* |
| adenosinmonofosfato | **adenosine monophosphate** *A nucleotide, it is produced when ATP is converted to ADP.* |
| adenovirus | **adenovirus** *A type of a virus that can cause upper respiratory tract infections.* |
| aderenza | **adhesion** *The abnormal adherence of tissue exposed to inflammation or after surgery.* |
| adiadococinesia | **adiadochokinesia** *The inability to perform rapid alternating movements.* |
| adiposo | **adipose** *Referring to fat. (adipose tissue)* |
| adiposo | **fatty** *Greasy or oily.* |
| adipsie | **adipsia** *Absence of thirst which can be caused by SIADH, hydrocephalus or injury/tumor to/of the hypothalamus.* |
| adito | **aditus** *The entrance to an organ or part.* |
| adiuvante | **adjuvant** *Term used to describe the medical treatment after initial therapy, as in adjuvant radiation therapy after initial chemotherapy.* |
| adolescenza | **adolescence** |
| adrenalina | **adrenaline (epinephrine)** *A hormone secreted by the adrenal glands and a synthetic medication used for treatment of allergic reactions and cardiac arrest.* |
| adrenalina | **epinephrine** *A hormone secreted by the adrenal gland.* |
| adrenalinico | **adrenergic** *That which is activated or transmitted by epinephrine.* |
| aeroba | **aerobe** *An organism that grows in the presence of oxygen.* |
| aerodontalgia | **aerodontalgia** *The dental pain that occurs with low atmospheric pressure, like during airflight.* |
| aerofagia | **aerophagy or aerophagia** *A condition associated with hysteria in which one swallow repeatedly swallows air and then belches.* |
| afachìa | **aphakia** *The congenital absence of the lens of the eye.* |
| afagia | **aglutition** *The inability to swallow.* |
| afagia | **aphagia** *The lack of eating.* |
| afasia | **aphasia** *Diminished ability to communicate via speech or writing.* |
| afasia anomica | **anomia** *Inability to name or recognize familiar objects.* |
| afasia anosmica | **anosmia** *Lack of the sense of smell.* |
| afebbrile | **afebrile** *Absence of fever.* |
| affaticato | **tired** *Fatigued.* |
| afferente | **afferent** *Moving toward the center.* |

| Italian | English |
|---|---|
| affettato | **affected** |
| affetto | **affect** *The expression of emotions or feelings.* |
| affezione erutiva o pustolosa | **pox** *A general term for fluid filled papules that upon rupturing leave pockmarks.* |
| affinità | **affinity** *To have a natural liking for.* |
| afflizione fetale | **fetal distress** *Term used to describe an abnormal heart rate or rhythm in a fetus indicating the need for urgent childbirth.* |
| afibrinogenemia | **afibrinogenemia** *Marked deficiency of fibrinogen in the blood.* |
| afide | **aphid** *A minute insect that feeds on plants.* |
| aflatossina | **aflatoxin** *A toxin produced by Aspergillus flavus.* |
| afonia | **aphonia** *The loss of voice.* |
| afta epizootica | **foot and mouth disease** *A contagious viral disease exhibited by oral and digital vesicles.* |
| agar | **agar** *Media used for bacterial cultures.* |
| agenesia | **agenesis** *The absence of an organ. (cerebellar agenesis)* |
| agente sialagogo | **sialogogue** *A substance that increase salivary flow.* |
| aggiungere | **add, to** *To count.* |
| agglutinazione | **agglutination** *The process of adherence of a mass.* |
| aggressione | **aggression** *Violent or hostile behavior.* |
| agitazione | **agitation** *A state of extreme emotional disturbance.* |
| agnazia | **agnathia** *Congenital abnormality characterized by the absence of the mandible.* |
| agnoscia | **agony** *Anguish or torment.* |
| agnosia | **agnosia** *A condition exhibited by the loss of sensory stimuli.* |
| agnosia acustico | **auditory agnosia** *Caused by a temporal lobe lesion, it is characterized by inability to recognize sounds as words.* |
| agnosia digitale | **finger agnosia** *The inability to distinguish which finger is being touched.* |
| agnosia gustativa | **gustatory agnosia** *The loss of the sense of taste.* |
| ago | **needle** *The slender cylindrical device attached to a syringe.* |
| ago biopsia | **needle biopsy** *Use of a needle to aspirate body contents for microscopic or pathologic examination.* |
| ago per puntura lombare | **needle for lumbar puncture** |
| agonista | **agonist** *A synthetic compound that activates cells normally activated by natural chemicals.* |
| agopuntura | **acupuncture** *Traditionally an aspect of Chinese medicine involving insertion of needles into the skin.* |
| agorafobia | **agoraphobia** *The fear of being in a large open space.* |
| agrafia | **agraphia** *The inability to express one's thoughts in writing.* |
| agranulocitosi | **agranulocytosis** *A condition characterized by leukopenia and neutropenia.* |
| agro | **sour** *An acid or bitter taste.* |
| aids | **AIDS** *Acquired Immunodeficiency Syndrome* |
| al cardiopalma | **nail biting** *A habit of chewing on one's fingernails.* |
| alattasia | **lactose intolerance** *The inability of the small bowel to digest lactose.* |
| albinismo | **albinism** *Congenital absence of pigment in the eyes, skin and hair.* |
| albino | **albino** *A person who lacks pigment in the eyes, skin and hair.* |
| albumina | **albumin** *A protein that is soluble in water and coagulates if heated.* |
| albuminuria | **albuminuria** *The presence of albumin in the urine.* |
| alcali | **alkali** *A class of compounds that form soluble carbonates.* |
| alcalino | **alkaline** *Referring to something with properties of an alkali.* |
| alcalinuria | **alkalinuria** *The urine in an alkaline state.* |

| Italian | English |
|---|---|
| alcaloide | **alkaloid** *Plant derived nitrogenous organic compound.* |
| alcalosis | **alkalosis** *A condition in which the pH is increased.* |
| alcaptonuria | **alkaptonuria** *A condition exhibited by the urine turning dark upon standing because of the presence of alkapton bodies in it.* |
| alcol | **alcohol** *Ethanol or ethyl alcohol.* |
| alcolismo | **alcoholism** *An addiction to alcohol.* |
| alcolizzato | **alcoholic** *A person with alcohol dependence.* |
| aldeidico | **aldehyde** *A substance derived by oxidizing and containing a CHO group from alcohol.* |
| aldosterone | **aldosterone** *A steroid secreted by the adrenal cortex that regulates electrolytes.* |
| aldosteronismo | **aldosteronism** *A condition characterized by the excessive secretion of aldosterone.* |
| alessia | **alexia** *Inability to read due to a central brain lesion.* |
| alfa-fetoproteina | **alpha-fetoprotein** *A glycoprotein that has a high serum level in hepatocellular and nonseminomatous germ cell tumors.* |
| alghe | **algae** *Nonflowering plants containing chlorophyll but without stems, roots, or leaves.* |
| algida | **algid** *cold* |
| algofobia | **algophilia** *Sexual perversion; getting pleasure in giving or receiving pain.* |
| algoritmo | **algorithm** *Any procedure designed to solve a problem in a step-by-step or mechanical fashion.* |
| alienato | **insane** *A term not used in formal medical evaluations that when used by a layperson means a serious mental illness.* |
| alienazione mentale | **insanity** *Referring to a serious mental illness.* |
| alienazione mentale | **madness** *Common term for insanity.* |
| alimentare | **alimentary** *Referring to the gastrointestinal tract.* |
| alimentazione enterico | **enteral feeding** *Nutrition supplied via the alimentary canal.* |
| alimentazione per sondaggio gastrico | **gavage** *The instillation of food into the stomach with use of a tube.* |
| alitosi | **halitosis** *Foul odor emanating from the mouth.* |
| allantoide | **allantois** *A posterior portion of the hind-gut of an embryo.* |
| allattamento al seno | **breast feeding** *The process of giving milk to a baby via the nipple.* |
| allattare al seno | **suckle, to** *An infant taking to his mother's nipple.* |
| allele | **allele** *A type of a gene; in humans there are two alleles per chromosome pair.* |
| allergene | **allergen** *Compound that causes an allergic reaction.* |
| allergia | **allergy** *An immune response by the body to a compound it is hypersensitive to.* |
| allettato | **bedridden** *Term used to indicate one is so ill they cannot get out of bed.* |
| alleviare | **alleviate, to** |
| alleviare | **relieve, to (pain)** *To make less severe.* |
| allopatia | **allopathy** *Treatment of disease with minute amounts of natural substances.* |
| alluce valgo | **hallux valgus** *Also called bunion, it is the lateral deviation of the great toe.* |
| alluce varo | **hallux varus** *Medial deviation of the great toe.* |
| allucinazione | **hallucination** *A perception that is not based on reality.* |
| allucinogeno | **hallucinogen** *A substance that elicits hallucinations.* |
| allungamento | **lengthening** *Becoming longer.* |
| alopecia | **alopecia** *The absence of hair in areas where it normally exists.* |

| Italian | English |
|---|---|
| alta pressione sanguigna | **high blood pressure** *Elevated arterial blood pressure.* |
| altezza | **height** *Distance between the bottom of the foot and top of the head.* |
| alto, elevato | **high** *Elevated.* |
| alveolare | **alveolar** *Referring to the alveolus.* |
| alveolo | **alveolus** *A small sac like structure commonly used for the pulmonary alveolus.* |
| amalgama | **amalgam** *An alloy that includes mercury as one ingredient.* |
| amalgamare | **amalgamate,to** *To make an amalgam by dissolving a metal in mercury.* |
| amaro | **bitter (taste)** *Having a harsh, unpleasant taste.* |
| amartoma | **hamartoma** *A nodule of superfluous tissue.* |
| amastia | **amastia** *A development condition exhibited by the absence of breasts.* |
| amaurosi | **amaurosis** *Blindness that occurs without an ocular lesion but may include the optic nerve.* |
| amaurosi fugax | **amaurosis fugax** *This transient monocular blindness is considered a sign of an impending stroke.* |
| ambidestro | **ambidextrous** *Ability to use both hands equal ability.* |
| ambientamento | **acclimatization** *The process of becoming adapted to a new environment.* |
| ambisessuale | **ambisexual** *Referring to both sexes.* |
| ambliopia | **amblyopia** *Decreased vision without an ocular lesion.* |
| ameba | **ameba** *A one-celled protozoan.* |
| amebiasi | **amebiasis** *A condition in which one is infected with amebae, mostly commonly Entamoeba histolytica.* |
| amebicida | **amebicide** *A compound used to treat amebiasis.* |
| amelia | **amelia** *A congenital anomaly exhibited by the absence of limbs.* |
| amenorrea | **amenorrhea** *The absence of menses.* |
| amenza | **amentia** *The absence of mental ability.* |
| ametra | **ametria** *Obsolete term for congenital uterine agenesis.* |
| ametropia | **ametropia** *Abnormal refractive ability of the eyes resulting in hypermetropia, myopia or astigmatism.* |
| amianto | **asbestos** *A heat resistant silicate material.* |
| amilase | **amylase** *An enzyme involved in the hydrolysis of starch.* |
| amiloidosi | **amyloidosis** *The accumulation of amyloid in body tissues.* |
| amiotonia | **amyotonia** *A condition associated with the lack of muscle tone.* |
| amiotrofia | **amyotrophy** *Atrophy of muscle tissue.* |
| ammalato | **patient** *The client being treated for a medical or surgical condition.* |
| ammiccamento | **blinking** *To open and close the eyelid rapidly.* |
| amminoacido | **amino acid** *A compound containing a carboxyl and an amino group.* |
| ammoniaca | **ammonia** *A colorless alkaline gas.* |
| amnesia | **amnesia** *The inability to remember past events.* |
| amnesia anterograda | **amnesia, antegrade** *The inability to remember events which occurred after the insult that caused the condition.* |
| amnio | **amnion** *The membrane lining the placenta which produces the amniotic fluid.* |
| amniocentesi | **amniocentesis** *Transabdominal aspiration of amniotic fluid.* |
| amniografia | **amniography** *X-ray of the gravid uterus after insertion of opaque dye.* |
| amorfo | **amorphus** *A fetus with no heart and no definitive shape.* |
| ampolla | **ampulla** *The dilated end of a duct.* |
| ampolla chyli | **ampulla chyli** *Also called cisterna chyli; it is a dilated area of the thoracic duct that collects lymph from several areas.* |
| amputazione | **amputation** *Typically referring to the surgical removal of a limb.* |

| Italian | English |
|---|---|
| anabolismo | **anabolism** *The formation of molecules in organisms from simpler molecules.* |
| anacroto | **anacrotic** *Referring to a prominent bulge on the ascending portion of a pulse recording.* |
| anaerobico | **anaerobe** *An organism that lives in the absence of oxygen.* |
| anafase | **anaphase** *A stage in mitosis following metaphase.* |
| anafilassi | **anaphylaxis** *An exaggerated response to a foreign substance.* |
| anale | **anal** *Near or referring to the anus.* |
| analettico | **analeptic** *A medication used as a stimulant to the central nervous system.* |
| analgesia | **analgesia** *The absence of pain.* |
| analgesico | **analgesic** *A medication used to remove pain.* |
| analisi del seme | **semen analysis** *Evaluation of semen used as part of a fertility workup.* |
| analizzatore del respiro | **breath test (for alcohol)** *A check of alcohol level by testing exhaled air.* |
| analogo | **analogous** *To resemble or be similar to.* |
| anaplasia | **anaplasia** *The loss of normal differentiation of tumor cells.* |
| anastomosi | **anastomosis** *Surgical formation of a connection between two previously separate parts.* |
| anatomia | **anatomy** *The study of body structure.* |
| anatomico | **anatomical** *Referring to the anatomy.* |
| anca; coscia | **hip** *The lateral eminence of the pelvis from the waist to the thigh; it is formed by the iliac crest and greater trochanter.* |
| anchiloglossia | **ankyloglossia** *Limitation of tongue motion because of a short frenulum.* |
| anchilosi | **ankylosis** *Abnormal immobility of a joint.* |
| anchilostoma | **hookworm** *A parasitic infection of the family Strongylidae that can cause anemia.* |
| anchilostomiasi | **ancylostomiasis** *A type of nematode parasite, also called hookworm.* |
| andare (all'ospedale) | **admission (to hospital)** |
| andatura | **gait** *The way one walks.* |
| andatura festinazione | **festinating gait** *Walking with increased speed involuntarily; often seen in Parkinson's disease.* |
| andatura ondeggiante | **waddling gait** *Walking in short steps in a swaying fashion.* |
| androgeno | **androgen** *A compound that produces masculinizing characteristics.* |
| androgino | **androgynous** *Referring to a female pseudohermaphroditism (a genetic female with masculine characteristics).* |
| androsterone | **androsterone** *A hormone excreted in the urine of men and women.* |
| anello | **ring** *A small circular band.* |
| anello inguinale profondo | **inguinal ring (deep)** *Indirect inguinal hernias exit the abdominal cavity via the deep inguinal ring.* |
| anello pericorneale | **pericorneal ring** *Also known as Kayser-Fleischer rings exhibited by presence of brown or grey-green rings on the cornea. This is from the deposition of copper and seen in Wilson's disease.* |
| anemia | **anemia** *Lower than normal red blood cell count.* |
| anemia aplastica | **aplastic anemia** *Bone marrow failure causing a decrease in all types of blood cells.* |
| anemia da carenza di ferro | **iron-deficiency anemia** *A microcytic anemia.* |
| anemia drepanocitica | **sickle-cell anemia** *A hereditary type of anemia characterized by crescent shaped red blood cells.* |
| anemie emolitico | **hemolytic anemia** *Reduced number of erythrocytes due to shortened survival and inability of the bone marrow to compensate.* |
| anencefalia | **anencephaly** *The congenital absence of the cranial vault and cerebral hemispheres.* |

| Italian | English |
|---|---|
| aneroide | **aneroid** *The absence of liquid.* |
| anestesia | **anesthesia** *Loss of sensation.* |
| anestesia del guanto | **glove anesthesia** *Absence of sensation of the hand and wrist.* |
| anestesia epidurale | **epidural anesthesia** *Medication into this space produces analgesia for surgical procedures.* |
| anestesia locale | **nerve block anesthesia** *Locally administered anesthesia.* |
| anestetico | **anesthetic** *A chemical that produces anesthesia.* |
| anestetista | **anesthetist** *A person who administers anesthesia.* |
| aneurisma | **aneurysm** *A condition exhibited by the dilatation of the walls of an artery or vein to form a blood-filled sac.* |
| aneurisma disseccante | **dissecting aneurysm** *A condition in which blood is present between the layers of an artery.* |
| anforesi | **anaphoresis** *Reduced activity of the sweat glands.* |
| angina erpetica | **herpangina** *An infectious disease caused by Coxsackie virus exhibited by vesicular lesion on the soft palate.* |
| angina indotta da esercizio | **exercised induce angina** *Chest pain noted during exertion related to coronary artery disease.* |
| angina pectoris | **angina pectoris** *Exercise induced myocardial ischemia.* |
| angioedema; edema angioneurotico | **angioedema** *Also called angioneurotic edema, it is caused by a histamine reaction. It can produce welts in mild cases but in severe cases can cause swelling of the lips and tongue.* |
| angiofibroma giugulare | **juvenile angiofibroma** *A noncancerous growth in the nose or pharyngeal region.* |
| angiografia | **angiography** *Roentgenographic imaging of blood vessels.* |
| angiografia delle coronarie | **coronary angiography** *Roentgenographic visualization of the coronary vessels after injection of dye.* |
| angiogramma | **angiogram** *Radiologic imaging of blood vessels.* |
| angioite | **angitis or angiitis** *The inflammation of a lymph or blood vessel.* |
| angioma | **angioma** *A tumor comprised of blood or lymph vessels.* |
| angioneurotico | **angioneurotic** *Caused by a neurosis affecting the blood vessels, like vasospasm.* |
| angioplastica | **angioplasty** *Surgical alteration of blood vessels.* |
| angiosarcoma | **angiosarcoma** *A sarcoma comprised of blood vessels.* |
| angiospasmo | **angiospasm** *A spasm of a blood vessel.* |
| angiotensina | **angiotensin** *A blood protein that increases aldosterone secretion.* |
| angoscia | **anguish** *Significant mental or physical pain.* |
| angoscia | **grief** *Deep sorrow.* |
| angoscia lancinante | **twitch** *A sudden jerking movement.* |
| anidro | **anhydrous** *Lacking water.* |
| anidrosi | **anhidrosis** *A condition exhibited by reduced quantity of sweat.* |
| anidrotico | **anhidrotic** *Something the reduces the quantity of sweat.* |
| animale domestico | **pet** *An animal kept for companionship.* |
| animale roditore | **rodent** *A gnawing mammal that includes rats and mice.* |
| aniseiconia | **aniseikonia** *A condition in which the ocular image of an object is viewed differently by each eye.* |
| anisocitosi | **anisocytosis** *Variation in size of erythrocytes.* |
| anisocoria | **anisocoria** *Pupillary diameter inequality.* |
| anisomelia | **anisomelia** *Unequal size of arms or legs.* |
| anisometropia | **anisometropia** *Refractive power inequality between the two eyes.* |
| annesso | **adnexa** *The appendages, for example, of the uterus are the ovaries, fallopian tubes and the ligaments of the uterus.* |
| anno | **year** *A time period that covers 365 days.* |
| annualmente | **yearly** *Occurring once each year.* |

| Italian | English |
|---|---|
| ano | **anus** *The body opening distal to the rectum.* |
| ano-perianale | **anoperineal** *Referring to the anus and perineum.* |
| anomalo | **aberrant** *Different than normal.* |
| anonichia | **anonychia** *Congenital absence of fingernails or toenails.* |
| anorchidismo | **anorchous** *The absence of testicles.* |
| anoressia | **anorexia** *The loss of appetite.* |
| anorettale | **anorectal** *Referring to the anus and rectum.* |
| anormale | **abnormal** |
| anossia | **anoxia** *Reduced oxygen levels in body tissues.* |
| anossiemia | **anoxemia** *Reduction in blood oxygen concentration.* |
| anovulazione | **anovulatory** *Lack of ovulation.* |
| ansia | **anxiety** *Nervousness or unease.* |
| ansimante | **wheezing** *A whistling or musical sound made by air passing through a narrowed airway.* |
| ansioso | **anxious** *Experiencing nervousness or unease.* |
| antagonista | **antagonist** *A muscle or agent that acts in counteract to effects of another muscle or agent.* |
| antelmintico; vermifugo | **anthelmintic** *An agent used to destroy worms.* |
| antepartum | **antenatal** *Refers to events before birth.* |
| anteriore | **anterior** *Toward the front.* |
| anterogrado | **anterograde** *Moving forward.* |
| anteroinferiore | **anteroinferior** *Toward the front and lower part.* |
| anterolaterale | **anterolateral** *Toward the front and away from the midline.* |
| anteromediana | **anteromedian** *Toward the front and toward the midline.* |
| anteroposteriore | **anteroposterior** *From front to the back. (An AP x-ray has the beam directed from the front to the back.)* |
| anterosuperiore | **anterosuperior** *Toward the front and the upper part.* |
| antiacido | **antacid** *A medication, usually with a calcium or magnesium base that binds with acid in the stomach.* |
| antibiotico | **antibiotic** *A medication that inhibits or kills microorganisms.* |
| anticoagulante | **anticoagulant** *Medication used to inhibit coagulation.* |
| anticodon | **anticodon** *A series of three nucleotides that form a unit of genetic code for transfer RNA.* |
| anticolinergico | **anticholinergic** *Parasympathetic blocker.* |
| anticolinesterasi | **anticholinesterase** *Cholinesterase blocker.* |
| anticonvulsivante | **anticonvulsant** *Medication used to treat seizures.* |
| anticorpo | **antibody** *A protein that combines with and counteracts foreign substances.* |
| antidepressivo | **antidepressant** *Medication used to treat depression.* |
| antidoto | **antidote** *A medication that neutralizes a toxin.* |
| antiemetico | **antiemetic** *A medication used to control nausea.* |
| antiemicrania | **antimigraine** *Medication used to treat headaches.* |
| antigene | **antigen** *A foreign substance, like bacteria, that induces an immune response.* |
| antiinfiammatorio | **anti-inflammatory** *Medication used to reduce inflammation.* |
| antiistamina | **antihistamine** *Medication used to treat conditions exhibited by a histamine response* |
| antilinfocito | **antilymphocyte** *A serum globulin that has antibodies to lymphocytes.* |
| antimalariale | **antimalarial** *Medication used to treat malaria.* |
| antimetabolita | **antimetabolite** *A substance that impedes metabolism.* |
| antimicotico | **antimycotic** *Inhibition of fungal growth.* |
| antimitotico | **antimitotic** *Impeding mitosis.* |

| Italian | English |
|---|---|
| antiperistaltico | **antiperistaltic** *An agent that impedes normal peristalsis.* |
| antipiretico | **antipyretic** *Medication used to treat fever.* |
| antiprurito | **antipruritic** *Medication used to treat pruritus.* |
| antisettico | **antiseptic** *A substance that inhibits microorganism growth.* |
| antisiero | **antiserum** *A substance that contains antibodies to specific antigens.* |
| antispastico | **antispasmodic** *Medication used to treat muscle spasm.* |
| antitiroide | **antithyroid** *A substance inhibiting the effect of the thyroid.* |
| antitosse | **antitussive** *Medication used to diminish a cough.* |
| antitossina | **antitoxin** *A substance that inhibits the effect of a toxin.* |
| antitreponemico fluorescente | **fluorescent antibody test (FTA test)** |
| antitreponemico fluorescente | **FTA test** *Fluorescent treponemal antibody test for syphilis.* |
| antitrombina | **antithrombin** *A substance that inhibits thrombin, thus decreasing the body's ability to coagulate.* |
| antiveleno | **antivenin** *An antitoxin formulated for various types of snake bites.* |
| antiversione | **anteversion** *The forward leaning of an organ.* |
| antrace | **anthrax** *An infectious disease caused by Bacillus anthracis; there are cutaneous, inhalation and gastrointestinal syndromes.* |
| antro | **antrum** *Referring to a cavity or chamber.* |
| antrotomia | **antrotomy** *To cut open the antrum.* |
| anulare | **annular** *Referring to a ring.* |
| anuria | **anuria** *The lack of urine excretion.* |
| anziano | **elderly** *Advanced in years.* |
| aorta | **aorta** *The large artery originating at the left ventricle and going to the pelvis where it bifurcates.* |
| aortico | **aortic** *Referring to the aorta.* |
| apatia | **apathy** *Lack of interest in one's environment or indifference.* |
| aperatura | **aperture** *An opening or hole, as in the hole the light passes through in a camera.* |
| apice | **apex** *The highest point of something.* |
| apice cardiaco | **apex of heart** *Normally found 8cm to the left of the midsternal line in the 5th intercostal space.* |
| apice della lingua | **proglottis** *Any segment of a tapeworm.* |
| apicectomia | **apicectomy** *Removal of the apex of the petrous portion of the temporal bone.* |
| aploide | **haploid** *Either a single set of chromosomes or a set of nonhomologous chromosomes.* |
| apnea | **apnea** *Absence of respiration.* |
| apnea del sonno | **sleep apnea** *Episodic apnea during sleep that is exhibited by daytime symptoms of fatigue, difficulty concentrating and sleepiness.* |
| apofisi | **apophysis** *Generally a bony outgrowth that forms a process or tubercle.* |
| apofisi coracoide | **coracoid** *A prominence on the scapula to which the biceps is attached.* |
| aponeurosi | **aponeurosis** *A tendinous expansion that connects with muscle to move a part.* |
| apoplexy | **apoplexy** *Extravasation of blood within an organ. For example, neonatal apoplexy is consistent with intracranial hemorrhage.* |
| apparecchio acustico | **hearing aid** *A device that fits in the ear used to amplify sound.* |
| apparecchio giustaglomerulare | **juxtaglomerular apparatus** *Cells located in the tunica media of the afferent glomerular arterioles.* |
| apparecchio ortopedico | **brace** *A splint.* |
| apparentemente | **ostensibly** *Synonym of apparently and seemingly.* |

| Italian | English |
|---|---|
| apparizione | **emergence** *Coming into prominence.* |
| appendice | **appendix** *An appendage of the cecum.* |
| appendicectomia | **appendectomy** *Surgical excision of the appendix.* |
| appendicite | **appendicitis** *Inflammation of the appendix.* |
| appercezione | **apperception** *The ability to interpret sensory impressions.* |
| appiattimento del'aspetto superiore del naso | **low nasal bridge** *A flattening of the top part of the nose.* |
| appiattire | **flatten, to** *To make even.* |
| applicatore | **applicator** *A device used to apply a topical medication.* |
| apprendimento | **learning** *The intentional acquisition of knowledge.* |
| apprensivo | **apprehensive** *A fear that something unpleasant will happen.* |
| appropriato | **apt** *Suitable in the circumstances.* |
| approssimarsi | **approximate, to** *To bring together, as in wound margins.* |
| approssimativamente | **approximately** *Nearly but not completely.* |
| approssimativo | **approximate** *Nearly but not totally accurate.* |
| approvazione | **approval** *Accepting something as satisfactory.* |
| appuntamento | **appointment** *A previously scheduled time to see a person.* |
| appurare | **ascertain, to** *Synonym of "to determine".* |
| aprassia | **apraxia** *The inability to carry out intentional movements when paralysis is not present.* |
| aptene | **hapten** *The molecular component that determines immunologic specificity.* |
| aptialismo | **aptyalism** *Diminished or absence of saliva.* |
| aracnodattilia | **arachnodactyly** *A condition exhibited by abnormally long and slender fingers.* |
| aracnoide | **arachnoid** *Refers to that which resembles a spider web.* |
| arbovirus | **arbovirus** *Virus that is transmitted by arthropods; responsible for diseases such as Yellow fever and dengue fever.* |
| archenteron | **gastrocele** *Protrusion of part of the stomach in the form of a hernia.* |
| archivio | **file** *Patient record or folder.* |
| arco | **arcus** *Narrow opaque band.* |
| arco sopracciliare | **superciliary arch** *The area superior to the upper border of each orbit.* |
| areola | **areola** *The pigmented skin surrounding a nipple.* |
| argento | **silver** *A precious metal with atomic number 47.* |
| argininosuccinicadiduria | **argininosuccinicaciduria** *Presence of arginosuccinic acid in the urine; associated with mental retardation.* |
| argiria | **argyria** *The greyish discoloration of the skin and conjunctiva.* |
| aria | **air** |
| aritmia | **arrhythmia** *An abnormal heart rhythm.* |
| aritmia sinusale | **sinus arrhythmia** *Cardiac dysrhythmias related to sinoatrial nodal dysfunction.* |
| arrenoblastoma | **arrhenoblastoma** *An ovarian tumor that results in masculine secondary sex characteristics.* |
| arresto cardiaco | **cardiac arrest** *Cessation of function of the heart.* |
| arrossare | **blush, to** *To have an increased volume of blood flow to one's face causing a red tint to the skin.* |
| artefatto | **artifact** *An aberration from the normal.* |
| arteria | **artery** *Vessel that carries oxygenated blood from the heart to the periphery.* |
| arteria brachiale | **brachial artery** *A continuation of the axillary artery and branches into the radial and ulnar among others.* |
| arteria carotide | **carotid** *Referring to the large artery on each side of the neck.* |
| arteria coronaria | **coronary vessel** *Referring to a coronary artery.* |

| Italian | English |
|---|---|
| arteria femorale | **femoral artery** *Continuation of the external iliac to the popliteal artery.* |
| arteria innominata | **innominate artery** *The first branch off the aortic arch that branches into the right common carotid and right subclavian arteries.* |
| arteriectomia | **arteriectomy** *Surgical excision of an artery.* |
| arteriografia | **arteriography** *Roentgenography of an artery after infusion of contrast media.* |
| arterioplastica | **arterioplasty** *Surgical repair of an artery.* |
| arteriosclerosi | **arteriosclerosis** *Hardening and thickening of arterial walls.* |
| arterioso | **arterial** *Referring to an artery.* |
| arteriotomia | **arteriotomy** *Creation of an opening in an artery.* |
| arterite | **arteritis** *Inflammation of an artery.* |
| articolare | **articular** *Referring to a joint.* |
| articolazioine tibioastragalica | **ankle joint** *The articulation of the tibia/fibula and talus.* |
| articolazione acromioclavicolare | **acromioclavicular joint** *Referring to the junction of the acromion and clavicle.* |
| articolazione dell'anca | **hip joint** *The lateral eminence of the pelvis from the waist to the thigh; it is formed by the iliac crest and greater trochanter.* |
| articolazione sella | **saddle joint** *A joint that exhibits two saddle type surfaces at a 90 degree angle to each other, such as the carpometacarpal joint.* |
| articolazione; giuntura | **joint** *Articulation of two adjacent bones.* |
| articulazione temporomandibolare | **temporomandibular joint** *The hinged joint of the temporal bone and mandible.* |
| artificiale | **artificial** *Not natural produced.* |
| artralgia | **arthralgia** *Joint pain.* |
| artralgia | **arthrodynia** *Joint pain.* |
| artrite | **arthritis** *Joint inflammation.* |
| artrite gonococcico | **gonorrheal arthritis** *A type of arthritis caused by the gram negative diplococcus Neisseria gonorrhoeae.* |
| artrite reumatoide | **rheumatoid arthritis** *A symmetric peripheral polyarthritis.* |
| artrodesi | **arthrodesis** *Surgical fusion of a joint.* |
| artrografia | **arthrography** *Joint roentgenography.* |
| artropatia emofilico | **hemophilic arthropathy** *The permanent joint disease caused by recurrent bleeding into the joint.* |
| artroplastica | **arthroplasty** *Plastic surgery involving a joint.* |
| artroscopia | **arthroscopy** *Viewing of the inside of a joint with a specially designed scope.* |
| artrotomia | **arthrotomy** *Surgical opening of a joint.* |
| asbestosi | **asbestosis** *Lung disease caused by the inhalation of asbestos.* |
| ascaris lumbricoides | **ascaris** *A nematode from genus intestinal lumbricoid parasite, also called round worm.* |
| ascella | **armpit** *A common term for axilla.* |
| ascella | **axilla** *The hollow beneath the arm.* |
| ascellare | **axillary** *Referring to the axilla.* |
| ascesso | **abscess** *A localized collection of pus.* |
| ascesso del fegato piogeno | **pyogenic liver abscess** *A pus filled fluid collection in the liver.* |
| ascesso del midollo spinale | **spinal cord abscess** *A localized collection of purulent material in or adjacent to the spinal cord.* |
| ascesso epatico amebico | **amebic liver abscess** *A pus filled fluid collection within the liver caused by amoebe.* |
| ascesso fegato | **liver abscess** *A localized collection of pus in the liver.* |

| Italian | English |
|---|---|
| ascesso gengivale sottoperiosteo | **gumboil** *Swelling noted on the gingiva over a dental abscess.* |
| ascesso intra-addominale | **intraabdominal abscess** *A collection of pus in the abdomen.* |
| ascesso peritonsillare | **peritonsillar abscess** |
| ascesso peritonsillare | **quinsy** *Peritonsillar inflammation or abscess.* |
| ascesso retrofaringeo | **retropharyngeal abscess** *A collection of purulent material posterior to the pharynx.* |
| ascesso subareolare | **subareolar abscess** *A purulent fluid collection in the areolar gland.* |
| ascite | **ascites** *Serous fluid in the abdominal cavity.* |
| asepsi | **asepsis** *Lack of infection.* |
| asessuale | **asexual** *Without sex or sex organs.* |
| asettico | **aseptic** *Being free of septic matter.* |
| asfissia | **asphyxia** *A condition exhibited by a lack of oxygen and subsequent loss of consciousness or death.* |
| asimmetria | **asymmetry** *Lack of symmetry.* |
| asinclitismo | **asynclitism** *Oblique presentation of the head during delivery.* |
| asintomatico | **asymptomatic** *The absence of symptoms.* |
| aspermatismo | **aspermia** *Absence of sperm.* |
| aspetto | **appearance** *The way someone looks or presents.* |
| aspetto generale | **general appearance** *The overall look of a patient.* |
| aspiratore | **aspirator** *A device used to remove fluid from a cavity.* |
| aspirazione di meconio | **meconium aspiration** *Presence of meconium on the newborn indicating there was fetal distress in-utero.* |
| aspirina | **aspirin** *Common name for acetylsalicylic acid.* |
| asportazione | **removal** *The act of removing something.* |
| assesta-ossa | **bonesetter** *A person who sets bones without being a physician.* |
| assistenza | **assistance** *The act of helping.* |
| assistenza infermieristica | **nursing care** *The assessment and treatment provided by nurses.* |
| associato; imparentato | **related to** *Causally connected.* |
| assone | **axon** *The structure along which nerve impulses are transmitted from the cell body to other cells.* |
| assorbente | **sanitary napkin** *Cloth or synthetic material used to absorb menstrual blood.* |
| assorbimento | **absorption (intestinal absorption)** |
| assunzione | **intake** *An amount of food taken into the body.* |
| assunzione di cibo | **food intake** *Quantitative record of nutritional intake.* |
| assunzione di liquidi | **fluid intake** *The amount of oral consumption plus the amount of intravenous fluids administered.* |
| asteatosi | **asteatosis** *A condition exhibited by diminished sebaceous secretion.* |
| astenia | **asthenia** *Diminished strength and energy.* |
| astenopia | **asthenopia** *Visual fatigue accompanied by ocular pain.* |
| astereognosi | **astereognosis** *Lack of ability to recognize objects by touching them.* |
| asterissi | **asterixis** *Commonly known as a flapping tremor, it is characterized by involuntary jerking movements of the hands and is seen commonly in hepatic encephalopathy.* |
| astragalo | **astragalus** *Synonym of talus.* |
| astringente | **astringent** *An agent causing contraction of the skin.* |
| astrocitoma | **astrocytoma** *A tumor comprised of astrocytes.* |
| atassia | **ataxia** *Lack of muscular coordination.* |
| atavismo | **atavism** *The inheritance of characteristics from remote rather than immediate ancestors.* |
| atelectasia | **atelectasis** *Incomplete expansion or collapse of a lung.* |

| Italian | English |
|---|---|
| aterogenico | **atherogenic** *Something that causes atheromatous lesions in arterial walls.* |
| ateroma | **atheroma** *Degenerative arteriosclerosis.* |
| atetosi | **athetosis** *An involuntary symptom exhibited by continuous slow, writhing movements, mostly in the hands.* |
| atipico | **atypical** *Not usual.* |
| atlante | **atlas** *The first cervical vertebra.* |
| atomizzatore | **atomizer** *A device for propelling a fine mist.* |
| atonia | **atony** *Absence of normal muscle tone.* |
| atresia | **atresia** *Closure of a body orifice as in atresia ani in which there is a congenital imperforate anus.* |
| atresia di coana | **choanal atresia** *A congenital condition characterized by blockage of the nasal passages by tissue.* |
| atriale | **atrial** *Referring to the atrium.* |
| atrio | **atrium** *Referring to a chamber used as an entrance, as in the entrance to the heart.* |
| atrioventricolare | **atrioventricular** *Referring to the atrium and ventricle.* |
| atrofia | **atrophy** *A diminution in the size of a part.* |
| atrofia peroneale | **peroneal atrophy** *Progressive muscle atrophy in the peroneal region.* |
| atrofico | **atrophic** *Referring to atrophy.* |
| atropina | **atropine** *A parasympathetic agent derived from Atropa belladonna.* |
| attacco di panico | **panic attack** *Sudden, profound anxiety.* |
| attaco; crisi epilettica | **seizure** *An episode of tonic/clonic movement noted in epilepsy.* |
| attendibile | **reliable** *Trustworthy.* |
| attenuazione | **relief** *Alleviation from pain or discomfort.* |
| attinon | **actinon** *A radioactive element, radon-219; short lived isotope of radon.* |
| attitudine | **aptitude** *A natural talent for something.* |
| attività | **activity** |
| atto dell'annusare | **sniffing** *Short, rapid nasal inhalation.* |
| attrito, sfegamento | **friction** *Grating or rasping.* |
| attualmente | **currently** *Presently.* |
| audiogramma | **audiogram** *The recording of a one's hearing in decibels.* |
| audiologo | **audiologist** *A specialist in the field of hearing.* |
| audiometro | **audiometer** *A device used to measure hearing.* |
| auricola | **auricle** *The external portion of the ear.* |
| auricolare | **auricular** *Referring to the auricle.* |
| auricolotemporale | **auriculotemporal** *The area of the ear and temple.* |
| auscultazione | **auscultation** *The act of listening to sounds emanating from the body.* |
| autismo | **autism** *A mental condition exhibited by difficulty in forming relationships, communicating and uses abstract thought.* |
| autistico | **autistic** *Referring to autism.* |
| autoanticorpo | **autoantibody** *An antibody that acts against the organism's own tissue.* |
| autoantigene | **autoantigen** *A normal tissue constituent that prompts a cell-mediated response.* |
| autoclave | **autoclave** *A device used for sterilization with the use of steam under pressure.* |
| autogeno | **autogenous** *Self-generated.* |
| autoimmunizzazione | **autoimmunization** *The body's ability to promote an immune response without external resources.* |
| autoipnosi | **autohypnosis** *Self-hypnosis.* |
| autolisi | **autolysis** *A state of self destruction of cells within a body.* |

| Italian | English |
|---|---|
| autopsia | **autopsy** *Examination of a body post-mortem in an attempt to determine cause of death.* |
| autosomico | **autosomal** *Referring to an autosome.* |
| autotransfusione | **autotransfusion** *The reinfusion of one's own blood.* |
| avambraccio | **forearm** *Segment of the arm from the elbow to wrist.* |
| avere la raucedine | **frog in the throat, to have** *An expression describing hoarseness.* |
| aviaria | **avian** *Referring to birds.* |
| avitaminosi | **avitaminosis** *A state of vitamin deficiency.* |
| avulsione | **evulsion** *Forcible extraction.* |
| avvelenamento da monssido di carbonio | **carbon monoxide poisoning** *This tasteless, odorless gas causes constitutional symptoms but can lead to death upon inhalation.* |
| avvelenamento da piombo | **lead poisoning** *The ingestion of lead, exhibited in severe cases by paralysis, encephalopathy, purple gingiva, and colic.* |
| avventato; esantema | **rash** *Exanthema or urticaria.* |
| avventizio | **adventitia** *Outermost.* |
| azoospermia | **azoospermia** *The absence of spermatozoa in the semen.* |
| azotemia | **azotemia** *Prerenal disease.* |
| azoto | **nitrogen** *A colorless, odorless gas used as a coolant in the liquid form.* |
| azoturia | **azoturia** *An excess of urea in the urine.* |
| bacillare | **bacillary** *Referring to bacilli.* |
| bacillo | **bacillus** *A rod-shaped bacterium.* |
| bacino | **basin** *A small bowl used for washing.* |
| bagassosi | **bagassosis** *A pulmonary disorder contracted from inhalation of the waste of sugar cane (bagasse dust).* |
| balanite | **balanitis** *Inflammation of the glans of the penis.* |
| balbuzie | **stammering** *The impulse to repeat the first letter of words and involuntary pauses while speaking.* |
| balbuziente | **stuttering** *Involuntary repetition of the first consonant.* |
| ballottamento | **ballottement** *Presence of movement of a floating object by palpation.* |
| balsamo | **balm** *A topical medical preparation.* |
| bambino, bambina | **child** *A person aged 1 to 8 years old. (male, female)* |
| banda | **bandage** *A strip of gauze used to immobilize or support.* |
| barriera ematoencefalica | **blood brain barrier** *A matrix of capillaries that move blood between the blood and brain, as well as, limiting some substances from passing.* |
| basale | **basal** *Referring to the base.* |
| basilare | **basilar** *Referring to the base or lower segment.* |
| basino di memtismo | **emesis basin** *A small bowl used to catch vomitus.* |
| basofilo | **basophil** *A polymorphonuclear granulocyte.* |
| basso addome | **abdomen, lower** |
| basso contenuto di grassi alimentari | **low-fat foods** *Nutrients with lower than normal fat content.* |
| bastoncino di nitrato d'argento | **silver nitrate stick** *A medical device used to treat hypergranulation tissue.* |
| battere | **throb, to** *The beat with strong regular rhythm.* |
| battericida | **bactericidal** *An agent that destroys bacteria.* |
| batterico | **bacterial** *Referring to bacteria.* |
| batteriemia | **bacteremia** *The presence of bacteria in the blood.* |
| batterio | **bacteria** *Plural for any organism of the order Eubacteriales.* |
| batteriostatico | **bacteriostatic** *An agent that impedes bacterial growth.* |
| batteriuria | **bacteriuria** *The presence of bacteria in the urine.* |
| battito | **beat** *As in heart beat.* |
| battito cardiaco | **heart beat** *A single contraction of the heart.* |

| Italian | English |
|---|---|
| batuffolo di cotone (utilizzato per raccogliere le mestruazioni | **tampon** *Disposable intravaginal product used to collect blood from menstruation.* |
| bendaggio | **banding** *The process of encircling with a thin piece of material.* |
| bendaggio a fionda o a triangolo | **sling** *A device used to give support to an injured extremity.* |
| bendaggio a spiga | **spica** *A figure of eight bandage.* |
| bendaggio elastico | **elastic bandage** *A stretch gauze used for compression of an extremity.* |
| benigno | **benign** *Not harmful.* |
| bere | **drink, to** *To imbibe.* |
| berilliosi | **berylliosis** *A lung exhibited by granulomas and caused by inhalation of beryllium.* |
| beta-bloccante | **betablocker** *A substance that inhibits adrenergic stimulation. It is used to reduce pulse, blood pressure and to treat angina.* |
| bezoar | **bezoar** *A concretion composed of either hair, vegetable/fruit fibers or hair and vegetable/fruit fibers that is found in the stomach.* |
| bianco | **white** *Of the color of snow.* |
| biauricolare | **binaural** *Referring to both ears.* |
| biblioteca | **library** |
| bicuspide | **bicuspid** *Having two points as in bicuspid valve or a premolar tooth.* |
| bifido | **bifid** *Presence of two branches.* |
| biforcuto | **bifurcate** *When one branch divides into two branches.* |
| bilance neonati | **baby-scale** *A device used to weigh an infant.* |
| bilancio acido-base | **acid-base balance** *The equilibrium of the electrolytes in the body.* |
| bilaterale | **bilateral** *Referring to both sides.* |
| bile | **bile** *An alkaline fluid secreted by the liver to aid digestion.* |
| biliare | **biliary** *Referring to bile, bile ducts or gallbladder.* |
| bilioso | **bilious** *Something that contains bile.* |
| bilirubina | **bilirubin** *A pigment found in bile that is responsible for the yellow color seen in patients with elevated serum levels of bilirubin.* |
| biliuria | **biliuria** *The presence of bile in the urine.* |
| biliverdina | **biliverdin** *A green pigment formed by oxidation of bilirubin.* |
| bimanuale | **bimanual** *Use of two hands, as in bimanual pelvic examination in which the right hand touches the cervix uteri and the left hand presses above the mons pubis.* |
| binoculare | **binocular** *Referring to both eyes.* |
| biochimica | **biochemistry** *The study of chemistry and physiochemical processes in living organisms.* |
| biodisponibilità | **bioavailability** *The portion of a drug that is able to be utilized by the body after it is introduced to the body.* |
| biologia | **biology** *The study of living organisms.* |
| biopsia | **biopsy** *The removal and examination of bodily tissues or fluids.* |
| biopsia del midollo osseo | **bone marrow puncture** *The aspiration of marrow to look for pressure of disease.* |
| biopsia del spazzola | **brush biopsy** *The process of tissue sampling using a brush.* |
| biopsia escissionale | **excisional biopsy** *Surgical removal of tissue for pathologic examination.* |
| biopsia per aspirazione | **aspiration biopsy** *Removal of fluid from a cavity for pathologic analysis.* |
| biossido | **dioxide** *A compound containing two oxygen atoms.* |
| biotina | **biotin** *A vitamin involved in the synthesis of fatty acids and glucose.* |
| biovulare | **binovular** *Derived from two different ova.* |
| bisbigliare; sussurrare | **whisper, to** *To speak in a volume that is barely discernible.* |

| Italian | English |
|---|---|
| bisogno | **need** *A want or obligation.* |
| bissinosi | **byssinosis** *A disease caused by inhalation of cotton dust; a type of pneumoconiosis.* |
| bisturi | **bistoury; scalpel** *A surgical knife.* |
| blastomicosi | **blastomycosis** Infection caused by organisms of genus Blastomyces. |
| blatta | **cockroach** *A beetle-like insect with long legs and antennae.* |
| blefarite | **blepharitis** *Inflammation of the eyelids.* |
| blefarospasmo | **blepharospasm** *A spasm of the orbicularis oculi muscle that causes closure of the eyelid.* |
| blenorragia | **blennorrhea** *Discharge from the mucous membranes, usually referring to gonorrhea.* |
| bloccante i canali del calcio | **calcium channel blocker** *A medication used to treat angina, supraventricular arrhythmias and hypertension; it works by blocking calcium influx into myocytes and vascular smooth muscle cells.* |
| blocco atrioventricolare | **atrio-ventricular block** *An interruption of the electrical conduction at the atrio-ventricular node.* |
| blocco cardiaco di conduzione | **heart block** *An alteration in the cardiac electrical conduction system.* |
| blocco di branca | **bundle branch block** *A cardiac dysrhythmia produced by a blockage of a branch of the bundle of His.* |
| blu | **blue** *A color between green and violet.* |
| bocca | **mouth** *The orifice on the lower part of the face.* |
| boccata | **mouthful** *A large quantity of something in one's mouth.* |
| bolla | **bulla** *A large cutaneous serous filled vesicle.* |
| bolo | **bolus** *A fluid bolus is a phrase used for rapid infusion of fluid.* |
| borbottare | **mumble, to** *To speak quietly and indistinctly.* |
| bordo, margine | **border** *Margin.* |
| borsite | **bursitis** *Inflammation of the bursa.* |
| borsite e periborsite dell'alluce | **bunion** *Swelling of the bursa of the metatarsal head of the first metatarsal.* |
| borsite achille | **achillobursitis** *Inflammation around the calcaneal tendon.* |
| braccio | **arm** *One of two upper extremities.* |
| braccio rotto | **broken (arm)** *Fracture of the arm.* |
| brachiale | **brachial** *Referring to the arm.* |
| brachicefalia | **brachycephaly** *The presence of a short broad skull.* |
| bradicardia | **bradycardia** *Lower than normal cardiac rate measured in beats per minute.* |
| bradichinina | **bradykinin** *A peptide that causes contraction of smooth muscle and dilation of blood vessels.* |
| branchiale | **branchial** *Referring to or resembling the gills of a fish.* |
| bregma | **bregma** *Located at the convergence of the coronal and sagittal sutures.* |
| brillante | **bright** *Giving out a lot of light.* |
| brivido non intenso | **shiver** *A trembling.* |
| bromidrosi | **bromidrosis** *Foul smelling perspiration.* |
| bromismo | **bromism** *Poisoning caused by excessive intake of bromine.* |
| bronchiale | **bronchial** *Referring to the bronchus.* |
| bronchiettasia | **bronchiectasis** *The presence of abnormally wide bronchi or branches.* |
| bronchiolite | **bronchiolitis** *Inflammation of the pulmonary bronchioles.* |
| bronchiolo | **bronchiole** *A small branch that a bronchus divides into.* |
| bronchite | **bronchitis** *Inflammation of the mucous membranes of the bronchioles that causes bronchospasm and cough.* |
| bronco | **bronchus** *The major air channels that bifurcate from the distal trachea.* |

| Italian | English |
|---|---|
| broncogeno | **bronchogenic** *Referring to the bronchi.* |
| broncografia | **bronchography** *Roentgenography of the bronchi after administration of contrast media.* |
| broncopolmonite | **bronchopneumonia** *Pneumonia that starts in the distal bronchioles.* |
| broncoscopia | **bronchoscopy** *Use of a scope to visualize the bronchi.* |
| broncospasmo | **bronchospasm** *Bronchial smooth muscle spasm.* |
| brucellosi | **brucellosis** *A gram-negative bacteria in cattle that causes persistent fever in humans.* |
| bruno | **brown** *Coffee-colored.* |
| bubbone | **bubo** *An inflamed, swollen lymph node in the axilla or inguinal region.* |
| bucato | **cribriform** *Like a sieve; the olfactory nerves pass through the cribriform plate of the ethmoid bone.* |
| bulimia | **bulimia** *Pathologic increase in hunger.* |
| cachessia | **cachexia** *Generalized weakness and severe wasting.* |
| cadavere | **cadaver** *A dead body.* |
| caduceo | **caduceus** *An ancient herald's wand with two serpents twined around that is a symbol of the medical arts.* |
| caffè macinato emesi | **coffee-ground emesis** *Bloody vomitus with appearance of ground coffee.* |
| calamita | **magnet** *A piece of iron with atoms ordered to make it magnetic.* |
| calazio | **chalazion** *A chronic granuloma of a meibomian gland.* |
| calcagno | **calcaneus** *Commonly called the heel bone.* |
| calcagno | **heel** *Proximal portion of the plantar aspect of the foot.* |
| calcareo | **calcareous** *Referring to something containing lime or calcium.* |
| calce | **calyx** *A cup shaped organ or cavity.* |
| calciferolo | **calciferol** *It is formed when egesterol is exposed to ultraviolet light; a D vitamin.* |
| calcificazione | **calcification** *Deposition of calcium salts causing hardening of an organic tissue.* |
| calcinazione | **calcitonin** *A thyroid hormone that lowers serum calcium levels.* |
| calcio | **calcium** *A chemical element that is an essential component in teeth and bone.* |
| calcoli biliari | **gallstone** *Calculus produced in the bile duct or gallbladder.* |
| calcolo | **calculus** *A stone of minerals that can lead to the blockage of the bile duct or ureters.* |
| calibrare | **calibrate, to** *To adjust an instrument using a standard.* |
| calibrazione | **calibration** *The process of calibrating an instrument.* |
| calibro | **gauge** *The size or thickness of something. An 18gauge needle.* |
| callo | **callus** *Thickened hardened skin.* |
| callosità | **callosity** *Callus; thickened hardened skin.* |
| callosità | **clavus** *A corn or horny protrusion.* |
| calore | **heat** *The quality of being hot.* |
| caloria | **calorie** *A unit of heat.* |
| calvaria; volta cranica | **calvaria** *The portion of the skull that is composed of the superior aspects of the occipital, parietal and frontal bones.* |
| calzino | **socks** *Worn on the feet before one puts on shoes.* |
| camera posteriore | **posterior chamber of the eye** *An aqueous filled space between the cornea and the lens.* |
| camicia di forza | **strait-jacket** *A device used to temporarily restrain the arms of patients who are psychotic and violent.* |
| camminando ingessatura | **walking cast** *A cast used for simple fractures of the lower leg.* |
| camminata piede cadente | **drop foot gait** *A gait characterized by dragging the foot, as there is no ankle dorsiflexion; usually associated with steppage gait.* |

| Italian | English |
|---|---|
| camminatore | **walker** *A metal frame used to facilitate walking.* |
| campi allo stomaco | **stomach cramps** *Sensation of muscle contraction in the epigastric area.* |
| campionatura | **sampling** *The taking of samples.* |
| campione | **specimen** *A sample for medical testing.* |
| campo visivo | **visual field** *The complete area a person can see with their eyes in a fixed position.* |
| canale inguinale superficiale | **superficial inguinal ring** *The opening of the aponeurosis of the external oblique muscle for the round ligament or spermatic cord.* |
| canale ionico | **ion channel** *A selectively permeable cell membrane to certain ions.* |
| canale sacrale | **sacral canal** *The portion of the vertebral canal that progresses into the sacrum.* |
| canale semicircolare | **semicircular canal** *The anterior, posterior and lateral canals in the inner ear that assist in balance control.* |
| canalicolo | **canaliculus** *A term for various small channels.* |
| canapa | **cannabis** *A plant from the Cannibidaceae family that is known for its psychotropic effects.* |
| cancellare | **cancel, to** *To stop or revoke.* |
| cancerogeno | **carcinogenic** *That which causes cancer.* |
| cancro | **cancer; carcinoma** *A disease of uncontrolled abnormal cell growth.* |
| cancroide | **cancroid** *A tumor occurring in the stomach, small or large bowel.* |
| candeggina | **bleach** *A solution that includes sodium hypochlorite.* |
| candela | **candle** *A cylindrical piece of wax with a central wick.* |
| cannula | **cannula** *A tube inserted into the body.* |
| capacità di resistenza | **stamina** *Ability to maintain physical or mental exertion for a long period.* |
| capacità polmonare totale | **lung capacity, total** *The amount of air in the lungs after a maximal inhalation.* |
| capacità vitale | **vital capacity (VC)** *The maximal amount of air exhaled after a maximal inhalation.* |
| capacità vitale forzata | **forced vital capacity** *Vital capacity measured as the patient is exhaling as rapidly as possible.* |
| capelli | **hair (of head)** |
| capezzolo | **nipple** *The small projection on the breast thru which milk is secreted.* |
| capillare | **capillary** *A vessel that connects arterioles to venules.* |
| capo | **caput** *The head.* |
| capogiro | **giddiness** *A tendency to fall or dizziness.* |
| capsula per medicamenti | **capsule** *Medication in the form of a capsule.* |
| capsula, tunica | **capsule** *A membranous sheath that covers an organ or structure.* |
| capsulite | **capsulitis** *Inflammation of a capsule.* |
| capsulotomia | **capsulotomy** *Incision of a capsule as in with eye surgery.* |
| caput succedaneum | **caput succedaneum** *Edema that occurs in the scalp of an infant during child-birth.* |
| carboidrati | **carbohydrate** *A group of organic compounds including sugar and starch.* |
| carbossiemoglobina | **carboxyhemoglobin** *A compound formed from hemoglobin when it is exposed to carbon monoxide.* |
| carcinoide | **carcinoid** *A tumor occurring in the stomach, intestine and colon.* |
| carcinoma bronchiale | **bronchial carcinoma** *A general term for a malignancy of the bronchi.* |
| carcinoma, cancro | **carcinoma** *A malignant growth.* |
| carcinomatosi | **carcinomatosis** *Dissemination of cancer throughout the body.* |
| cardiaco | **cardiac** *Referring to the heart.* |

| Italian | English |
|---|---|
| cardias | **cardia** *The superior aspect of the stomach at the opening of the esophagus.* |
| cardiologia | **cardiology** *A specialty of medical practice involve treatment and prevention of heart disease.* |
| cardiopatia ischemica | **ischemic heart disease** *Inadequate blood supply to the heart.* |
| cardiovascolare | **cardiovascular** *Referring to the heart or circulatory system.* |
| cardite | **carditis** *Inflammation of the heart.* |
| cardite reumatica | **rheumatic heart disease** *A manifestation of rheumatic fever, frequently causing valvular dysfunction.* |
| carena | **carina** *The protrusion of the lowest tracheal cartilage.* |
| carie | **caries** *Referring to decay or death of a tooth.* |
| carie dentaria | **dental caries** *Decay of teeth.* |
| cariocinesi | **karyokinesis** *A part of mitosis involving the cell nucleus division.* |
| cariotipo | **karyotype** *The arrangement of chromosomes in a single cell.* |
| carne | **flesh** *The tissue between the skin and bones.* |
| carnoso | **carneous** *Synonym of fleshy.* |
| carotene | **carotene** *A hydrocarbon that can be converted to vitamin A.* |
| carpo | **carpus** *The joint between the hand and wrist.* |
| carpometacarpico | **carpometacarpal** *Referring to the carpus and metacarpus.* |
| carpoptosi | **wrist drop** *The inability to hyperextend the wrist due to radial nerve injury.* |
| cartella clinica | **clinical record** *The ongoing medical summary.* |
| cartella clinica | **medical record** *The electronic or paper report on a patient.* |
| cartelle colori | **color chart** *A card used to check for color blindness.* |
| cartilagine aritenoide | **arytenoid** *Referring to the cartilage in the posterior larynx.* |
| cartilagine cricoidea | **cricoid cartilage** *The ring-shaped cartilage of the larynx.* |
| cartografia | **mapping** *A collection of data points showing spatial distribution.* |
| caruncola | **caruncle** *A small fleshy protuberance.* |
| caseina | **casein** *The principal protein in milk, a phospholipid.* |
| castrazione | **castration** *Excision of the gonads.* |
| catabolismo | **catabolism** *The reduction of complex molecules to more simple ones in living organisms.* |
| cataforesi | **cataphoresis** *The use of an electric field to move charged particles in fluid.* |
| catalessia | **catalepsy** *A condition exhibited by rigidity and the person maintains the same position if he is moved by another.* |
| cataplessia | **cataplexy** *A condition exhibited by rigidity and immobility.* |
| cataratta | **cataract** *An opacity of an eye lens or the capsule.* |
| catarro | **catarrh** *Inflammation of a mucous membrane.* |
| catarsi | **catharsis** *The act of cleansing or purging, usually referring to thought.* |
| catartico | **cathartic** *To be cleansed or evacuated, referring to thought or the cleansing of the bowels.* |
| catatonia | **catatonia** *Seen in schizophrenia, it is a state of stupor or excitability and abnormal movements.* |
| caterere urinario a tre vie | **three way foley** *A urinary tube used for irrigation of the bladder.* |
| catetere | **catheter** *A flexible tube inserted into the body.* |
| catetere a permanenza | **indwelling catheter** *Continuous use tube usually referring to a tube in the urinary bladder.* |
| catetere urinario di Foley | **Foley catheter** *A drainage tube placed in the urinary bladder via the urethra.* |
| cateterismo a scopo dilatante | **bougienage** *Passage of a bougie through a body orifice with the goal of increasing the diameter of the orifice.* |
| caudale | **caudal** *Referring to a cauda.* |

| Italian | English |
|---|---|
| caudato | **caudate** *Referring to the caudate nucleus.* |
| caustico | **caustic** *Abrasive or corrosive.* |
| cauterio | **cautery** *Application of an electric current to cut something.* |
| caviglia | **ankle** *The area of the ankle joint.* |
| cavità | **cavity** *Pouch or chamber.* |
| cavo | **hollow** *An indentation.* |
| cecità | **blindness** *Absence of visual perception.* |
| cecità per i colori | **color blindness** *The inability to distinguish colors.* |
| ceco | **cecum** *The portion of the bowel between the ileum and and the ascending colon.* |
| cefalea | **headache** *Cephalgia.* |
| cefalea a grappolo | **cluster headache** *A unilateral, severe, recurrent headache.* |
| cefalico | **cephalic** *Towards the head.* |
| celiaco | **celiac** *Referring to the abdominal cavity.* |
| cellula calice | **goblet cell** *Aids in the secretion of respiratory and intestinal mucous.* |
| cellula capello | **hair cell** *Epithelial cells with hairlike projections.* |
| cellula parietale | **parietal cell** *Acid secreting cells of the stomach.* |
| cellula plasma | **plasma cell** *A cell that produces only one type of antibody.* |
| cellulare | **cell** *The smallest functional unit of an organism.* |
| cellule a bersaglio | **target cell** *An abnormal cell that is present in liver disease and certain hemoglobinopathies.* |
| cellule ematiche | **blood cells** *A common term that does not differentiate between erythrocyte or leukocyte.* |
| cellulosa | **cellulose** *A polysaccharide that occurs naturally in fibrous products.* |
| centigrado | **centigrade** *A scale with 100 gradations, usually referring to a temperature scale.* |
| centimetro | **centimeter** *One hundredth of a meter.* |
| centre | **center** *A point equidistant from all sides.* |
| centrifuga | **centrifuge** *Machine used to separate substances of different weights.* |
| centripeto | **centripetal** *The movement toward the center.* |
| cera | **wax** *Cerumen.* |
| cercaria | **cercaria** *Larval trematode worm that live in a molluscan.* |
| cerebrale | **cerebral** *Referring to the cerebrum.* |
| cerebrazione | **cerebration** *Operating activity of the cerebrum.* |
| cerottoreazione | **patch test** *A test used to determine which substances provoke an allergic response in a patient.* |
| certificato di vaccinazione | **vaccine certificate** *A document that denotes what vaccines have been received by the holder.* |
| cerume | **cerumen** *Waxy substance found normally in the external ear canals.* |
| cervelletto | **cerebellum** *The part of the brain in the posterior portion of the skull that controls muscle coordination and movement.* |
| cervello | **brain** *A common term for cerebrum.* |
| cervicale | **cervical** *Referring to the neck or the cervix.* |
| cervice | **cervix uteri** *The narrow end of the uterus.* |
| cervicectomia | **cervicectomy** *Excision of the cervix uteri.* |
| cervicite | **cervicitis** *Inflammation of the cervix.* |
| cestodi | **cestode** *A class of parasitic flatworms.* |
| che sta sotto | **underlying** *Causative, unexposed, or fundamental.* |
| cheilite | **cheilitis** *Inflammation of the lip.* |
| chelazione | **chelation** *The process used to bind a compound with metal typically used in the treatment of poisoning.* |

| Italian | English |
|---|---|
| cheloide | **keloid** *Hypertrophic scar tissue that forms after a minor cut or surgical procedure.* |
| chemiorecettore | **chemoreceptor** *A sense organ that responds to stimuli.* |
| chemiotassi | **chemotaxis** *The response of an organism to chemical agents.* |
| chemioterapia | **chemotherapy** *Use of medication (chemical agents) in the treatment of disease. This term is commonly used to refer to the treatment of cancer patients with medication.* |
| chemosi | **chemosis** *Swelling of conjunctival tissue adjacent to the cornea.* |
| cheratectasia | **keratectasia** *Obtrusion of the cornea.* |
| cheratectomia | **keratectomy** *Excision of a portion of the cornea.* |
| cheratina | **keratin** *A protein found in the skin, hair, nails and enamel of the teeth.* |
| cheratoma | **keratoma** *A protuberance of horny tissue.* |
| cheratomalacia | **keratomalacia** *Softening of the cornea.* |
| cheratosi | **keratosis** *A growth of keratin such as a wart or callosity.* |
| chetoacidosi | **ketoacidosis** *Usually referring to diabetic ketoacidosis in which ketones are broken down, causing a decrease in blood pH.* |
| chetonemia | **ketonemia** *Presence of ketone in the blood.* |
| chetonuria | **ketonuria** *Presence of ketone in the urine.* |
| chetosi | **ketosis** *The presence of an abnormally high level of ketones in the blood and body tissues.* |
| chi presta soccorso medico | **caregiver** *A person who provides care to another.* |
| chiamare | **yell, to** *To speak in a loud tone.* |
| chiaro | **overt** *Not hidden.* |
| chiasma | **chiasma** *The optic chiasma is the area inferior to the hypothalamus where the optic nerves cross.* |
| chilo | **chyle** *A combination of lymph fluid and fat that enters the blood via the thoracic duct.* |
| chilomicrone | **chylomicron** *A one micron particle of emulsified fat.* |
| chiloso | **chylous** *Referring to chyle.* |
| chimera | **chimera** *A mixture of genetically distinct tissues.* |
| chimo | **chyme** *The gruel produced by gastric digestion.* |
| chinasi | **kinase** *An enzyme that facilitates movement of phosphate from ATP to another molecule.* |
| chinetosi | **motion sickness** *Nausea associated with travel.* |
| chiocciola | **cochlea** *The essential organ of hearing which is in a spiral form.* |
| chiodo intramidollare | **pin, intramedullary** *Hardware used for fracture management or during joint replacement.* |
| chiropratica | **chiropractic** *Referring to the medical practice of adjusting malaligned joints.* |
| chiropratico | **chiropractor** *A medical practitioner who is involved with the treatment of disease by manipulating malaligned joints.* |
| chirurgico | **surgical** *Referring to surgery.* |
| chirurgo | **surgeon** *A physician who performs surgery.* |
| chiuso | **closed** |
| cianocobalamina | **cyanocobalamin** *Also called B12; used to treat pernicious and other macrocytic anemias.* |
| cianosi | **cyanosis** *Bluish discoloration of the skin and mucous membranes.* |
| cicatrice | **cicatrix (scar)** *New tissue in a healed wound.* |
| cicatriziale | **cicatricial** *Referring to cicatrix.* |
| ciclite | **cyclitis** *Inflammation of the ciliary body.* |
| ciclo anovulare | **anovulatory cycle** *A menstrual cycle in which no ovum is released.* |

| Italian | English |
|---|---|
| ciclo di Kreb | **Krebs cycle** *The process of aerobic respiration by which living cells generate energy.* |
| ciclo di vomito | **cyclical vomiting** *Periods of recurrent vomiting with no apparent pathologic cause and the person has a normal state of health between the episodes.* |
| ciclodialisi | **cyclodialysis** *The surgical creation of a communication between the anterior chamber of the eye and the suprachorodial space for the purpose of treating glaucoma.* |
| cicloplegia | **cycloplegia** *Paralysis of the ciliary muscle.* |
| ciclotimia | **cyclothymia** *Manic-depressive tendencies.* |
| ciclotomia | **cyclotomy** *Surgically creating an opening in the ciliary body.* |
| cieco | **blind** *Absence of sight.* |
| cifoscoliosi | **kyphoscoliosis** *An abnormal outward and lateral curvature of the spine.* |
| cifosi | **hunchback** *Synonym of kyphosis.* |
| cifosi | **kyphosis** *Abnormal outward curvature of the spine.* |
| ciglia | **cilia** *The hairs growing on the eyelid or a motile extension of a cell surface.* |
| ciglia | **eyelash** *Each of the short hairs on the eyelid.* |
| cilindro renale epiteliale | **epithelial cast** *Debris found in the urine composed of columnar renal epithelium.* |
| cilindro urinario | **urinary casts** *A protein precipitated from renal tubules and excreted in the urine.* |
| Cimex lectularius; cimice | **bedbug Cimex lectularius.** *A small insect that is parasitic and hides in clothing or bedding.* |
| cinconismo | **cinchonism** *The toxic effects induced by ingestion of cinchona bark; it is exhibited by tinnitus, deafness and cognitive changes.* |
| cineplastica | **kineplasty** *An amputation done in a fashion to facilitate ambulation.* |
| cinesi | **kinesis** *Movement of a part in response to a stimulus* |
| cinto erniario | **truss** *A synthetic device for containing a hernia within the abdomen.* |
| cintura | **belt** *A strap used to hold clothing up.* |
| circadiano | **circadian** *Referring to a 24 hour period.* |
| circoncisione | **circumcision** *Surgical excision of the foreskin.* |
| circonferenza | **circumference** *The distance around an object or part.* |
| circonferenza addominale | **abdominal girth** *Waist circumference.* |
| circonvoluzione | **gyrus** *Convolutions of the brain where there is infolding.* |
| circoscritto | **circumscribed** *To have well defined borders.* |
| cirrosi | **cirrhosis** *A liver disease characterized by destruction of liver cells and increased connective tissue.* |
| ciste ovarico | **ovarian cysts** *Generally used to describe benign tumors.* |
| ciste pilonidale | **pilonidal cyst** *A small cone-shaped cluster of tissue situated posterior to the third ventricle of the brain.* |
| cistectomia | **cystectomy** *Surgical removal of a cyst or the bladder.* |
| cisti Bartholin | **Bartholin's cyst or abscess** *This is a purulent fluid collection in the Bartholin cysts which are located in the perivaginal area.* |
| cisti di meibomio | **meibomian cyst** *An enclosed fluid collection along a sebaceous gland of the eyelid.* |
| cisti idatidea | **hydatid cyst** *A cyst produced by and containing tapeworm larvae.* |
| cisti poplitea | **Baker cyst** *A synovial fluid collection in the popliteal fossa.* |
| cisticercosi | **cysticercosis** *The state of being infected with a type of tapeworm.* |
| cistico | **cystic** *Referring to a cyst.* |
| cistifellia | **gallbladder** *The organ adjacent to the liver that stores bile and secretes it into the duodenum.* |

| Italian | English |
|---|---|
| cistinosi | **cystinosis** *A congenital disorder of increased cystine that leads to renal insufficiency, rickets and dwarfism.* |
| cistinuria | **cystinuria** *The presence of cystine in the urine.* |
| cistite | **cystitis** *Inflammation of the urinary bladder.* |
| cisto dermoide | **dermoid cyst** *An abnormal growth containing hair follicles, skin and sebaceous glands.* |
| cisto tireoglosso | **thyroglossal cyst** *A common congenital growth in the thyroglossal duct.* |
| cistocele | **cystocele** *Protrusion of the urinary bladder through the vaginal wall.* |
| cistografia | **cystography** *Roentgenographic visualization of the urinary bladder after insertion of contrast media.* |
| cistografia svuotamento | **voiding cystography** *Roentgenography of the bladder and urethra after administration of contrast media.* |
| cistolitiasi | **cystolithiasis** *Presence of a calculus in the urinary bladder.* |
| cistoscopia | **cystoscopy** *Direct visualization of the urinary bladder with a cystoscope.* |
| cistoscopio | **cystoscope** *A device used to visualized the urinary bladder.* |
| citologia | **cytology** *The study of cells, their function and structure.* |
| citoplasma | **cytoplasm** *The protoplasm of the cell except for the nucleus.* |
| citotossico | **cytotoxic** *Referring to being harmful to cells.* |
| citotossina | **cytotoxin** *That which is harmful to cells.* |
| claudicazione | **claudication** *Intermittent claudication is a phrase used to describe pain experienced in the leg from arterial insufficiency.* |
| claustrofobia | **claustrophobia** *An unreasonable fear of being in an enclosed environment.* |
| clavicola | **clavicle** *A bone that articulates with the sternum and scapula.* |
| clavicola | **collarbone** *Common term for the clavicle.* |
| cleidotomia | **cleidotomy** *A procedure used in difficult deliveries in which the clavicle is broken to facilitate childbirth.* |
| clinico | **clinic** *A building where patients are evaluated.* |
| clisma | **enema** *A procedure involving insertion of fluid into the rectum.* |
| clisma baritato | **barium enema** *Administration of barium into the rectum followed by roentgenography to check for rectal or colon abnormalities.* |
| clitoride | **clitoris** *A small erectile body in the anterosuperior aspect of the vulva.* |
| cloasma | **chloasma** *Brown or black macula that occur on the face during pregnancy or when there is ovarian dysfunction.* |
| clonico | **clonic** *Referring to a spasm that alternates in rigidity and relaxation.* |
| clono del palato | **palatal myoclonus** *An involuntary, persistent, rapid regular tremor of the soft palate and face.* |
| clono del piede | **ankle clonus** *An abnormal response exhibited by alternating plantar- and dorsiflexion noted after the examiner rapidly dorsiflexes the foot.* |
| cloridrato | **hydrochloride** |
| cloroformio | **chloroform** *A colorless, sweet smelling liquid formerly used as a general anesthetic.* |
| cloroma | **chloroma** *A malignant tumor associated with myelogenous leukemia.* |
| coagulazione | **coagulation** *The formation of a clot.* |
| coagulo | **clot** *A thrombus or embolus.* |
| coagulo sanguigno | **blood clot** *A mass of coagulated blood.* |
| coana | **choanae** *The two openings between the nasal cavity and the nasopharynx.* |
| coartazione dell'aorta | **coarctation of the aorta** *A stricture, as in narrowing of the aorta.* |
| cobalto | **cobalt** *A metal that with causes polycythemia with increased ingestion.* |
| cocaina | **cocaine** *A highly addictive opiate derivative.* |

| Italian | English |
|---|---|
| coccige | **coccyx** *The small bone formed by the natural fusion of rudimentary vertebrae.* |
| coccigodinia | **coccydynia** *Coccygeal pain.* |
| cocco | **coccus** *A spherical shaped bacterium.* |
| codeina | **codeine** *A morphine derived analgesic.* |
| codone | **codon** *A series of three nucleotides that form a unit of genetic code.* |
| cognome | **surname** *One's given "last" name that generally changes for women upon marriage to that of the man's surname.* |
| coilonichia | **koilonychia** *Thin and concave fingernails.* |
| coito | **coitus** *Sexual intercourse between members of the opposite sex.* |
| colagogo | **cholagogue** *A compound used to stimulate flow of bile from the liver.* |
| colangiogramma | **cholangiogram** *Radiologic imaging of the gallbladder and bile ducts.* |
| colangite | **cholangitis** *Inflammation of the bile ducts.* |
| colare | **weep, to** *To ooze fluid, such as from a wound.* |
| colecistectomia | **cholecystectomy** *Surgical excision of the gallbladder.* |
| colecistite | **cholecystitis** *Inflammation of the gallbladder.* |
| colecistoenterostomia | **cholecystenterostomy** *Creation of a surgical anastomosis between the intestine and the gallbladder.* |
| colecistolitiasi | **cholecystolithiasis** *The presence of gallstones in the gallbladder.* |
| colectomia | **colectomy** *Surgical removal of part of the colon.* |
| coledocolitotomia | **choledocholithotomy** *Creation of an incision in the bile duct for the purpose of removing a stone.* |
| colelitiasi | **cholelithiasis** *Presence or creation of gallstones.* |
| colemia | **cholemia** *Bile or bile products in the blood.* |
| colera | **cholera** *An infectious disease exhibited by vomiting and diarrhea and caused by Vibrio cholerae.* |
| colesteatoma | **cholesteatoma** *A cystic mass that has a lining made of keratinizing material and cholesterol.* |
| colesterolo | **cholesterol** *A compound or its derivatives are found in cell membranes and precursors to hormones but high levels can cause atherosclerosis.* |
| colesterolo alto | **high cholesterol** *Elevated serum cholesterol.* |
| colica | **colic** *Acute abdominal pain.* |
| colica renale | **renal colic** *Pain caused by passage of a calculus through the ureter.* |
| colinergico | **cholinergic** *Referring to the stimulation, activation or transmission of acetylcholine.* |

| Italian | English |
|---|---|
| colinesterasi | **cholinesterase** *An esterase used to cleave acetylcholine into choline and acetic acid.* |
| colite | **colitis** *Inflammation of the colon.* |
| colite ulcerativo | **ulcerative colitis** *Recurrent episode of inflammation of the membranous layer of the colon.* |
| colla | **glue** *Plastic cements* |
| collageno | **collagen** *The principal supportive protein bone, skin, tendon and cartilage.* |
| collasso | **collapse** *A physical or mental breakdown.* |
| collasso da calore | **heat exhaustion** *A condition that occurs secondary to prolonged exposure to high ambient temperature; it is exhibited by subnormal temperature, dizziness and nausea.* |
| collirio | **eye drops** *Liquid applied to eyes for various medical problems.* |
| collo | **neck** *The part of the body that connects the body to the head.* |
| collo del femore | **neck of the femur** *The portion of the femur between the shaft and head.* |
| collodio | **collodion** *A product of the breakdown of colloid.* |
| colloidale | **colloid** *A solution used for infusion, such as albumin or hetastarch, that are more likely to remain in the intravascular space than crystalloids.* |
| coloboma | **coloboma** *A congenital defect that involves a fissure of the eye.* |
| colon | **colon** *The portion of the large intestine that goes from the cecum to the rectum.* |
| colon ascendente | **ascending colon** *The portion of the colon between the cecum and the right colic flexure.* |
| colonna spinale posteriore | **posterior columns** *The dorsal portion of the gray matter of the spinal cord.* |
| colonna vertebrale | **vertebral column** *The cervical, thoracic and lumbar vertebrae.* |
| colorante di Ziehl-Neelsen | **Ziehl-Neelsen carbolfuchsin stain** *A stain used to detect acid-fast bacilli that appear red on the methylene blue background.* |
| colore | **flushing** *Transient erythema due to heat, stress or disease.* |
| colori di congiuntiva | **color of conjunctiva** *A point of assessment to check for pallor.* |
| coloscopia | **colonoscopy** *Inspection the color, ideally to the cecum, with a lighted scope.* |
| colostomia | **colostomy** *Surgically creating an opening in the colon that is extended to outside the abdominal wall.* |
| colostro | **colostrum** *The fluid secreted by the mammary glands a few days around parturition.* |
| colpo apoplettico | **stroke** *Common term for cerebrovascular accident.* |
| colpo di calore | **heat stroke** *A condition caused by excessive exposure to high ambient temperature; it is exhibited by dry skin, thirst, vertigo, muscle cramps and nausea. The three forms are heat exhaustion, heat cramps and sunstroke.* |
| colpo di frusta | **whiplash** *Common term for cervical strain following a sudden deceleration.* |
| colpocele | **colpocele** *A hernia into the vagina.* |
| colporrafia | **colporrhaphy** *A surgical procedure that involves suturing the vagina.* |
| colposcopia | **colposcopy** *Use of a scope to visualize the vagina and cervix.* |
| colposcopio | **colposcope** *A scope used to visualize the vagina.* |
| coltura | **culture** *The growth of bacteria in artificial medium.* |

| Italian | English |
|---|---|
| coluria | **choluria** *Term indicating the presence of bile in the urine.* |
| coma | **coma** *A state of unconsciousness.* |
| comatoso | **comatose** *Referring to a coma.* |
| comedone | **comedone** *The medical term (singular) for blackheads.* |
| commensale | **commensal** *Living in or on another organism without being a detriment.* |
| commozione cerebrale | **concussion** *Head trauma resulting in temporary loss of consciousness.* |
| compatibile | **compatible** *To coexist without problems.* |
| compatibile con | **consistent** *Compatible with something or congruous with.* |
| compendio | **compendium** *A concise summary about a subject.* |
| compiacenza | **compliance** *The act of going along with a plan.* |
| compiere | **accomplish, to** *Achieve.* |
| completamente a termine | **full-term** *A normal length pregnancy.* |
| comportamento di alimentazione | **feeding behavior** *How a child is tolerating breast or cup feeding.* |
| composti | **compound** *A substance formed by covalent union of two or more atoms.* |
| compressa preparati ritardo | **sustained release tablet** *Describes a medicine that is slowly dispersed so it has a lasting effect.* |
| compressione | **compression** *Squeezing together.* |
| compressione di midollo spinale | **cord compression** *Pressure being applied to the spinal cord.* |
| comune | **common** *That which is usual.* |
| conato di vomito | **retching** *Spasm of the stomach without presence of gastric material.* |
| conca | **concha** *A part of the body that is spiral shaped. Nasal concha are the small bones in the sides of the nasal cavity.* |
| concavità | **acetabular** *Referring to the acetabulum.* |
| concavità | **concavity** *The state of being concave.* |
| concentrazione | **concentration** *The quantity of a substance per unit volume.* |
| concentrico | **concentric** *Referring to circles or arcs that share the same center.* |
| concepimento | **conception** *The act of an egg being fertilized by sperm.* |
| concrescenza | **accretion** *The expected growth of tissue from the intake of nutrients.* |
| concrezione | **concretion** *A hard solid mass.* |
| condilo | **condyle** *A rounded protrusion of a bone.* |
| condiloma acuminato | **condyloma** *A warty papule near the anus or vulva.* |
| condotto lattifero | **lactiferous duct** *A canal that carries milk.* |
| condotto uditivo esterno | **external ear canal** *Auditory canal.* |
| condrite | **chondritis** *Cartilaginous inflammation.* |
| condrodinia | **chondralgia** *Cartilaginous pain.* |
| condroma | **chondroma** *Cartilaginous hyperplastic growth.* |
| condromalacia | **chondromalacia** *Excessive softening of the cartilages.* |
| condromalacia patellare | **chondromalacia of the patella** *Softening of the articular cartilage of the patella.* |
| condrosarcoma | **chondrosarcoma** *Cartilaginous tumor which exhibits rapid growth.* |
| conffabulazione | **confabulation** *The fabrication of experiences to compensate for memory loss.* |
| confidenza | **confidence** *Self-assurance.* |
| confinamento | **confinement** *As in confined to bed.* |
| conflitto | **conflict** *Dispute or disagreement.* |
| confusione | **confusion** *Disorientation.* |
| congelamento | **freezing (as in ambient temperature)** *Below 0 Celsius.* |
| congelamento | **frostbite** *Local tissue destruction after exposure to cold.* |

| Italian | English |
|---|---|
| congenito | **congenital** *A disease or anomaly present from birth.* |
| congestizio | **congestive** |
| congiuntiva | **conjunctiva** *The membrane that lines the eyelid.* |
| congiuntivite | **conjunctivitis** *Inflammation of the conjunctiva.* |
| cono | **cone** *A light sensitive cell in the retina.* |
| conoscenza | **cognition** *The process of acquiring thought or understanding.* |
| conoscere | **acquaint, to** *To make someone familiar with something.* |
| conosciuto | **known** *Recognized or familiar.* |
| consanguineità | **consanguinity** *The relationship by blood.* |
| conscio | **conscious** *Being award and being able to respond to one's surroundings.* |
| conseguire | **achieve, to** *To complete something one was striving for.* |
| conservativo | **conservative** *Control rather than elimination of a disease.* |
| consigliabile maritale | **marital counseling** *Therapy aimed at marriage reconciliation.* |
| consigliare | **advise, to** *To give counsel.* |
| consulenza genetica | **genetic counseling** *A discussion of the concerns related to genetic testing.* |
| contagio | **contact** *The touching of two bodies or a person who has been exposed to a contagious disease.* |
| contagioso | **contagious** *Description of a disease that can be spread by direct or indirect contact.* |
| contagocce | **dropper** *A device used to administer medicines one drop at a time.* |
| contaminazione | **contaminate, to** *To make impure by exposing to an polluted agent.* |
| contare | **count, to** *To determine a number.* |
| contento | **content** *What something is made up of.* |
| continuo | **on going** *Continuing,* |
| conto | **bill** *A financial statement that indicates how much one owes.* |
| contraccettivo orale | **oral contraceptive** *Tablet taken by mouth to prevent pregnancy.* |
| contraccezione | **contraceptive** *A device or medication used to prevent pregnancy.* |
| contraccezione; controllo delle nascite | **birth control** *Any method of limiting contraception.* |
| contraddittorio | **contradictory** *Two elements that are inconsistent.* |
| contraddizione | **contraindication** *A situation in which two elements are inconsistent.* |
| contrattura ischemico | **ischemic contracture** *A muscle's resistance to passive stretch that is related to a decrease in arterial flow from any reason.* |
| controllare per | **check for, to** |
| contusione | **bruise** *Common term for ecchymosis.* |
| contusione | **contusion** *An area of broken capillaries in the skin causing discoloration; commonly called a bruise.* |
| conveniente | **convenient** *Opportune or well-timed.* |
| convesso | **convex** *Having an exterior curved the outside of a sphere.* |
| convulsione epilettico | **epileptic seizure** *A convulsion related to abnormal brain activity (as opposed to being precipitated by hypoglycemia.)* |
| convulsioni | **convulsion** *An involuntary series of tonic and clonic movements.* |
| copulazione | **copulation** *Sexual relations.* |
| corda | **chorda** *A cord or sinew.* |
| corde vocali | **vocal cords** *Paired folds of mucous membranes stretched across the larynx.* |
| cordite | **chorditis** *Inflammation of a vocal or spermatic cord.* |
| cordone anteriore del midollo spinale | **funiculus of the spinal cord** *The white matter of the spinal cord that is further defined by location.* |
| cordone umbelicale | **umbilical cord** *The stalk between the placenta and the unborn infant.* |

| Italian | English |
|---|---|
| corea | **chorea** *Involuntary, continuous rapid, jerking movements.* |
| corea degenerativa di Huntington | **Huntington's chorea** *A neurodegenerative disease characterized initially by behavioral changes and later by a movement disorder. Called Huntington's disease now.* |
| corea di Sydenham | **Sydenham chorea** *Historically known as Saint Vitus' dance, it is a childhood chorea associated with rheumatic fever.* |
| corea minor | **Saint Vitus' dance** *Historic name for chorea minor characterized by hypotonia and emotional lability months after a streptococcal infection.* |
| corizza | **coryza** *An acute condition exhibited by copious nasal discharge.* |
| cornea | **cornea** *The transparent segment located at the anterior part of the eye.* |
| corneale | **corneal** *Referring to the cornea.* |
| corneo | **keratic** *Referring to the cornea.* |
| corno | **horn** *A keratinized outgrowth.* |
| coroideo | **choroid** *Similar to the chorion (fertilized ovum or zygote)* |
| coroidite | **choroiditis** *Inflammation of the choroid.* |
| coroidociclite | **choroidocyclitis** *Inflammation of the ciliary processes and choroid.* |
| coroner | **coroner** *A person who investigates sudden or suspicious deaths.* |
| coronoide | **coronoid** *Crown-shaped.* |
| corpi quadrigemino | **quadrigeminal bodies** *The cranial and caudal colliculi.* |
| corpo calloso | **corpus callosum** *A point of connection between the two cerebral hemispheres.* |
| corpo capelli | **hair (of body)** |
| corpo cellulare | **cell body** *The portion of the cell containing the nucleus.* |
| corpo chetone | **ketone body** *One ketone with a decarboxylation product of acetone.* |
| corpo ciliare | **ciliary body** *The connection between the iris and the choroid.* |
| corpo estraneo | **foreign body** *Term used to describe an object found in a body orifice that is not part of the body.* |
| corpo genicolato | **geniculate body** *Protrusions on the thalamus that relay visual and auditory signals to the brain.* |
| corpo inclusione | **inclusion body** *Variably shaped bodies in the nuclei of cells found in infections such as rabies and herpes.* |
| corpo luteo | **corpus luteum** *A structure that is discharged from an ovary; it degenerates if it is not impregnated.* |
| corpulenza | **corpulence** *Fatness.* |
| corpuscolo | **corpuscle** *A red or white blood cell.* |
| corpuscolo terminale | **end organ** *The encapsulated end of a sensory nerve.* |
| corrente | **current** *Flow or stream.* |
| corrente | **stream** *The flow of a liquid.* |
| corrente sanguigna | **blood stream** *Common term or the arterial or venous systems.* |
| corrispondente in stile | **matching** *Corresponding in pattern or style.* |
| corsetto gessato | **cast; plaster cast** *Use of plaster of paris to immobilize an extremity.* |
| corteccia | **cortex** *An external layer.* |
| corteccia surrenale | **adrenal cortex** *The outer layer of the adrenal gland.* |
| corticale | **cortical** *Referring to the cortex.* |
| corticosteroide | **corticosteroid** *A hormone developed in the adrenal cortex.* |
| corticotropina | **corticotropin** *A hormone of the adrenal cortex.* |
| cortisolo | **cortisol** *An adrenal cortical hormone, also called hydrocortisone.* |
| cortisone | **cortisone** *An adrenal cortical hormone responsible for carbohydrate regulation.* |
| cortocircuito | **shunt** *An alternate path for blood or fluid.* |
| coscia | **thigh** *The body region between the inguinal crease and knee.* |
| costo, prezzo | **cost** *The fee or penalty.* |

| Italian | English |
|---|---|
| costocondrite | **costochondritis** *Inflammation of the rib and or its cartilage.* |
| costole | **rib** *A series of curved paired boney articulations protecting the thorax.* |
| costrizione | **constriction** *Circumferential tightening* |
| cotto; canale; tubo | **duct** *Hollow tubular tissue used to carry fluid from a secretory organ.* |
| cotton grezzo | **cotton wool** *Raw cotton.* |
| crampo | **cramp** *A painful contraction of muscles.* |
| craniale | **cranial** *Referring to the skull.* |
| cranio | **cranium** *The skeleton of the head.* |
| cranioclasto | **cranioclast** *An instrument used to crush a fetal skull.* |
| craniofaringioma | **craniopharyngioma** *A tumor that originates in the hypophyseal stalk.* |
| craniostosi | **craniosynostosis** *Closure of the sutures of the skull that occurs prematurely.* |
| craniotabe | **craniotabes** *Softening of the skull bones causing widened sutures; this occurs in rickets.* |
| craniotomia | **craniotomy** *Surgical creation of a hole in the skull.* |
| craurosi vulvare | **kraurosis vulvae** *Dryness and shrinkage of the vulva.* |
| craw-craw | **craw-craw** *A pruritic papular skin eruption sometimes caused by Onchocerca.* |
| creatina | **creatine** *A compound involved with muscle contraction.* |
| creatinina | **creatinine** *A compound excreted in the urine that is produced by the metabolism of creatine.* |
| crenoterapia | **crenotherapy** *A form of treatment from mineral springs.* |
| crepa; fessura | **crevice** *A narrow opening.* |
| crepitio | **crepitus** *A noise heard when one auscultates the lungs that is similar to the sound of rubbing hair between one's fingers. It is also considered the sound of two broken bones rubbing together.* |
| crescita | **growth** *The increase in physical size.* |
| cresta acustico | **acoustic crest** *A prominence on ampulla of the semicircular ducts.* |
| cresta iliaca | **iliac crest** *The upper border of the ilium.* |
| cresta tibiale | **cnemial** *Referring to the shin.* |
| cresta tibiale | **shin** *Refers to the anterior tibial region.* |
| cretinismo | **cretinism** *A chronic condition caused by diminished thyroid hormone secretion.* |
| criochirurgia | **cryosurgery** *The application of extreme cold to destroy tissue.* |
| crioestesia | **cryesthesia** *Abnormal sensitivity to cold.* |
| crioterapia | **cryotherapy** *The use of cold for therapeutic purposes.* |
| criptorchidismo | **cryptorchism** *A condition characterized by the failure of the testes to descend into the scrotum.* |
| criptosporidiosi | **cryptosporidiosis** *A parasitic related diarrhea seen in AIDS.* |
| crisi | **crisis** *A turning point in the treatment of a disease.* |
| cristalloide | **crystalloid** *A substance that can pass through a semipermeable membrane; not a colloid.* |
| cristalluria | **crystalluria** *The presence of crystals in the urine.* |
| cromatina | **chromatin** *A desocyribose nucleic acid that carries the genes of inheritance.* |
| cromosoma | **chromosome** *A structure in the nucleus of living cells that carries genetic information.* |
| cronico | **chronic** *When referring to an illness, it means recurring or persistent.* |
| crosta | **crust** *Dried serous exudate covering a wound.* |
| croup | **croup** *An acute laryngeal condition that is accompanied by a hoarse, barking cough.* |
| crurale | **crural; femoral** *Referring to the femur or leg.* |

| Italian | English |
|---|---|
| cucchiaiata | **spoonful** *A measurement that does not specify teaspoon or tablespoon.* |
| cucchiaino da tè | **teaspoon** *A measure instrument that holds 5 milliliters of fluid.* |
| cucchiaio da tavola | **tablespoon** *An eating utensil that holds 15milliliters of fluid.* |
| cucciaio per raschiamento | **curette** *The instrument used during a curettage.* |
| cuffia dei muscoli rotatori | **rotator cuff** *The structure around the capsule of the shoulder joint formed by the infraspinatus, supraspinatus, teres minor and subscapularis muscles.* |
| culdoscopia | **culdoscopy** *Examination of the female pelvic viscera with a scope inserted through the posterior vaginal fornix.* |
| culla | **cradle** *A bed for an infant.* |
| cuneiforme | **cuneiform** *The three bones between the navicular bone and the metatarsals.* |
| cuoio capelluto | **scalp** *The skin covering the head except for the face.* |
| cuore | **heart** *Muscular organ that pumps blood thru the circulatory system.* |
| cuore pulmonare | **cor pulmonale** *Heart disease that is secondary to lung disease.* |
| cura della ferita | **wound care** *The treatment applied to a tissue injury.* |
| cura di una malattia | **cure** *A remedy for a medical illness.* |
| curaro | **curare** *A toxic botanical substance used at one time in poison darts in South America. Curare derivatives have been used in general anesthesia.* |
| curativo | **curative** *A remedy capable of healing completely.* |
| curettage | **curettage** *Removal of tissues from a cavity.* |
| cuscinetto | **pad** *A thick piece of soft clothing.* |
| cuscino | **cushion** *A pillow or stuffed pad used to sit on.* |
| cuscino | **pillow** *An encased fabric covering soft material used for a cushion.* |
| custodia a lungo termine | **long-term care** *Generally referring to nursing home care.* |
| cutaneo | **cutaneous** *Referring to the skin.* |
| cuticola | **cuticle** *The dead skin at the base of the toenail or fingernail, also called the eponychium.* |
| dacrioadenite | **dacryoadenitis** *Inflammation of the lacrimal gland.* |
| dacriocistite | **dacryocystitis** *Inflammation of a lacrimal sac.* |
| dacriocistorinostomia | **dacryocystorhinostomy** *Surgical reaction of a communication between the lacrimal sac and nasal cavity.* |
| dacriolito | **dacryolith** *A stone in the lacrimal sac or duct.* |
| dannoso | **detrimental** *Harmful.* |
| dare alla luce | **bear, to** *To give birth to a child.* |
| dare un calcio a | **kick, to** *To strike an object with one's foot.* |
| data di ingresso ospedale | **date of admission** *Beginning date of hospitalization.* |
| data di licenziamento ospedal | **discharge date** *The day a patient is released from the hospital.* |
| data di nascita | **date of birth** |
| data di scadenza | **expiration date** *The date when a medication should no longer be used.* |
| debole | **weak** *Feeble or deconditioned.* |
| debolezza | **debility** *Physical weakness.* |
| debolezza | **weakness** *Feebleness.* |
| debolezza muscolare | **muscle weakness** *Decreased muscular function.* |
| decapitare | **decapitate, to** *The physical separation of the head from the body.* |
| decerebrare | **decerebrate** *The removal of the brain.* |
| decibel | **decibel** *A unit used in the measurement of sound.* |
| decidua | **decidua** *The mucous membrane lining the uterus during pregnancy.* |
| decina | **decade** *Ten years.* |

| Italian | English |
|---|---|
| declino | **decline** *As in a decrease in status or health.* |
| decompressione | **decompression** *The surgical procedure relieving pressure on a part.* |
| decussazione | **decussation** *An area of intersection.* |
| defecazione | **defecation** *The discharge of feces from the rectum.* |
| defibrillatore | **defibrillator** *A device used to convert an abnormal cardiac rhythm (ventricular fibrillation) into a normal rhythm with use of electrical stimulation.* |
| deformità | **deformity** *A malformation or imperfection.* |
| deglutizione | **deglutition** *The process of swallowing.* |
| delirante | **delusional** *Referring to a delusion.* |
| delirio | **delirium** *An acute mental state exhibited by altered thought processes and restlessness.* |
| delirio | **delusion** *A belief that is contradictory to rational thought.* |
| delirium tremens | **delirium tremens** *A condition seen when alcohol is withdrawn which is exhibited by restlessness, hallucinations and tremors.* |
| dell'arto superiore | **upper limb** *Referring to either arm.* |
| dell'occhio di gatto | **cat's eye pupil** *A pupil in the shape of an oval.* |
| dell'orecchio | **aural** *Referring to the ear.* |
| deltoide | **deltoid** *A term referring to "three". The deltoid muscle has its origin at three areas: clavicle, acromion, and spine of the scapula.* |
| demarcazione | **demarcation** *Having a fixed boundary.* |
| demenza | **dementia** *A chronic brain disorder exhibited by memory loss, personality changes and faulty reasoning.* |
| demografia | **demography** *The study of the structure of human populations.* |
| dendrite | **dendrite** *Impulses are transmitted along a dendrite to a nerve cell body.* |
| denervazione | **denervation** *The removal of nerve supply.* |
| dengue | **dengue** *A mosquito-borne viral disease exhibited by fever and joint pain.* |
| densità | **density** *The denseness of an object.* |
| dentale | **dental** *Referring to teeth.* |
| dente | **tooth** *One of a set of hard, bony enamel coated structure in the jaw.* |
| dente canino | **canine teeth** *Located between the incisors and premolars.* |
| dente del giudizio | **wisdom tooth** *Third molar.* |
| dente molare | **molar tooth** *Any of the most posterior teeth bilaterally which includes 8 deciduous and usually 12 permanent teeth.* |
| denti deciduo | **deciduous teeth** *The first teeth.* |
| denti permanenti | **permanent teeth** *Dentition that comes in after the primary teeth.* |
| dentiera | **denture** *A frame that holds artificial teeth.* |
| dentizione | **dentition** *The natural teeth.* |
| depilatorio | **depilatory** *An agent used to remove hair.* |
| depilazione | **epilation** *Removal of hair and the roots.* |
| deposito | **sludge** *A viscous fluid.* |
| depressione | **depression** *A medical condition exhibited by profound despondency.* |
| depressione, incisione | **incisure** *A notch or incision.* |
| depresso | **depressed** *Melancholy.* |
| deprivazione | **deprivation** *The lack of a necessity.* |
| derivazione precordiali | **chest leads (precordial)** *Leads going from the skin to an electrocardiographic device.* |
| derma | **dermis** *The "true skin" that lies beneath the epidermis.* |
| dermatie vescicolosa da embrione di anchilostoma | **ground itch** *Marked pruritus caused by a hookworm larvae, known otherwise as cutaneous larva migrans.* |

| Italian | English |
|---|---|
| dermatite | **dermatitis** *Non-specific inflammation of the skin.* |
| dermatite da pannolino | **diaper rash** *Macular rash in the inguinal/perineal region related to exposure to urine.* |
| dermatite di disidrosi | **dyshidrotic eczema** *A dermatitis characterized by vescicobullous lesions.* |
| dermatite pruriginosa | **itch** *A sensation that makes one want to scratch.* |
| dermatofito | **dermatophyte** *A fungal parasite living on the skin.* |
| dermatografia | **dermatography** *A description of the skin.* |
| dermatologia | **dermatology** *The medical profession involving the treatment of skin conditions.* |
| dermatologo | **dermatologist** *A physician specializing in dermatology.* |
| dermatomicosi | **dermatomycosis** *An infection of the skin by Trichophyton, Microsporum or Epidermophyton fungi.* |
| dermatomiosite | **dermatomyositis** *Inflammation of the skin, subcutaneous tissue and adjacent muscle.* |
| dermatomo | **dermatome** *The area of sensation of the skin supplied by a single posterior spinal root.* |
| dermatosi | **dermatosis** *Any skin disease.* |
| dermatosi da Pediculoides ventricosus della paglia | **straw itch** *Pruritus associated with exposure to straw that is infested with the mite Pyemotes ventricosus. Also referred to as dermatitis pediculoides ventricosus.* |
| dermografismo | **dermographia** *A raised, pale line with hyperemic borders is elicited upon scratching the skin with a dull instrument, in this condition.* |
| desensibilizzare | **desensitize, to** *To gradually expose a person to an offending agent to prevent an abnormal response upon a secondary exposure.* |
| desiderio insaziabile | **craving** *An unusually strong urge for something.* |
| desmoide | **desmoid** *A tumor typically found in the abdomen which contains muscle and connective tissue.* |
| desquamazione | **desquamation** *The shedding of skin in flakes or sheets.* |
| destra | **right** *Opposite of left.* |
| destrano | **dextran** *A high glucose polymer used as a plasma substitute.* |
| destrimane | **right-handed** *Having a preference to use the right hand.* |
| destro | **dexter**; *right; straight; erect* |
| destrocardia | **dextrocardia** *Location of the heart in the right hemithorax.* |
| destrorso | **clockwise** *Movement in the same direction as a normal clock.* |
| deterioramento | **deterioration** *Worsening in one's medical condition.* |
| deteriorare | **worsen, to** *To deteriorate.* |
| detrito | **detritus** *Particulate matter produced by the decomposition of an organic substance.* |
| deuteranomalia | **deuteranomaly** *Abnormal color vision sometimes called "green weakness".* |
| deviazione (caduta verso destra) | **deviation** *Away from the norm. (deviation to the right)* |
| di essere nato | **born, to be** *Being present as a result of birth.* |
| di qua, di qui, per cui | **hence** *Thus.* |
| diabete insipido | **diabetes insipidus** *Caused by a deficiency in vasopressin, it is exhibited by great thirst and large volume urine output (and normal blood sugar).* |
| diabete mellito | **diabetes mellitus** *A disease exhibited by a deficiency of the pancreatic hormone insulin.* |
| diabetico | **diabetic** *A person who has diabetes mellitus.* |
| diafisi | **diaphysis** *The central part of a long bone.* |
| diaforetico | **diaphoretic** *Exhibited by profuse perspiration.* |

| Italian | English |
|---|---|
| diaframma | **diaphragm** *The muscular separation between the thoracic and abdominal cavities.* |
| diagnosi differenziale | **differential diagnosis** *A term used to refer to the various options for diagnoses.* |
| diagnostico | **diagnostic** *A specific symptom or characteristic.* |
| diagramma anatomico | **anatomical chart** *A pictorial diagram of part of the anatomy.* |
| diametro coniugata | **conjugate diameter** *A pelvic inlet measurement used to determine whether a woman is capable of delivering a fetus vaginally.* |
| diapason | **tuning fork** *A device used to distinguish between perceptive and conductive hearing loss.* |
| diapedesi | **diapedesis** *The outward passage of blood elements through an intact vessel wall.* |
| diarrea | **diarrhea** *Increase in frequency and a loose consistency of the stools.* |
| diartrosi | **diarthrosis** *An articulation allowing free movement.* |
| diastasi | **diastase** *Amylase.* |
| diastole | **diastole** *The period of dilatation of the heart; between the first and second heart sounds.* |
| diatermia | **diathermy** *The use of heat produced from high-frequency electric currents to medically or surgically treat someone.* |
| diatesi | **diathesis** *A medical tendency to develop a specific condition.* |
| dichiarazione | **statement** *A written or oral commentary.* |
| dieta | **diet** *The kinds of food a person eats.* |
| dietista | **dietitian** *A professional who works with diet and nutrition.* |
| difetto congenito | **birth defect** *A congenital anomaly.* |
| difetto del setto atriale | **atrial septal defect** *An abnormal communication between the atria of the heart.* |
| difetto del setto ventricolare | **ventricular septal defect** *An abnormal communication between the right and left ventricles via a hole in the septum.* |
| differenziale contegio dei leucociti | **differential leukocyte count** *The percentage of different types of leukocytes.* |
| difterite | **diphtheria** *A contagious bacterial disease characterized by a grey membrane on the pharynx along with respiratory or cutaneous symptoms; caused by Corynebacterium diphtheriae.* |
| digestione | **digestion** *The process of enzymatic breakdown of food in the alimentary canal.* |
| digitalis | **digitalis** *Cardiac medication derived from the leaf of Digitalis purpurea.* |
| digiunectomia | **jejunectomy** *Surgical removal of the jejunum.* |
| digiuno | **fasting** *Absence of caloric intake for a specified period.* |
| digiunotomia | **jejunostomy** *Surgical creation of an opening in the jejunum.* |
| dilatatore | **dilator** *An instrument that dilates.* |
| dilatazione | **dilatation** *The process of becoming wider or larger.* |
| diluizione | **dilution** *The process of making a weaker solution.* |
| dimensioni | **size** *The dimensions of something.* |
| dimercaprolo | **dimercaprol** *A medication used as a binding agent for heavy metal poisoning.* |
| diminuzione | **decrease** *Becoming smaller or fewer.* |
| diottria | **dioptre** *Referring to refraction or transmitted and refracted light.* |
| dipendenza da cocaina | **cocaine addiction** *Physical habituation to cocaine.* |
| dipendenza di l'annusar colla | **glue sniffing addiction** *Habituation of plastic cement fumes inhalation which includes toluene, xylene and benzene.* |
| diplegia | **diplegia** *The paralysis of both arms or both legs.* |
| diplococcus | **diplococcus** *A bacterium that occurs in pairs including pneumococcus and Neisseria gonorrhoeae and Neisseria meningitidis.* |

| Italian | English |
|---|---|
| diploide | **diploid** *A nucleus containing two complete sets of chromosomes.* |
| diplopia | **diplopia** *Double vision.* |
| dipsomania | **dipsomania** *Compulsion to drink alcoholic beverages.* |
| diretto verso la guancia | **buccal** *Referring to the cheek.* |
| disaccaride | **disaccharide** *A type of sugar that yields two monosaccharides upon hydrolysis.* |
| disafia | **dysaphia** *Altered sense of touch.* |
| disagio | **discomfort** *A feeling of physical or mental unease.* |
| disarticolazione | **disarticulation** *The separation or amputation of a joint.* |
| disartria | **dysarthria** *Difficulty in articulation of speech.* |
| disbarismo | **dysbarism** *Condition caused by a change in pressure, noted most commonly among scuba divers.* |
| discendente | **descending** *Moving toward the inferior portion.* |
| dischezia | **dyschezia** *Pain experienced during defecation.* |
| discinesia | **dyskinesia** *Abnormal movement.* |
| disco ottico | **optic disk** *The area of the retina where the optic nerve enters.* |
| discondroplasia | **dyschondroplasia** *The formation of cartilaginous and bony tumors near the epiphyses.* |
| discoria | **dyscoria** *A discordance in pupillary reaction.* |
| discrasia | **dyscrasia** *An abnormal condition, mostly referring to the blood.* |
| disdiadococinesia | **dysdiadocokinesia** *The inability to arrest one motor response and substitute its opposite.* |
| disestesia | **dysesthesia** *1. Impairment of the sense of touch. 2. The presence of persistent pain upon receiving a light touch.* |
| disfagia | **dysphagia** *Difficulty in swallowing.* |
| disfasia | **dysphasia** *Difficulty in speaking caused by cerebral dysfunction.* |
| disfunzione | **dysfunction** *Abnormal function in a gland or body organ.* |
| disgenesi gonadico | **gonadal dysgenesis** *The lack of complete development of the gonads.* |
| disidratazione | **dehydration** *The status of having a decrease in total body water.* |
| disidrosi | **dyshidrosis** *Disregulation of sweating* |
| disinfettante | **disinfectant** *A substance that kills bacteria.* |
| disintossicazione | **detoxification** *The process of removing toxins from the body.* |
| disintubazione | **extubation** *The removal of a tube that was in a body orifice.* |
| dislalia | **dyslalia** *The absence of comprehensible speech articulation.* |
| dislessia | **dyslexia** *Difficulty in learning or reading written language with no effect on intelligence.* |
| dismenorrea | **dysmenorrhea** *Pain during menstruation.* |
| disordine | **disorder** *Impairment.* |
| disorientamento | **disorientation** *Mental confusion.* |
| dispareunia | **dyspareunia** *Pain during sexual intercourse.* |
| dispepsia | **dyspepsia** *Indigestion.* |
| dispersione | **scatter** *The degree to which repeated measurements differ.* |
| displasia | **dysplasia** *The increase in organ size due to an increase in the number of abnormal cell types.* |
| dispnea | **dyspnea** *Difficult breathing.* |
| dispnea indotta da esercizio | **exercise-induced dyspnea** |
| disponibile | **available** *Attainable, obtainable.* |
| disponibilità | **availability** *A person or thing that is available.* |
| dispositivo di prelievo | **fingerstick device** *A device used to project a lancet into the skin so a drop of blood can be obtained for analysis.* |
| disseminato | **widespread** *Encompassing or spanning.* |

| Italian | English |
|---|---|
| disseminazione | **dissemination** *To be spread or dispersed widely.* |
| dissenteria | **dysentery** *A severe form of diarrhea with blood and mucous in the stool.* |
| dissolvimento | **dissolution** *Disintegration.* |
| distacco retinico | **retinal detachment** *A tear or hole in the retina caused by vitreous traction.* |
| distale | **distal** *Situated away from the center of the body.* |
| distensione | **distension** *Swollen.* |
| distichiasi | **distichiasis** *Presence of two rows of eyelashes on one eyelid which are turned inward toward the globe.* |
| distocie | **dystocia** *Difficult birth caused by fetal position, narrow pelvis or lack of opening of the cervix.* |
| distonia muscolare deformante progressiva | **torsion spasm** *Also called dystonia musculorum deformans, a genetic condition exhibited by twisting contortions sideways and forward while walking.* |
| distorsione | **sprain** *A joint injury without fracture.* |
| distribuzione | **distribution** *The manner in which something is shared or spread out.* |
| distrofia muscolare | **muscular dystrophy** *A hereditary condition exhibited by progressive muscular weakness and muscle atrophy.* |
| disturbo alimentare | **eating disorder** *General term for pathologic eating habits.* |
| disturbo cognitivo | **cognitive disorders** *Any disease process that involves altered cognition.* |
| disuria | **dysuria** *Difficulty or pain upon urination.* |
| dito a grilletto | **trigger finger** *A condition in which one's finger gets stuck in the flexed position and when extended it snaps like a trigger. Also called stenosing tenosynovitis.* |
| dito a martello | **hammer toe** *A condition characterized by extension of the proximal phalanx and flexion of the second and distal phalanges.* |
| dito a martello di una mano | **mallet finger** *Flexion contracture of the distal phalanx.* |
| dito del piede | **toe** *Any of the digits of of the feet.* |
| dito della mano | **finger** *Any of the five digits on the hand.* |
| dito della mano o di un piede | **digit** *Finger or toe.* |
| diuresi | **diuresis** *Increased excretion of urine.* |
| diuretico | **diuretic** *Medication which causes an increased excretion of urine.* |
| diurno | **diurnal** *Occurring during the day.* |
| divaricatore chirurgico | **retractor** *A device for pulling back tissue during surgery.* |
| diverticolite | **diverticulitis** *Inflammation of the diverticulum.* |
| diverticolo | **diverticulum** *A sac or pouch created by herniation of a mucous membrane in the alimentary canal.* |
| diverticolo faringeo | **pharyngeal pouch** *A lateral diverticulum of the pharynx.* |
| diverticolosi | **diverticulosis** *Presence of diverticulum.* |
| divisione | **cleavage** *A sharp division or demarcation.* |
| doccia | **douche** *Cleansing of a canal; unless otherwise specified it refers to cleansing of the vaginal canal.* |
| dolorabilità di rimbalzo | **rebound** *A term used to describe a type of tenderness found with peritonitis.* |
| dolore | **pain** *Physical suffering or discomfort.* |
| dolore all'arto fantasma | **phantom limb pain** *Pain sensed in an area where one has had an amputation as though the limb is still present.* |
| dolore del secondamento | **after-pains** *The pain experienced after childbirth caused by uterine contractions.* |
| dolore eterotopico | **referred pain** *Pain felt in an area distinct from the original source.* |

| Italian | English |
|---|---|
| dolore trafittura | **stabbing pain** *A sharp piercing quality to pain.* |
| doloroso | **painful** *Affected with pain.* |
| donatore | **donor** *Referring to a person who donates tissue or an organ.* |
| dopamina | **dopamine** *An intermediate product in the creation of norepinephrine.* |
| doppia | **double** *Twice the size, quantity or strength.* |
| dorsale | **dorsal** *Referring to the back or back surface.* |
| dorsalgia | **back pain** *Discomfort on the dorsal surface of the torso.* |
| dorsiflessione | **dorsiflexion** *Backward bending of the foot or hand.* |
| dorso | **dorsum** *The back part.* |
| dosaggio | **dosage** *The amount and frequency a medication is given.* |
| dose | **dose** *The quantity of a medication.* |
| dose di mantenimento | **dose, maintenance** *The chronic dose given after the initial bolus.* |
| dose letale | **lethal dose** *The amount of a drug required to cause death.* |
| dotti biliari | **bile ducts** *The structures that are conduits for passage of bile from the liver and gallbladder to the duodenum.* |
| dotto arterioso pervio | **ductus arteriosus** *A fetal artery that communicates between the pulmonary artery and the descending aorta.* |
| dotto epatico | **hepatic duct** *The right and left hepatic ducts join the cystic duct to form the common bile duct.* |
| dovuto a | **owing to** *On account of.* |
| drappo di sala operatoria | **drape** *The fabric used as a sterile covering in the OR.* |
| drastico | **drastic** *Having significant effect.* |
| dritto | **upright** *Vertical or standing.* |
| ducto cistico | **cystic duct** *The duct connecting the gallbladder to the common bile duct.* |
| ductus arteriosus persistens | **patent ductus arteriosus** *A condition exhibited by failure of the ductus arteriosus (communication between the aorta the the pulmonary artery normally noted in a fetus) to close.* |
| due volte | **two times** *One action being done on two occasions.* |
| duodenale | **duodenal** *Referring to the duodenum.* |
| duodenectomia | **duodenectomy** *Excision of the duodenum.* |
| duodenite | **duodenitis** *Inflammation of the duodenum.* |
| duodeno | **duodenum** *The portion of the small bowel between the stomach and jejunum.* |
| duplicazione | **duplication** *The process of duplicating something.* |
| dura madre | **dura mater** *The outermost covering of the brain and spinal cord.* |
| durata della vita | **lifetime** *Duration of a person's life.* |
| durata presumibile della vita | **life expectancy** *The length of time a person is anticipated to live.* |
| duro | **hard** *Rigid or very firm.* |
| duro di udito | **hard of hearing** *Decreased sense of hearing.* |
| duro; rigido | **stiff** *Not easily bent.* |
| ebbrezza | **inebriation** *Intoxication with drugs or alcohol.* |
| ebefrenia | **hebephrenia** *A type of schizophrenia exhibited by hallucinations and inappropriate laughter.* |
| eccesso | **excess** *Surplus or overabundance.* |
| ecchimosi | **ecchymosis** *Skin discoloration caused by bleeding beneath the epidermis.* |
| eccipiente | **excipient** *An inactive substance used to deliver an active substance.* |
| eccondroma | **ecchondroma** *Hyperplastic growth of cartilage on the surface of other cartilage.* |
| echinococco | **Echinococcus** *A tapeworm of the family Taeniidae that can cause hydatid cysts.* |

| Italian | English |
|---|---|
| eclampsia | **eclampsia** *A maternal condition characterized by convulsions and hypertension that can lead to maternal and fetal death.* |
| ecmnesia | **ecmnesia** *Memory loss for recent events but retained memory of remote events.* |
| ecocardiografia | **echocardiography** *The use of ultrasound waves to visualize the heart and its structures.* |
| ecografia transvaginale | **transvaginal ultrasound** *Insertion of an ultrasound probe in the vagina to view adjacent structures.* |
| ecolalia | **echolalia** *The meaningless repetition of the words spoken by another person.* |
| ectasia | **ectasia** *Expansion or distension.* |
| ectoderma | **ectoderm** *The outermost layer of the three layers of the embryo.* |
| ectopico | **ectopic** *Abnormal position.* |
| ectrodattilia | **ectrodactylia** *A congenital anomaly exhibited by absence of one digit or part of a digit.* |
| ectropion | **ectropion** *Eversion of the eyelid, usually the lower lid.* |
| eczema | **eczema** *A medical condition exhibited by pruritic, red, scaly patches on the scalp, cheeks and extensor surfaces.* |
| edema | **edema** *Extravascular fluid accumulation.* |
| edema angioneurotico | **angioneurotic edema** *A condition exhibited by sudden edema of skin and mucous membranes.* |
| edema caviglia | **ankle edema or dependent edema** *Extracellular fluid volume noted by swelling or pitting.* |
| edema dell'arto inferiore | **lower extremity edema** *Interstitial edema of the legs.* |
| edema plastico | **pitting edema** *Edema of the lower extremities characterized by an indentation being left when the examiner applies pressure with their thumb.* |
| edema polmonare | **pulmonary edema** *Characterized by abnormal fluid buildup in the lungs.* |
| edematoso | **edematous** *Referring to the presence of edema.* |
| edonismo | **hedonism** *Devoting oneself to being happy.* |
| educazione | **education** *Instruction or guidance.* |
| efedrina | **ephedrine** *A chemical used to treat asthma because it expands bronchial passages and used to control spinal anesthesia associated shock because it constricts blood vessels.* |
| effetto collaterale | **side effect** *An expected but unwanted effect of a medication.* |
| effetto cumulativo | **cumulative effect** *A consequence of successive additions.* |
| effetto indesiderato | **adverse effect** *In reference to medication use, it is an undesirable consequence of the drug.* |
| effettore | **effector** *An organ that responds to a stimulus.* |
| effettuare uno striscio | **smear** *Used to refer to a specimen smeared on a slide.* |
| efficace | **efficacious** *Effective.* |
| effusione | **effusion** *The accumulation of fluid in a body cavity.* |
| effusione pleurico | **pleural effusion** *An abnormal collection of fluid between the internal chest wall and the pleura.* |
| egocentrico | **egocentric** *Thinking of self without considering the feelings or thoughts of others.* |
| ehrlichiosi | **ehrlichiosis** *A tickborne infectious disease.* |
| eiaculazione | **ejaculation** *The emission of semen at the moment of sexual climax in a male.* |
| elastina | **elastin** *A connective tissue-based glycoprotein.* |
| elefantiasi | **elephantiasis** *A condition caused by nematode parasites leading to lymphatic obstruction and limb or scrotal swelling.* |
| elettivo | **elective** *Non-urgent and not life-saving.* |

| Italian | English |
|---|---|
| elettrocardiogramma | **electrocardiogram** *Display of a person's heart beat that can be used in the diagnosis of cardiac disorders.* |
| elettrodo | **electrode** *A device used to facilitate conduction of electricity to or from a body.* |
| elettroencefalogramma | **electroencephalogram (EEG)** *A display of brain waves used in the diagnosis of brain disorders, especially epilepsy.* |
| elettroforesi | **electrophoresis** *The movement of charged particles in a fluid that is under the influence of an electric field. This is used in testing for various maladies in the form of serum protein electrophoresis.* |
| elettrolito | **electrolyte** *The ionized constituents including potassium, sodium, chloride and others.* |
| elettromiografia | **electromyography** *The display of the electrical activity of muscle.* |
| elio | **helium** *An inert gas that is the lightest of the noble gases.* |
| elioterapia | **heliotherapy** *Treatment of disease with sunlight.* |
| elisir | **elixir** *A medical solution.* |
| ellettuario | **lincture** *A medicine mixed with a sweet substance.* |
| elmintiasi | **helminthiasis** *Being infected by a helminth.* |
| elmintico | **verminous** *Referring to presence of worms.* |
| elminto | **helminth** *A fluke, tapeworm or nematode.* |
| emaciazione | **emaciation** *Abnormally thin and weak.* |
| emangioma | **hemangioma** *A benign tumor composed of blood vessels.* |
| emangioma cavernoso | **cavernous hemangioma** *A tumor composed of connective tissue with blood filled areas.* |
| emartro | **hemarthrosis** *Presence of intra-articular blood.* |
| ematemesi | **hematemesis** *Vomiting blood.* |
| ematina | **hematin** *The insoluble iron protoporphyrin component of hemoglobin.* |
| ematocele | **hematocele** *A mass or area of swelling caused by the accumulation of blood.* |
| ematochezia | **hematochezia** *Presence of blood in the excrement.* |
| ematocrito | **hematocrit** *The measurement of the volume of red blood cells compared to the total volume of blood; recorded in percent.* |
| ematoma | **hematoma** *A mass containing blood.* |
| ematoma epidurale | **epidural hematoma** *Formation of a collection of blood outside the dural layer of the brain; usually caused by trauma.* |
| ematoma subdurale | **subdural hematoma** *Formation of a blood clot between the dura mater and the arachnoid membrane.* |
| ematomielia | **hematomyelia** *Accumulation of blood in the spinal cord.* |
| ematoporfirina | **hematoporphyrin** *A derivative of heme that does not contain iron.* |
| ematrometra | **hematometra** *The accretion of blood in the uterus.* |
| ematuria | **hematuria** *The presence of blood in the urine.* |
| embolectomia | **embolectomy** *The removal of an embolus.* |
| embolia gassosa | **air embolism** *The blockage of an artery or vein by an air bubble.* |
| embolia grassa | **fat embolism** *A deposit of fat that obstructs a vessel.* |
| embolia polmonare | **pulmonary embolism** *A sudden blockage of a lung artery frequently emanating from a blood clot in one's leg.* |
| embolo | **embolus** *A blood clot, air bubble or fatty deposit that cause obstruction of a vessel.* |
| embriologia | **embryology** *The study of the embryo.* |
| embrione | **embryo** *The term used to describe a fertilized ovum in the first 8 weeks of development.* |
| eme | **heme** *A constituent of hemoglobin that is an insoluble iron protoporphyrin.* |
| ementomia | **hymenotomy** *Surgically creating an opening in the hymen.* |

| Italian | English |
|---|---|
| emeralopia | **hemeralopia** *Night blindness.* |
| emergenza | **emergency** *An urgent, life-threatening situation.* |
| emetico | **emetic** *An agent that induces vomiting.* |
| emianopia a quadrante | **quadranic hemianopia** *Loss of a quarter of the visual field in one or both eyes. If bilateral, it may be further described as homonymous, heteronymous, binasal, bitemporal, or crossed.* |
| emianopsia | **hemianopsia** *Blindness over half the field of vision.* |
| emianopsia bitemporale | **bitemporal hemianopsia** *A visual defect seen commonly in pituitary tumors in which the visual defect is in the temporal portion of each eye.* |
| emiballismo | **hemiballismus** *Severe motor restlessness unilaterally, usually from a subthalamic lesion.* |
| emicolectomia | **hemicolectomy** *Surgical removal of part of the colon.* |
| emicrania | **hemicrania** *1. Pain on one side of the head. 2. Incomplete anencephaly.* |
| emicrania | **migraine** *An episodic, unilateral headache accompanied by nausea.* |
| eminenza ipotenar | **hypothenar eminence** *The prominence on the palm at the base of the fingers adjacent to the ulna.* |
| eminenza tenar | **thenar eminence** *Formed by the bellies of the abductor pollicis brevis, flexor pollicis brevis and opponens pollicis.* |
| emiparesi | **hemiparesis** *Unilateral muscle weakness (half the body).* |
| emiplegia | **hemiplegia** *Paralysis of one side of the body.* |
| emisfero | **hemisphere** *Referring to either the right or left portion of the cerebrum.* |
| emivita | **half-life** *The time a drug decreases its effect in half over time.* |
| emizigote | **hemizygote** *A cell with only one set of genes.* |
| emmetropia | **emmetropia** *The normal correlation between eye refraction and the axial length of the eyeball.* |
| emoagglutinina | **hemagglutinin** *An antibody that facilitates the agglutination of blood.* |
| emobanca | **blood bank** *An area where blood products are stored for later use.* |
| emocitometro | **hemocytometer** *A device used for counting cells from a blood sample.* |
| emoconcentrazione | **hemoconcentration** *Decrease in the total fluid content of the blood, leading at times to a falsely elevated hematocrit.* |
| emocromatosi | **hemochromatosis** *A hereditary condition exhibited by iron deposition in the tissue and leading to liver disease, bronze discoloration of the skin and diabetes.* |
| emodialisi | **hemodialysis** *The process of filtering blood outside the body to remove toxins normally excreted by functioning kidneys.* |
| emofilia | **hemophilia** *A hereditary bleeding disorder characterized by hemarthroses and deep tissue bleeding as a result of absence of a coagulation factor such as factor VIII.* |
| emofilico | **hemophiliac** *A person with hemophilia.* |
| emoftalmo | **hemophthalmia** *Bleeding within the eye.* |
| emoglobina | **hemoglobin** *An iron containing protein used for the transport of oxygen in blood.* |
| emoglobinuria | **hemoglobinuria** *Presence of free hemoglobin in the urine.* |
| emolisi | **hemolysis** *Breakdown of hemoglobin.* |
| emolitico | **hemolytic** *Something that causes hemolysis.* |
| emolliente | **emollient** *Having softening or soothing qualities.* |
| emopericardio | **hemopericardium** *Abnormal presence of blood in the pericardium.* |
| emoperitoneo | **hemoperitoneum** *Abnormal presence of blood in the peritoneum.* |
| emopneumotorace | **hemopneumothorax** *Accumulation of blood and air in the pleural space.* |
| emopoiesi | **hemopoiesis** *The production of blood cells from stem cells.* |

| Italian | English |
|---|---|
| emopoietico | **hemopoietic** Referring to *a hormone secreted by the kidneys that stimulates the bone marrow to produce erythrocytes.* |
| emorragia | **bleeding** *Loss of blood.* |
| emorragia | **hemorrhage** *Bleeding from a damaged blood vessel.* |
| emorroidectomia | **hemorrhoidectomy** *Surgical excision of a hemorrhoid.* |
| emorroidi | **hemorrhoids** *Engorgement of the veins in the anus or rectum.* |
| emosalpinge | **hematosalpinx** *Presence of blood in the fallopian tube.* |
| emostasi | **hemostasis** *The control of bleeding.* |
| emotorace | **hemothrorax** *The abnormal presence of blood in the pleural cavity.* |
| emottisi | **hemoptysis** *Expectoration of blood.* |
| emozione | **emotion** *An intense feeling.* |
| empatia | **empathy** *To be concerned for and share the feelings of another.* |
| empiema | **empyema** *A collection of purulent material in a body cavity, usually referring to a thoracic empyema.* |
| emulsione | **emulsion** *The dispersion of one liquid into another, but it is not dissolved.* |
| enartrosi | **enarthrosis** *The type of joint in which a spherical bone is set into the socket of another bone.* |
| encefalico | **encephalic** *Referring to the brain.* |
| encefaline | **enkephalin** *Peptide found in the brain that has similar effects as the endorphins.* |
| encefalite | **encephalitis** *Inflammation of the brain.* |
| encefalocele | **encephalocele** *The protrusion of the brain through a defect in the skull.* |
| encefalografia | **encephalography** *Roentgenography of the brain.* |
| encefalomalacia | **encephalomacia** *Abnormal softness of the brain.* |
| encefalomielite | **encephalomyelitis** *Inflammation of the brain and spinal cord.* |
| encefalopatia | **encephalopathy** *Degeneration of cerebral function.* |
| encondroma | **enchondroma** *An abnormal increase in cartilage growth on the inside of bone or of other cartilage.* |
| encopresi | **encopresis** *Involuntary defecation.* |
| endemico | **endemic** *When a disease is commonly found in a location or in a people group.* |
| endoaddominale | **intraabdominal** *Within the abdominal cavity.* |
| endoarterite | **endarteritis** *Tunica intima inflammation.* |
| endocardite | **endocarditis** *Inflammation of the endocardium.* |
| endocrino | **endocrine** *Referring to glands that secrete hormones and other chemicals into the blood.* |
| endocrinologia | **endocrinology** *The study of endocrine glands and hormones.* |
| endogeno | **endogenous** *Originating from within.* |
| endolinfa | **endolymph** *The fluid collection the labyrinth of the ear.* |
| endometrio | **endometrium** *The mucous membrane lining of the uterus.* |
| endometrioma | **endometrioma** *An isolated benign mass containing endometrial tissue.* |
| endometriosi | **endometriosis** *Presence of uterine mucosal tissue in the pelvis in abnormal locations.* |
| endometrite | **endometritis** *Inflammation of the endometrium.* |
| endometrite cervicale | **endocervicitis** *Inflammation of the mucosal lining of the cervix.* |
| endonervio | **endoneurium** *The tissue in a peripheral nerve that separates the individual nerve fibers.* |
| endorfine | **endorphin** *Hormone secreted that activates the body's opiate receptors and acts as an analgesic.* |

| Italian | English |
|---|---|
| endoscopio | **endoscope** *A device used to view the interior of a hollow organ (sigmoidoscope, gastroscope)* |
| endotelioma | **endothelioma** *A mass that propagates from the endothelium of blood vessels, lymphatics or serous cavities.* |
| endotracheale | **endotracheal** *Within the trachea.* |
| enfisema | **emphysema** *Abnormal enlargement of the airspaces distal to the terminal bronchioles.* |
| enoftalmo | **enophthalmos** *Posterior displacement of the eyeball in the orbit.* |
| enorme | **enormous** *Very large.* |
| enostosi | **enostosis** *The abnormal bony growth inside a bone or on the cortex.* |
| enterectomia | **enterectomy** *Surgical resection of part of the intestine.* |
| enterico | **enteric** *Referring to the intestines.* |
| enterite | **enteritis** *Inflammation of the intestines.* |
| enterococco | **enterococcus** *A gram positive cocci that occurs naturally in the intestine but is pathogenic elsewhere in the body.* |
| enterolito | **enterolith** *A calculus of the intestine.* |
| enteroptosi | **enteroptosis** *Inferior displacement of the intestines in the abdomen.* |
| enterotomia | **enterotomy** *A surgical opening of the intestines.* |
| entoderma | **endoderm** *The innermost layer of the embryonic germ cell layers.* |
| enucleazione | **enucleation** *Surgical removal of a globe.* |
| enuresi | **enuresis** *Involuntary urination.* |
| enzima | **enzyme** *A compound that acts as a catalyst for reactions within cells as assists with digestion outside of cells.* |
| eosinofilia | **eosinophilia** *An increased number of eosinophils in the blood.* |
| eosinofilo | **eosinophil** *A cell with eosin stain used to designate a type of leukocyte that is elevated during allergic reactions.* |
| eparina | **heparin** *A polysaccharide that occurs naturally in the liver and is used as a medication to induce a hypocoagulable state.* |
| epatectomia | **hepatectomy** *Partial or complete surgical resection of the liver.* |
| epatico | **hepatic** *Referring to the liver.* |
| epatite | **hepatitis** *Inflammation of the liver.* |
| epatite colostatica | **cholestatic hepatitis** *Liver inflammation caused by obstruction of bile flow from the liver to the duodenum.* |
| epatocito | **hepatocyte** *A liver cell.* |
| epatoma | **hepatoma** *A tumor of the liver.* |
| epatomegalia | **hepatomegaly** *Enlargement of the liver.* |
| epatosplenomegalia | **hepatosplenomegaly** *Enlargement of the spleen and the liver.* |
| ependima | **ependyma** *The glial lined covering of the cerebral ventricles and the central portion of the spinal cord.* |
| ependimoma | **ependymoma** *A tumor composed of cells that line the ventricles of the brain.* |
| epiblefaron | **epiblepharon** *A condition exhibited by the eyelashes pressing against the eyeball.* |
| epicardio | **epicardium** *The serous membranous, innermost lining of the pericardium.* |
| epicondilite | **epicondylitis** *Inflammation of the epicondyle.* |
| epicondilo | **epicondyle** *A protrusion at the distal end of the humerus.* |
| epicranio | **epicranium** *The skin, fibrous layer (aponeurosis), and muscles lining the scalp.* |
| epidemia | **outbreak (of a disease)** *A sudden start of a disease in a population.* |
| epidemico | **epidemic** *Ubiquitous development of an infectious disease.* |
| epidemiologia | **epidemiology** *The study of the incidence, development and control of disease.* |

| Italian | English |
|---|---|
| epidermide | **epidermis** *The skin cells overlying the dermis.* |
| epidermofitosi | **epidermophytosis** *A fungal skin infection caused by an organism from the genus Epidermophyton.* |
| epidermomicosi eritmatosquamosa | **ringworm** *A fungal skin infection exhibited by pruritic well circumscribed patches on the scalp or feet.* |
| epididimite | **epididymitis** *Inflammation of the duct that moves sperm from the testis to the vas deferens.* |
| epidurale | **epidural** *The space around the dura of the spinal cord.* |
| epifisi cerebrale | **epiphysis cerebri** *A small structure situated on the mesencephalon between the two sections of the thalamus.* |
| epifisite | **epiphysitis** *Inflammation of the end of a long bone that is separated from the shaft by a cartilaginous disc.* |
| epigastrio | **epigastrium** *The section of the abdomen that overlies the stomach.* |
| epiglottide | **epiglottis** *Tissue at the base of the tongue that covers the trachea when one swallows.* |
| epilessia | **epilepsy** *A condition associated with abnormal brain activity and exhibited by sudden, recurrent convulsions, sensory disturbances and loss of consciousness.* |
| epilettiforme | **epileptiform** *Being similar to epilepsy.* |
| epilettogeno | **epileptogenic** *That which induces seizures.* |
| episclerite | **episcleritis** *Inflammation of the tissue lying above the sclera.* |
| episiotomia | **episiotomy** *A surgical incision of the vagina used to aid childbirth.* |
| epispadia | **epispadias** *A congenital condition characterized by the urethral meatus being at the superior aspect of the penis* |
| epistassi | **epistaxis** *Bleeding emanating from the nose.* |
| epistassi | **nosebleed** *Common term for epistaxis.* |
| epiteliale | **epithelial** *Referring to the epithelium.* |
| epitelio | **epithelium** *The tissue lining the skin and the gastrointestinal tract that is derived from the embryonic ectoderm and endoderm..* |
| epitelioma | **epithelioma** *A malignant tumor composed of epithelial cells.* |
| epitrocleare | **epitrochlea** *The medial condyle of the humerus.* |
| epulsione prematura del cordone ombelicale durante il parto | **prolapse of the umbilical cord** *Refers to the umbilical cord protruding from the cervix during active labor.* |
| equilibrio | **equilibrium** *When opposing forces are in balance.* |
| equilibrio dinamico | **steady state** *In equilibrium.* |
| equipaggiamento | **equipment** *Apparatus or instrument.* |
| equivalente | **equal** *The same or uniform.* |
| ereditario | **hereditary** *That which is transmitted genetically* |
| ergometro | **ergometer** *A device that measures energy expenditure.* |
| ergonomia | **ergonomics** *The study of workplace design that focuses on reducing work-related injuries.* |
| ergosterolo | **ergosterol** *A compound converted to vitamin D2 upon exposure to ultraviolet light.* |
| erisipela | **erysipelas** *An acute infection caused by Streptococcus pyogenes that causes fever along with swelling and inflammation. The infection frequently effects the face or one leg.* |
| eritema multiforme | **erythema mutliforme** *A skin condition exhibited by purpuric lesions and bullae usually on the distal parts of extremities but can affect the face and trunk.* |
| eritema nodoso | **erythema nodosum** *The presence of red or purple nodules on the pretibial area.* |
| eritroblasto | **erythroblast** *A nucleus containing immature erythrocyte.* |
| eritroblastosi fetale | **erythroblastosis fetalis** *A hemolytic disease of the newborn.* |

| Italian | English |
|---|---|
| eritrocianosi | **erythrocyanosis** *A condition exhibited by purple patches with asymmetric swelling, pruritus and burning.* |
| eritrocito | **erythrocyte** *Called a red blood cell, it transports oxygen and carbon dioxide to and from the tissues.* |
| eritrocitosi | **erythrocytosis** *A higher than normal level of erythrocytes in the blood stream.* |
| eritropenia | **erythrocytopenia** *Low level of erythrocytes in the blood stream.* |
| eritropoiesi | **erythropoiesis** *The production of red blood cells.* |
| ermafrodita | **hermaphrodite** *A person possessing gonadal characteristics of both sexes.* |
| ernia diaframmatica | **diaphragmatic hernia** *Protrusion of visceral contents through the diaphragm.* |
| ernia femorale | **hernia, femoral** *A bulge in the upper thigh/groin region because of bowel protruding through the muscle. Also called crural hernia.* |
| ernia iatale | **hiatus hernia** *Protrusion of part of the stomach through the esophageal hiatus of the diaphragm.* |
| ernia inguinale | **hernia, inguinal** *Protrusion of abdominal-cavity contents through the inguinal canal.* |
| ernia lombare | **hernia, lumbar** *Defect in the lumbar muscles or the posterior fascia, below the 12th rib and above the iliac crest.* |
| ernia ombelicale | **hernia, umbilical** *Protrusion of abdominal contents at the umbilicus.* |
| ernia strozzata | **hernia, incarcerated** *An irreducible hernia.* |
| erniorrafia | **herniorrhaphy** *The surgical repair of a hernia.* |
| eroina | **heroin** *A morphine derivative that is highly addictive.* |
| erosione | **erosion** *The gradual destruction of surface tissue.* |
| erpetico | **herpetic** *Referring to herpes.* |
| erpetiforme | **herpetiform** *Something that is characteristic of herpes.* |
| errore | **error** *Mistake or inaccuracy.* |
| eruttazione | **eructation** *Belch or burp.* |
| eruzione di droga | **drug eruption** *A diffuse rash caused by a medication.* |
| esacerbazione | **exacerbation** *Worsening of an existing problem.* |
| esame | **examination** *Assessment or evaluation.* |
| esame clinico | **clinical examination** *Physical assessment data.* |
| esame delle urine | **urinalysis** *Chemical and microscopic examination of the urine.* |
| esame delle urine (nel mezzo della corrente) | **clean catch urine specimen** *A urine specimen obtained by having a patient cleanse the perineal area prior to voiding in a collection device.* |
| esame fisico | **physical exam** *Examination of a client to assess their medical status.* |
| esame morfologico completo | **complete blood count** *An assay that includes white blood cell, red blood cell, platelet count, hemoglobin, hematocrit and white blood cell differential.* |
| esame rettale digitale | **rectal digital examination** *Use of a gloved finger to assess the rectal vault.* |
| esantema | **exanthema** *A rash that accompanies a disease or fever.* |
| escara | **eschar** *Dry, hard, dead tissue commonly seen with a chronic pressure ulcer or anthrax.* |
| escoriazione | **excoriation** *Superficial loss of skin.* |
| escremento | **excrement** *Feces.* |
| escreti | **excreta** *Fecal material.* |
| eserina | **eserine** *Physostigmine.* |
| esfoliazione | **exfoliation** *The shedding of scales.* |
| esigente | **demanding** *Requiring a lot of skill or requiring a lot of others.* |
| esito di malattia | **disease outcome** *The response obtained from treatment.* |

| Italian | English |
|---|---|
| esofagectomia | **esophagectomy** *Surgical removal of the esophagus.* |
| esofageo | **esophageal** *Referring to the esophagus.* |
| esofagite | **esophagitis** *Inflammation of the esophagus.* |
| esofago | **esophagus** *The muscular tube that connects the throat to the stomach.* |
| esofago di Barrett | **Barretts's esophagus** *A condition characterized by varying degrees of esophageal injury from gastric acid.* |
| esofagoscopia | **esophagoscopy** *Visual inspection the esophagus utilizing a scope.* |
| esoftalmo | **proptosis oculi** *Synonym of exophthalmos; bulging of the eye.* |
| esogeno | **exogenous** *Referring to external factors.* |
| esostosi | **exostosis** *A bony prominence growing from the surface of a bone.* |
| esotossine | **exotoxin** *A toxin released from a living cell.* |
| espansione | **expansion** *Enlargement or increase in size.* |
| espettorante | **expectorant** *A substance that promotes the secretion of sputum.* |
| espettorazione | **expectoration** *The presence of sputum that has been coughed out.* |
| espiratorio | **expiratory** *Referring to exhalation of air from the lungs.* |
| espressione del viso | **facies** *A facial expression that is typical for a particular disease.* |
| espulsione | **expulsion** *Evacuation or elimination.* |
| espulsione della placenta | **expulsion of placenta** *Passage of the placenta out the cervix after childbirth.* |
| espulsivo | **bearing down** *As in during labor.* |
| essenziale | **essential** *Crucial or necessary.* |
| essere bleso | **lisping** *A speech problem in which "s" and "z" are pronounced "th".* |
| essere compiacente | **comply, to** *Adhere to.* |
| essere strabico | **squint, to** *To look at something with the eyes partially closed.* |
| essicctivo | **desiccation** *The act of drying up.* |
| essudati cotonosi | **cotton wool spots** *Condition characterized by blue or white discoloration on the retina related to nerve ischemia.* |
| essudato | **exudate** *The fluid, cells, and debris found in the tissues or a cavity (like pleural space) during inflammation.* |
| essudazione dopo il parto vaginale | **discharge, postpartum vaginal** *The secretions noted after delivery.* |
| essudazione nasale | **discharge, nasal** *Nasal secretions.* |
| essudazione orecchio | **discharge, ear** *Otic secretions.* |
| estendere | **extend, to** *To expand or stretch out.* |
| estensione | **extension** *Going from a bent to straight position.* |
| estensore | **extensor** *Referring to the extension of an extremity or part of an extremity.* |
| esterno | **external** *Outside of the body.* |
| estirpare | **extirpate, to** *To totally destroy.* |
| estraneo, non pertinente | **irrelevant** *Not pertinent.* |
| estratto | **extract** *A substance in a concentrated form.* |
| estremità | **extremity** *Refers to one arm or one leg.* |
| estrinseco | **extrinsic** *Coming from outside or external sources.* |
| estrogeno | **estrogen** *A hormone involved with developing and maintaining female sexual characteristics.* |
| esumazione | **exhumation** *To remove a dead body from a grave.* |
| etanolo | **ethanol** *Synonym for ethyl alcohol.* |
| età | **age** *Length of life.* |
| eterocromia dell'iride; sindrome di Eric | **heterochromia iridis or syndrome of Eric** *Congenital anomaly in which the iris of each eye is of a different color.* |
| eterogeno | **heterogenous** *That which originates outside the organism.* |

| Italian | English |
|---|---|
| eterotrapianto | **allograft** *A tissue transplant of from someone of the same species but different genotype.* |
| eterotropia | **heterotropia** *Synonym of strabismus.* |
| eterozigotico | **heterozygous** *Having different alleles concerning a certain trait.* |
| eunuco | **eunuch** *A man who has been castrated.* |
| eurzione cutanea | **skin rash** *Dermal exanthema.* |
| eutanasia | **euthanasia** *Killing someone painlessly who is thought to have a terminal condition.* |
| evacuazione | **evacuation** *The emptying of an organ of fluids or gas.* |
| eversione | **eversion** *To turn outward.* |
| evidente | **evident** *Obvious.* |
| eviscerazione | **evisceration** *The removal of bowels from the body.* |
| eviscerazione | **exenteration** *Complete surgical removal of an organ.* |
| evitabile | **avoidable** *That which can be stopped or inhibited.* |
| exonfalo | **exomphalos** *Umbilical hernia.* |
| exotropia | **exotropia** *A type of strabismus that is characterized by the eyes turned outward.* |
| extracapsulare | **extracapsular** *Situated outside a capsule.* |
| extracellulare | **extracellular** *Outside the cell.* |
| extrasistole | **extrasystole** *Either a premature atrial or ventricular contraction.* |
| eziologia | **etiology** *The underlying cause of a problem.* |
| faccetta | **facet** *A small flat surface of a bone.* |
| faccia | **face** *Anterior aspect of the head from the forehead to the chin.* |
| faccia di Hutchinson | **Hutchinson's mask** *The sensation the face is covered in cobwebs, associated with tabes dorsalis.* |
| fagocito | **phagocyte** *A cell capable of surrounding and digesting microorganisms.* |
| fagocitosi | **phagocytosis** *The action of a phagocyte.* |
| falange | **phalanx** *One of the long bones of the fingers or toes.* |
| falcata | **stride** *Walk with long definitive steps.* |
| falce cerebri | **falx cerebri** *A fold in the dura that separates the two cerebral hemispheres.* |
| falciforme | **falciform** *Referring to something that is curved. The falciform ligament attaches the liver to the diaphragm.* |
| fame | **hunger** *A sense of discomfort caused by a lack of food.* |
| famiglia | **family** |
| familiare | **familial** *Referring to the family* |
| fanciullezza | **childhood** *The time between infancy and puberty.* |
| faradismo | **faradism** *The gradual increasing and decreasing of the amplitude of electricity.* |
| fare il solletico | **tickle, to** *To lightly touch a person to cause one to laugh.* |
| fare inclinare | **biased** *Prejudiced.* |
| fare ostruzionismo | **obstructed** *To be blocked or halted.* |
| fare scoppiare | **burst, to** *To rupture.* |
| fare un trattamento | **treat, to** *Medical care one receives for illness or injury.* |
| faringe | **pharynx** *The membranous cavity from the mouth to esophagus.* |
| faringectomia | **pharyngectomy** *Surgical excision of part of the pharynx.* |
| faringeo | **pharyngeal** *Referring to the pharynx.* |
| faringite | **pharyngitis** *Inflammation of the pharynx.* |
| faringolaringectomia | **pharyngolaryngectomy** *Surgical removal of part of the pharynx and larynx.* |
| farmacia | **pharmacy** *A business that sells prescription medication.* |

| Italian | English |
|---|---|
| farmacista | **pharmacist** *A professional who prepares and sells medicine through various systems, including governmental organizations like the Veterans Administration.* |
| farmaco-dipendenza | **drug dependence** *Addiction to a substance.* |
| farmaco; medicamento | **drug** *A medication, sometimes with negative connotation.* |
| farmacocinetica | **pharmacokinetics** *The study of the distribution, absorption and excretion of drugs within the body.* |
| farmacologia | **pharmacology** *The study of all aspects of medicines.* |
| fascia | **fascia** *The fibrous sheath enclosing a muscle or organ.* |
| fasciatura occlusivo | **occlusive dressing** *A synthetic covering for a wound that has a semipermeable membrane.* |
| fascicolazione | **fasciculation** *Involuntary contraction of muscle fibers.* |
| fascicolo | **fascicle** *A bundle of nerve or muscle fibers.* |
| fascio anteriore | **anterior root** *A motor nerve root that is in the anterior part of the spinal cord between the anterior and lateral funiculi.* |
| fascio di His | **atrioventricular bundle** *Also called bundle of His.* |
| fascio di His | **bundle of His** *The atrial contraction rhythm is facilitated by this bundle to the ventricles.* |
| fasciotomia | **fasciotomy** *Incision into a fascia.* |
| fascite | **fasciitis** *Inflammation of a fascia.* |
| fatica | **fatigue** *Tiredness and exhaustion.* |
| fattore antiemofilico | **antihemophilic factor** *Also called factor VIII. A deficiency of the factor causes hemophilia.* |
| fattore antinucleare | **antinuclear factor** *Also called antinucleic antibody (ANA); it is found in conditions such as lupus and rheumatoid arthritis.* |
| fattore di rilascio dell'ormone della crescita | **growth hormone-releasing factor** *Released by the hypothalamus, it induces the release of somatotropin.* |
| fattore natriuretico atriale | **atrial natriuretic factor** *A chemical secreted by the right atrium that promotes sodium excretion in the urine.* |
| febbre | **fever** *A temperature above the normal range.* |
| febbre da acaro | **mite fever** *Synonym of typhus fever.* |
| febbre da fieno | **hay fever** *An allergy exhibited by pruritus of the eyes and nose, rhinorrhea and excessive lacrimal secretion.* |
| febbre da morso di ratto | **rat bite fever** *As the name implies, it is a condition exhibited by fever, nausea and skin erythema after one is bitten by a rat.* |
| febbre dell'ematuria | **blackwater fever** *A term used to describe the fever associated with malaria when the urine is reddish-black.* |
| febbre di mosca della sabbia | **sandfly fever** *A febrile illness transmitted by a sandfly, from the genus Phlebotomus, and found in the Mediterranean.* |
| febbre di risaia | **rice-field fever** *An infection cause by a species of Leptospira, affecting rice workers in Italy and Sumatra.* |
| febbre di zecche | **tick-borne fever** *A relapsing fever caused by a spirochete of the genus Borrelia.* |
| febbre effimero | **ephemeral fever** *A fever lasting no more than 24-48 hours.* |
| febbre fossato tettonico | **Rift valley fever** *A human febrile illness that is an endemic disease in sheep, transmitted by mosquitos and direct contact and caused by a virus of the family Bunyaviridae.* |
| febbre gialla | **yellow fever** *A viral, hemorrhagic fever transmitted by mosquitos.* |
| febbre malarica | **ague** *A term used to describe recurrent fever and shivering typically associated with malaria.* |
| febbre ondulante | **undulant fever** *Wave-like variations in the fever, going from very high to normal and back again, as seen in Brucellosis.* |
| febbre Q | **Q fever** *A disease caused by rickettsiae from the ingestion of unpasteurized milk.* |

| Italian | English |
|---|---|
| febbre recidivante | **relapsing fever** *A recurrent bacterial infection, with fever, caused by Spirochetes.* |
| febbre reumatico | **rheumatic fever** *A febrile streptococcal disease causing pain and joint swelling.* |
| febbre terzana | **tertian fever** *A febrile syndrome caused by Plasmodium vivax which produces a fever spike every 48 hours.* |
| febbre tifo | **typhus fever** *A rickettsiae infection exhibited by rash, fever, headache and myalgia.* |
| febbrile | **febrile** *Presence of an supraphysiologic temperature.* |
| febroelastosi | **fibroelastosis** *The abnormal increase in growth of fibrous and elastic tissue.* |
| fecaloma | **fecal impaction** *The presence of hard excrement in the rectum that requires manual removal.* |
| feci | **feces** *Excrement.* |
| feci nere | **black stools** *Common term for melena.* |
| fecondazione | **fertilization** *The melding of male and female gametes to form a zygote.* |
| fecondità | **fecundity** *The capability of producing offspring quickly and frequently.* |
| fedeltà | **adherence** *To stick to something figuratively or literally.* |
| feerita di cervello contraccolpo | **injury, contrecoup of brain** *An injury to the brain on the side opposite of that which was struck.* |
| fegato | **liver** *A large glandular organ in the right upper quadrant that functions in digestive processes, as well as, neutralizing toxins.* |
| femminile | **female** *Feminine.* |
| femore | **femur** *The long bone in the thigh.* |
| fenestrazione | **fenestration** *Usually referring to a surgical window.* |
| fenilchetonuria | **phenylketonuria** *A hereditary condition in which a person cannot excrete phenylalanine; untreated it causes brain and spinal cord dysfunction.* |
| fenotipo | **phenotype** *The visual expression exhibited by a person from the association of the genotype with the environment.* |
| ferire | **injure, to** *To hurt or to wound.* |
| ferita | **wound** *A tissue injury of varying severity.* |
| ferita da arma bianca | **stab wound** *An injury occurring with a sharp object.* |
| ferita da arma da fuoco | **gunshot wound** *An penetrating injury sustained from a bullet.* |
| ferita fisica o psichica | **trauma** *A physical injury or emotional shock.* |
| fermo | **firm** *Hard or unyielding.* |
| ferro | **iron** *An element found in hemoglobin.* |
| fertilità | **fertility** *The ability of a person to contribute to contraception.* |
| fessura | **fissure** *A general term for a cleft or deep groove. An anal fissure, for example, is a small ulcer adjacent to the anus.* |
| fessura vulvare; rima pudendi | **vulval cleft** *The area between the labia majora where the vagina and urethra rest.* |
| fetale | **fetal** *Referring to the fetus.* |
| feticismo | **fetichism** *The glorification of an inanimate object.* |
| feto | **fetus** *Medical term for the infant prior to birth.* |
| fetore | **fetor** *A foul odor.* |
| fettina | **slice** *A sliver or shaving.* |
| fiacco | **faint** *Weak and dizzy.* |
| fiala | **vial** *A small cylindrical container typically used to hold liquid medicine.* |
| fiasco | **flask** *A narrow-necked container.* |

| Italian | English |
|---|---|
| fibre simili a muschio | **mossy fiber** *Nerve fibers that surround the nerve cells of the cerebellar cortex.* |
| fibrillatura | **fibrillation** *Uncoordinated, ineffective contraction as in atrial fibrillation.* |
| fibrina | **fibrin** *An insoluble protein formed when fibrinogen is acted upon by thrombin.* |
| fibroadenoma | **fibroadenoma** *A benign breast mass composed of fibrous and glandular tissue.* |
| fibroblasto | **fibroblast** *A collagen producing cell in connective tissue.* |
| fibrocondrite | **fibrochondritis** *The inflammation of a structure composed of cartilage and fibrous tissue.* |
| fibroide | **fibroid** *A benign mass, typically uterine, composed of fibrous and muscle tissue.* |
| fibroma uterino | **uterine fibroids** *Benign tumors made up of muscular and fibrous tissue in the uterus. This is an older term for what is now known as leiomyoma.* |
| fibromatose plantare | **plantar fibromatosis** *Deep fascia nodules on the plantar aspect of the feet.* |
| fibromioma; leiomioma | **fibromyoma** *A mass containing fibrous and muscle tissue.* |
| fibrosarcoma | **fibrosarcoma** *A sarcoma composed primarily of malignant fibroblasts.* |
| fibrosi cistica | **cystic fibrosis** *A congenital disorder exhibited by abnormal thick mucous which leads to problems in the intestines, pancreas and lungs.* |
| fibrosite | **fibrositis** *Fibrous connective tissue that is inflamed.* |
| fibroso | **fibrosis** *Connective tissue that is scarred and thickened after injury.* |
| fibula | **fibula** *The smaller of two bones in the lower leg.* |
| figlia | **daughter** |
| filaria | **filaria** *A parasitic nematode worm that is transmitted by flies and mosquitos causing filariasis.* |
| filiforme | **filiform** *Threadlike.* |
| filo terminale | **filum terminale** *The thin structure at the end of the conus medullaris which connects the spinal cord with the coccyx.* |
| filtro vena cava inferiore | **vena cava filter** *A screen placed in the inferior vena cava to prevent blood clots from causing a pulmonary embolism.* |
| fimbria | **fimbria** *A slender projection at the end of the fallopian tube near the ovary.* |
| fimosi | **phimosis** *Stricture of the prepuce preventing it from being pulled back over the glans penis.* |
| finale | **last** *Final.* |
| finestra terapeutica | **therapeutic range** *The highest to lowest value that will produce a desired effect.* |
| fischiare | **whistle, to** *To make a high pitch noise by forcing air through the lips.* |
| fisiologia | **physiology** *A subspecialty of biology that studies the normal functioning of the body.* |
| fisioterapia | **physiotherapy** *Physical therapy.* |
| fissazione | **fixation** *1. An obsessive interest. 2. The securing of a body part.* |
| fistola | **fistula** *An abnormal communication between two organs or an organ and the skin, as in rectovaginal fistula.* |
| fistola anale | **anal fistula** *An opening in the skin that tracts to the anal canal thus causing some fecal material to leak from the opening in the skin.* |
| flaccido | **flaccid** *Limp. A term applied to an extremity one cannot move actively.* |
| flacone | **bottle** *A container used for the storage of liquids.* |
| flagellazione | **flagellation** *1. The protrusion found on flagella. 2. Massage administered by tapping a body part with fingers.* |
| flagello | **flagellum** *A slender appendage that allows protozoa to swim.* |

| Italian | English |
|---|---|
| flatulenza | **flatulence** *The gas expulsed from the anus.* |
| flatulenza | **flatus** *Term for air that is expelled from the anus.* |
| flebectomia | **phlebectomy** *Surgical excision of a vein.* |
| flebite | **phlebitis** *Inflammation of a vein.* |
| flebotrombosi | **phlebothrombosis** *Presence of a clot in a vein, without associated inflammation.* |
| flegmasia | **phlegmasia** *Inflammation or fever.* |
| flessione epatica del colon | **hepatic flexure of the colon** *The junction of the ascending and transverse portion of the colon.* |
| flessura | **flexure** *The action of bending.* |
| flessura iliaca del colon | **sigmoid flexure** *The S shaped curve located between the descending colon and rectum.* |
| flessura splenico del colon | **splenic flexure of the colon** *The portion of the colon that turns from the transverse to the descending colon.* |
| flittenulare | **phlyctenular** *Related to the formation of small vesicles on the cornea or conjunctiva.* |
| flottante | **floating** *Buoyant or suspended.* |
| fluido intraoculare | **intraocular fluid** *Fluid within the globe.* |
| fluido lacrimale | **lacrimal fluid** *Fluid secreted by the lacrimal gland.* |
| fluoresceina | **fluoresceine** *A fluorane dye used to check for corneal ulcers.* |
| fluoro | **fluorine** *A chemical that causes severe burns if exposed to the skin.* |
| fluorurazione | **fluoridation** *The addition of fluorine to something.* |
| flusso | **flow** *Movement in a continuous stream.* |
| flussometro con indicatore limite di portata | **peak flow** meter *A devic used to measure lung function in asthma.* |
| flutter | **flutter** *Used to describe a cardiac rhythm disturbance, as in atrial flutter.* |
| flutter atriale | **atrial flutter** *Sawtooth waves on an electrocardiogram with atrial rate of 250-330 per minute.* |
| fobia | **phobia** *An profound fear of something.* |
| foglietto | **leaflet** *Cusp.* |
| follicolare | **follicular** *Referring to a small secretory gland.* |
| follicolo pilifero | **hair follicle** *Tubelike invagination of the epidermis that the hair shaft develops from.* |
| fonazione | **phonation** *The vocalization of sounds.* |
| fondo dell'occhio | **eyeground** *The fundus that is visualized with an ophthalmoscope.* |
| fondo dell'occhio | **fundus oculi** *Portion of the interior eyeball in the posterior aspect which can be viewed by an ophthalmoscope.* |
| fondo gastrico | **fundus of the stomach** *Referring to the part of the stomach above the cardiac notch.* |
| foniatria | **phoniatrics** *The treatment of speech abnormalities.* |
| fontanella | **fontanelle or fontanel** *The space between the bones in the skull that are separate at birth.* |
| forame | **foramen** *An opening in a bone.* |
| forame magno | **foramen magnum** *The hole in the skull that the spinal cord passes through.* |
| forame nutrient | **nutrient foramen** *A conduit for passage of nutrient vessels in the marrow of bone.* |
| forame ovale | **foramen ovale** *A hole in the atrial septal wall in a fetus.* |
| forame ovale pervio | **patent foramen ovale** *A congenital anomaly in which there is a defect in the wall between the right and left atria; this can be a benign condition or result in cryptogenic strokes.* |
| forbici | **scissors** *A cutting instrument with two blades, joined at the middle.* |

| Italian | English |
|---|---|
| forchetta | **fourchette** *The fork shaped fold of skin where the labia minora meet superior to the perineum.* |
| forcipe | **forceps** *A surgical instrument, commonly called tweezers.* |
| forense | **forensic** *Referring to the scientific method of studying crime.* |
| forfora | **dandruff** *Dead skin found in the hair.* |
| fori di trapanazione | **burr hole** *A treatment of subdural hematoma that involves drilling a hole into the cranium to release the hematoma.* |
| forma di croce | **cruciform** *Shaped like a cross.* |
| formazione di ernia del disco | **herniated disc** *Prolapse of the nucleus pulposus into the spinal cord.* |
| formazione di ernia del tronco cerebrale | **brainstem herniation** *Movement of the brainstem into the incisura because of increased intracranial pressure.* |
| formicolio | **tingling** *Prickling or stinging sensation.* |
| formulario | **formulary** *A list of medicines that are permissible to prescribe.* |
| fornice | **fornix** *A vaulted structure.* |
| forte | **strong** *Having the power to move heavy objects.* |
| foruncolosi | **furunculosis** *The presence of multiple furuncles.* |
| forunucolo | **furuncle** *A painful erythematous nodule with a central core.* |
| forza | **strength** *Force, might or vigor.* |
| forza prensile | **grip strength** *Quantitative measurement of the force of a hand grip.* |
| fosfatasi acida | **acid phosphatase** *A phosphate derived chemical that is optimally active in an acidic environment.* |
| fosfaturia | **phosphaturia** *Presence of phosphates in the urine.* |
| fosfolipide | **phospholipid** *A substance, such as lecithin, that when hydrolyzed produces fatty acids, glycerin, and a nitrogen compound.* |
| fosfonecrosi | **phosphonecrosis** *The breakdown of the mandible caused by excessive exposure to phosphorus.* |
| fossa | **fossa** *A shallow depression.* |
| fossa cubitale | **cubital fossa** *The bend at the elbow.* |
| fossa popliteo | **popliteal fossa** *The hollow in the posterior aspect of the knee joint.* |
| fossa, fovea | **fovea** *The area on the retina where the visual acuity is optimal.* |
| fotofobia | **photophobia** *Abnormal sensitivity to light.* |
| fotometro a fiamma | **flame photometer** *A device used to measure the intensity of light.* |
| fotosensibilizzazione | **photosensitization** *The process of reacting to sunlight by developing edema and dermatitis.* |
| framboesia | **framboesia; yaws** *An endemic tropical disease caused by Treponema pertenue.* |
| framboesia | **yaws** *A tropical disease characterized by ulcers on the extremities, caused by Treponema pertenue.* |
| fratello (m); sorella (f) | **sibling** *A brother or sister.* |
| frattura | **fracture** *A broken bone.* |
| frattura a legno verde | **fracture, greenstick** *A spiral fracture.* |
| frattura aperta | **fracture, open** *A fracture in which there is a break in the skin and bone is exposed.* |
| frattura comminuta | **fracture, comminuted** *A broken bone where one segment overrides the other.* |
| frattura composta | **compound fracture** *Open fracture.* |
| frattura da avulsione | **fracture, avulsion** *A broken bone associated with a ligament or tendon pulling a piece of the bone away.* |
| frattura da sforza | **stress fracture** *A long bone fracture caused by repetitive mechanical stress.* |
| frattura depressa | **fracture, depressed** *The presence of concavity associated with a fracture as in a depressed skull fracture.* |

| Italian | English |
|---|---|
| frattura depressa del cranio | **depressed skull fracture** *Concave fracture deformity of the skull.* |
| frattura ossea | **break** *A common term for a fracture in a bone.* |
| frattura pathologica | **fracture, pathologic** *A fracture due at least in part to another condition, such as a fracture at a location where there is bone cancer.* |
| frattura semplice | **fracture, closed** *A broken bone where there is no break in the skin.* |
| frattura sforzo | **fracture, stress** *A fracture associated with overuse.* |
| freddo | **chill** *Sensation of coldness.* |
| freddo | **cold** *Having a sense of being cold.* |
| fremito | **fremitus** *A vibration that is appreciated with palpation.* |
| frenicectomia | **phrenicectomy** *Surgical excision of the phrenic nerve.* |
| frenico | **phrenic** *Referring to the diaphragm.* |
| frenoplegia | **phrenoplegia** *Paralysis of the diaphragm.* |
| frenulo | **frenulum** *The tissue that connects the inferior portion of the tongue to the base of the mouth.* |
| frequenza | **frequency** *Rate of occurrence.* |
| frequenza cardiaca | **heart rate** *Number or cardiac contractions per minute.* |
| frequenza cardiaca fetale (FCF) | **fetal heart tone** *Refers to the cardiac rate and pattern of the fetus.* |
| frequenza respiratoria | **respiratory rate** *The number of breaths per minute.* |
| friabile | **friable** *Easily reduced to powder.* |
| frontale | **frontal** *Referring to the anterior aspect, as in frontal lobe.* |
| fronte | **forehead** *Section of the face from the hairline to the eyebrows.* |
| frugale | **sparing** *Economical.* |
| fruttosuria | **fructosuria** *Presence of fructose in the urine.* |
| FSH ormone follicolo stimolante | **follicle stimulating hormone (FSH)** *An anterior pituitary gland hormone responsible for production of sperm or ova.* |
| fuga delle idee | **flight of ideas** *Streams of unrelated ideas noted in a manic phase.* |
| fulminante | **fulminant** *Sudden and severe.* |

| Italian | English |
|---|---|
| fumare | **smoke, to** *To inhale on a cigarette.* |
| fungicida | **fungicide** *An agent that destroys fungus.* |
| fungo | **fungus** *A spore-producing organism that feeds on organic matter.* |
| funicolite | **funiculitis** *Inflammation of the funiculi.* |
| funicolo laterale | **funiculus, lateral** *The lateral white column of the spinal cord between the anterior and posterior nerve roots.* |
| funicolo spermatico | **spermatic cord** *The structure containing the ductus deferens, testicular artery, and nerves that goes from the inguinal ring to the testis.* |
| funzione | **function** *An activity natural to a person or thing.* |
| fuoriuscita | **leakage** *Unintentional escape of gas or fluid.* |
| fusiforme | **fusiform** *Spindle-shaped.* |
| fusiforme acromatico | **achromatic spindle** *The threads between the poles of the spindle in karyokinesis.* |
| galattocele | **galactocele** *A milk-filled cyst in the mammary gland.* |
| galattorrea | **galactorrhea** *Excessive production of milk.* |
| galattosemia | **galactosemie** *1. Galactose in the blood. 2. A congenital condition exhibited by impaired carbohydrate metabolism.* |
| galattosio | **galactose** *A sugar that is a constituent of lactose.* |
| galoppo | **gallop** *An abnormal heart sound.* |
| galvanismo | **galvanism** *The use of electric currents for medical treatment.* |
| galvanometro | **galvanometer** *A device used to measure small electric currents.* |
| gamba | **leg** *One of two lower extremities.* |
| gambe senza riposa | **restless legs** *Associated with a syndrome exhibited by continuous movement of the legs from uncertain etiology.* |
| gamete | **gamete** *A germ cell that is able to unite with another germ cell of the opposite gender to form a zygote.* |
| gammaglobulina | **gamma globulin** *A blood serum protein with little electrophoretic mobility.* |
| gancio | **clasp** *Holding onto something with one's hand.* |
| gangli basale | **basal ganglia** *Structures adjacent to the thalamus that are involved with coordination of movement.* |
| gangliectomia | **ganglionectomy** *The removal of a benign swelling on a tendon sheath.* |
| ganglio genicolato | **geniculate ganglion** *The sensory ganglion of the facial nerve.* |
| ganglio spinale | **spinal ganglion** *The ganglion located on the dorsal root of each spinal nerve.* |
| ganglio stellato | **stellate ganglion** *Formed by the seventh cervical, eighth cervical and first thoracic ganglia.* |
| gangrena | **gangrene** *Tissue death from either impaired blood flow or an infection.* |
| gangrena gassosa | **gas gangrene** *A life and limb threatening disorder caused associated with tissue death and caused by an anaerobic bacterium in the genus of Clostridium.* |
| garantire | **ensure, to** *To make certain of.* |
| gargarizzare | **gargle, to** *To rinse one's mouth out and exhale through the liquid.* |
| gargoilismo | **gargoylism** *A congenital defect, also known as Hurler syndrome, it is characterized by skeletal anomalies, mental retardation and gargoyle-like facial features.* |
| garza | **gauze** *A fabric used for dressing changes.* |
| gas ematici arterioso | **arterial blood gas** *Measurement of the arterial concentration of carbon dioxide and oxygen.* |

| Italian | English |
|---|---|
| gas monossido di carbonio | **carbon dioxide gas** *A gas expelled during exhalation.* |
| gastrectomia | **gastrectomy** *Complete or partial surgical resection of the stomach.* |
| gastrico | **gastric** *Referring to the stomach.* |
| gastrina | **gastrin** *Hormones that stimulates gastric secretions.* |
| gastrite | **gastritis** *Inflammation of the stomach.* |
| gastrodigiunostomia | **gastrojejunostomy** *A surgical procedure that directly connects the stomach to the jejunum.* |
| gastroenterite | **gastroenteritis** *A bacterial or viral infection that leads to vomiting and diarrhea.* |
| gastroenterostomia | **gastroenterostomy** *A surgical opening in the stomach or intestine.* |
| gastropessia | **gastropexy** *Securing the stomach to the abdominal wall.* |
| gastroscopia | **gastroscopy** *Use of an endoscope to directly visualize the stomach.* |
| gastrostomia | **gastrostomy** *A surgical creation of an opening in the stomach.* |
| gel | **gel** *A jellylike substance.* |
| gelato | **frozen** *Past participle of to freeze. Freeze: turn a liquid into a solid.* |
| gemelli | **twins** *Two infants born at the same birthing.* |
| gemelli dizigotici | **dizygotic twins** *Twins from two separate zygotes (non-identical twins).* |
| gemelli monozigotici | **identical twins** *Twins from the same zygote.* |
| gemente | **mourning** *A period of grieving.* |
| gemito | **groan** *A deep inarticulate sound made due to pain or despair.* |
| gene | **gene** *A unit of heredity that is passed on from parent to child.* |
| generale | **general** *Common or expected.* |
| genetico | **genetic** *Referring to genes or heredity.* |
| gengiva | **gingival** *Referring to the gums.* |
| gengiva | **gum** *Gingiva.* |
| gengivite | **gingivitis** *Inflammation of the gums.* |
| genicolato | **geniculate** *Bent at a sharp angle.* |
| genitale | **genitalia** *Genitals.* |
| genitali ambigui | **genital ambiguity** *A disorder of sexual development in which the genitalia are not sufficiently developed to tell clearly if the person is male or female.* |
| genitourinario | **genitourinary** *Referring to the urinary system through the organs or urine excretion.* |
| genoma | **genome** *A full set of genetic information for an organism.* |
| geriatria | **geriatrics** *The study of the health of old people.* |
| germe | **germ** *Microorganism.* |
| gerontologia | **gerontology** *The study of old persons.* |
| gesso | **plaster** *Dehydrated gypsum that has water added to it in order to immobilize fractured extremities.* |
| gestazione | **gestation** *The development of a fetus from conception until birth.* |
| ghaiandola pineale | **pineal gland** *A small body posterior to the third ventricle of the brain.* |
| ghiandola acinoso | **acinous gland** *The exocrine part of the pancreas.* |
| ghiandola endocrino | **endocrine gland** *A gland that secrete hormones and other substances into the blood.* |
| ghiandola mammaria | **mammary gland** *The mass of tissue posterior to the nipples which has the essential task of milk production.* |
| ghiandola sebaceo | **sebaceous gland** *A gland in the skin that secretes sebum.* |
| ghiandola sudoripara | **apocrine gland** *A gland that releases some of its cytoplasm in secretions; an example is axillary sweat glands.* |
| ghiandole salivari | **salivary gland** *The parotid, submandibular and sublingual glands that secrete saliva.* |
| giallo | **yellow** *A color between green and orange in the spectrum* |

| Italian | English |
|---|---|
| giardiasi | **giardiasis** *A flagellate protozoa, Giardia lamblia, that causes diarrhea.* |
| gigantesco | **giant** *Huge or massive.* |
| ginecologia | **gynecology** *The branch of medicine associated with the reproductive system of women.* |
| ginecomastia | **gynecomastia** *Enlargement of the breasts.* |
| ginglimo | **ginglymus** *A joint that allows movement in one direction only.* |
| ginocchio | **knee** *The joint at the distal femur and proximal tibia.* |
| ginocchio delle lavandaie; borsite prepatellare | **housemaid's knee** *Also referred to as prepatellar bursitis.* |
| ginocchio instabile | **unstable knee** *A condition with giving way of the knee due to ligamentous or cartilaginous dysfunction.* |
| ginocchio valgo | **genu valgum** *A condition exhibited by the knees turning inward, commonly referred to as knock-knee.* |
| ginocchio valgo | **knock knees** *Common term for genu valgum.* |
| ginocchio varo | **genu varum** *A condition exhibited by the knees turning outward, commonly referred to as bowleg.* |
| giovane | **young** *Having lived for a short period.* |
| giovinezza | **youth** *The time between childhood and being an adult.* |
| gittata cardiaca | **cardiac output** *Amount of blood pumped by the heart in liters per minute.* |
| gittata ventricolare sistolica | **stroke volume** *The amount of blood ejected from the ventricle with each contraction.* |
| giugulare | **jugular** *Referring to the neck, as in jugular vein.* |
| giunzione stretto | **tight junction** *An intercellular junction with an impermeable membrane.* |
| giuramento di Ippocrate | **Hippocratic oath** *An vow taken by doctors, indicating they will treat people properly.* |
| giusto | **fair** *Equitable.* |
| glabella | **glabella** *The area of the forehead above and between the eyebrows.* |
| glande del pene | **glans penis** *The distal aspect of the penis.* |
| glaucoma | **glaucoma** *A condition characterized by increased intraocular pressure.* |
| glenoideo | **glenoid** *Referring to the fossa that is a shallow depression, such as the hollow of the scapula where the humeral head sets.* |
| glicemia | **glycemia** *The amount of glucose in the blood.* |
| glicerina | **glycerin** *A byproduct in the manufacture of soap that is used as a laxative.* |
| glicogenesi | **glycogenesis** *The production of glycogen from glucose.* |
| glicogeno | **glycogen** *A compound that stores glucose and when it undergoes hydrolysis forms glucose.* |
| glicolisi | **glycolysis** *The production of energy and pyruvic acid when glucose is broken down by enzymes.* |
| glicoproteina | **glycoprotein** *A protein that has a carbohydrate attached to its polypeptide chain.* |
| glicosuria | **glycosuria** *Presence of glucose in the urine.* |
| glioma | **glioma** *A neural malignant tumor of glial cells.* |
| gliomioma | **gliomyoma** *A mass with gliomatous and myomatous characteristics.* |
| globulina antilinfocito | **antilymphocyte globulin** *The gamma globulin portion of antilymphocyte serum.* |
| globus pallidus | **globus pallidus** *A portion of the lentiform nucleus in the brain.* |
| glomerulo | **glomerulus** *A grouping of capillaries where waste is filtered from the blood.* |

| Italian | English |
|---|---|
| glomerulonefrite | **glomerulonephritis** *Inflammation of the renal glomeruli, usually from hemolytic streptococcus.* |
| glomo carotideo | **carotid body** *Carotid artery receptors that are sensitive to blood chemistry changes.* |
| glossectomia | **glossectomy** *Surgical resection of the whole or part of the tongue.* |
| glossite | **glossitis** *Inflammation of the tongue.* |
| glossodinia | **glossodynia** *Tongue pain.* |
| glossofaringeo | **glossopharyngeal** *The name for cranial nerve IX that supplies the tongue and pharynx.* |
| glottide | **glottis** *Essentially the vocal structure, including the true vocal cords and the opening between them.* |
| glucagone | **glucagon** *A pancreatic enzyme responsible for breakdown of glycogen to glucose.* |
| gluteale | **gluteal** *Referring to the gluteus.* |
| gnosia | **gnosia** *Ability to recognize things and people.* |
| gocce al minuto | **drops per minute** *Refers to iv fluid rate.* |
| goccia | **drop** *A single bit of fluid as in a drop seen while giving IV fluids.* |
| goccia a goccia | **drop by drop** *Expression meaning little by little.* |
| gocciolamento postnasal | **post-nasal drip** *The descent of sinus drainage.* |
| gocciolare | **dribble, to** *To slowly, drip-by-drip, release urine for example.* |
| gola | **throat** *The anterior aspect of the neck.* |
| gomito | **elbow** *The joint between the humerus and radius/ulna.(right elbow, left elbow)* |
| gomito del tennista; epicondilalgia omerale | **tennis elbow** *Inflammation at the lateral aspect of the epicondyle where the muscle and tendon join; lateral epicondylitis.* |
| gomma | **gumma** *A soft granulomatous tumor of the skin or cardiovascular system seen in tertiary syphilis.* |
| gomma da masticare | **gum (chewing gum)** |
| gonade | **gonad** *A testis or an ovary.* |
| gonadotropina | **gonadotrophin** *Pituitary hormone that promotes gonadal activity.* |
| gonfiore caviglia | **ankle swelling** *Enlargement of the ankle region with or without pitting.* |
| gonococco | **gonococcus** *A diploccocal bacteria that is the causative agent in gonorrhea, formally Neisseria gonorrhoeae.* |
| gonorrea | **gonorrhea** *A sexually transmitted disease that is exhibited by purulent discharge from the vagina or penis.* |
| gota | **gout** *Monosodium urate crystal deposition disease.* |
| gozzo | **goiter** *Swelling of the thyroid gland.* |
| grado | **grade** *A level of rank or quality.* |
| grammo | **gram** *A unit of mass, 1/1000th of a kilogram.* |
| grande labbro della vulva | **labium majus (plural= labia majora)** *The folds of skin forming the lateral borders of the pudendal cleft.* |
| granulocito | **granulocyte** *A white blood cell with cytoplasmic secretory granules.* |
| granuloma | **granuloma** *A mass of granulation tissue.* |
| grasso | **fat** *A greasy or oiling substance naturally occurring in the body.* |
| gravida, incinta | **gravida** *Pregnant.* |
| gravidanza | **pregnancy** *The period of being pregnant.* |
| gravidanza ectopica | **ectopic pregnancy** *A pregnancy that is not intrauterine.* |
| grifosi | **chordee** *Downward bending of the penis.* |
| grosso | **gross** *Distended; not well defined.* |
| grosso, voluminoso | **bulky** *Voluminous or substantial.* |
| gruccia | **crutch** *Long metal or wooden stick used for support while walking.* |

| Italian | English |
|---|---|
| grugnito | **grunting** *A low guttural sound used to describe a person with profound respiratory difficulty.* |
| gruppo sanguigno | **blood grouping** *Testing blood to determine which type should be used for transfusion.* |
| gruppo sanguigno | **blood type** *Determined and listed in the ABO system.* |
| guaiaco | **guaiac** *A substance derived from guaiacum trees used to test for trace amounts of blood, in stool for instance.* |
| guaina | **sheath** *A covering.* |
| guancia | **cheek** *Lateral facial tissue.* |
| guanto | **glove** *A covering for hand protection.* |
| gustativa | **gustatory** *Referring to sense of taste.* |
| gusto | **taste** *Sensation of flavor perceived in one's mouth.* |
| gutturale | **guttural** *Having a harsh quality; coming from the back of the throat.* |
| herpes genitale | **genital herpes** *A sexually transmitted infection caused by herpes simplex.* |
| herpes simplex | **cold sore** *A perioral blister caused by herpes simplex.* |
| herpes, erpete | **herpes** *A skin condition exhibited by formation of clustered vesicular lesions; herpes simplex is at times referred to, albeit incompletely, as herpes.* |
| HIV virus dell'immuno deficienza umana | **HIV** *Abbreviation for human immunodeficiency virus.* |
| ialino | **hyaline** *Having a glassy, transparent appearance.* |
| ialino, vitreo | **hyaloid** *Transparent.* |
| iatrogeno | **iatrogenic** *A problem caused by medical treatment.* |
| ibrido | **hybrid** *An animal or plant produced from two different species.* |
| ictus amnesico | **amnesic stroke** *Cerebral infarct exhibited by loss of memory.* |
| id est; cioè | **i.e.** *A latin derived abbreviation for "that is to say"(In latin: id est)* |
| idatidiforme | **hydatiform** *Referring to a hydatid cyst.* |
| idiopatico | **idiopathic** *Relating to a disease with an unknown cause.* |
| idrartro | **hydrarthrosis** *An accumulation of water-like fluid in a joint cavity.* |
| idratazione | **hydration** *Used to describe fluid balance.* |
| idrocefalo | **hydrocephalus** *The excessive accumulation of cerebral spinal fluid in the brain causing enlargement of the head.* |
| idrocele | **hydrocele** *The accumulation of fluid in a body sac.* |
| idrocele scrotale | **scrotal hydrocele** *A benign collection of fluid in the scrotum.* |
| idrocortisone | **hydrocortisone** *A natural steroid hormone secreted by the adrenal cortex and used in a synthetic formulation for treatment of various medical conditions.* |
| idrofobia | **hydrophobia** *Abnormal fear of water.* |
| idrolisi | **hydrolysis** *A reaction with water causing a compound to breakdown.* |
| idronefrosi | **hydronephrosis** *Enlargement of a kidney due to interruption of outflow of urine from that kidney.* |
| idrope | **hydrops** *The abnormal collection of fluid in a cavity.* |
| idrope fetalis | **hydrops fetalis** *The total body accumulation of fluid in a fetus; the result of a hemolytic reaction in a Rh neg mother.* |
| idropneumotorace | **hydropneumothorax** *Abnormal accumulation of fluid and air in the pleural space.* |
| idrosadenite | **hidradenitis** *Inflammation of a sweat gland. When there is purulent discharge it is called hidradenitis suppurativa.* |
| idrosalpinge | **hydrosalpinx** *Collection of fluid in a fallopian tube.* |
| idrotorace | **hydrothorax** *Accumulation of fluid within the thoracic cavity.* |
| ifema | **hyphema** *A blood collection in the front of the eye.* |
| igiene orale | **oral hygiene** *Cleansing of the mouth and associated structures.* |

| Italian | English |
|---|---|
| igroma | **hygroma** *A cyst or bursa filled with fluid.* |
| igroscopico | **hygroscopic** *The tendency to absorb moisture from the air.* |
| iipotensione | **hypotension** *Abnormally low blood pressure.* |
| ilare | **hilar** *Referring to a hilus.* |
| ileite | **ileitis** *Inflammation of the ileum.* |
| ileo | **ileum** *The portion of the small bowel from the jejunum to the cecum.* |
| ileo | **ileus** *A temporary obstruction in the intestine.* |
| ileo elmintico | **verminous ileus** *Obstruction due to masses of intestinal parasites.* |
| ileocolite | **ileocolitis** *Inflammation of the ileum and cecum.* |
| ileocolostomia | **ileocolostomy** *Creating a surgical opening between the ileum and colon.* |
| ileoproctostomia | **ileoproctostomy** *Creating a surgical opening between the ileum and the rectum.* |
| ileostomia | **ileostomy** *Surgical creation of an opening in the ileum that is placed at the skin surface.* |
| iliococcigeo | **iliococcygeal** *Referring to the ilium and coccyx.* |
| illetterato | **illiterate** *Unable to read or write.* |
| ilo | **hilum or hilus** *A depression where blood vessels and nerve fibers enter an organ.* |
| imene | **hymen** *A membrane in the vagina.* |
| immobilizzare (con ferula un osso fratturato) | **brace, to** *Application of a splint.* |
| immune | **immune** *Being resistant to an infection.* |
| immunizzazione | **immunization** *A medication given to provide immunity.* |
| immunochimica | **immunochemistry** *The study of immune response and biochemistry.* |
| immunodeficienza | **immunodeficiency** *An inadequate immune response.* |
| immunoelettroforesi | **immunoelectrophoresis** *A means of differentiating proteins and other compounds by comparing their mobility and antigenic specificities.* |
| immunoglobuline | **immunoglobulin** *Serum and cellular proteins of the immune system.* |
| immunosoppressione | **immunosuppression** *The inhibition of the immune response.* |
| impastamento | **petrissage** *Massage using a kneading action.* |
| imperfezione | **defect** *A shortcoming or imperfection.* |
| imperforato | **imperforate** *Lack of an opening. An infant with an imperforate anus has a congenital defect with no anal opening.* |
| impervio | **impervious** *Not affected by.* |
| impianto | **implant** *A device or prosthesis implanted in a person.* |
| implementazione | **implementation** *The process of putting a plan into effect.* |
| impotenza | **impotence** *Inability to act or inability to achieve a penile erection.* |
| imprevisto | **unexpected** *Unforeseen.* |
| improvviso | **abrupt** *Suddenly or hastily.* |
| impulso nervo | **nerve impulse** *A signal transmitted along a nerve fiber.* |
| in atto da lungo tempo | **long-standing** *Having existed for a long time.* |
| in avanti | **forwards** *Towards the front.* |
| in disparte | **apart** *Separated by a distance.* |
| inadattabilità | **maladjustment** *Having the trait of being unable to cope normally.* |
| inalazione | **inhalation** *The act of breathing in.* |
| inanizione | **inanition** *Generalized weakness from lack of nutrition.* |
| inanizione | **starvation** *Death related to starvation.* |
| inarticolato | **inarticulate** *Indistinct speech.* |
| incapacità lavorativa | **disability** *Decreased or impaired mental or physical ability.* |
| incavo | **socket** *An anatomical hollow that is part of an articulation. (eyeball socket)* |

| Italian | English |
|---|---|
| incerto | **unsteady** *Unstable or wobbly.* |
| incesto | **incest** *Sexual relations between related people.* |
| inchiodamento (di osso fratturato) | **nailing** *Referring to placement of an intramedullary rod in a long bone in order to treat a fracture.* |
| incipiente | **incipient** *Starting to happen.* |
| incisione | **incision** *An intentional surgical cut in the skin.* |
| incisivo | **incisor** *Sharp-edged tooth; humans have four incisors.* |
| incisura | **incisura** *A notch or indentation usually on the edge of a bone.* |
| incisura giugulare | **jugular notch** *The notch on the upper border of the sternum.* |
| incoerente | **incoherent** *Absence of intelligible speech.* |
| incompetenza cervicale | **Cervical insufficiency (formerly incompetent cervix)** *Painless changes in the cervix that result in recurrent second semester pregnancy loss.* |
| incontinenza | **incontinence** *Inability to control urination.* |
| incontinenza urinaria | **urinary incontinence** *Involuntary micturition.* |
| incoordinazione | **incoordination** *Absence of smooth, efficient body movement.* |
| incoscienza | **unconsciousness** *Unable to respond to sensory stimuli.* |
| incremento | **increment** *An increase on a fixed scale.* |
| incubatrice | **incubator** *A warming device for infants.* |
| incubo | **nightmare** *An unpleasant or frightening dream.* |
| incudine | **incus** *The middle ear bone between the stapes and malleus.* |
| incuneamento di un dente | **impaction, tooth** *A tooth that does not erupt because adjacent teeth prevent it.* |
| indagine di massa | **screening** *An evaluation as part of a methodical study.* |
| indagine urodinamica | **urodynamics** *A study done to determine whether a person has the contractile capacity in the bladder to void spontaneously.* |
| indigeno | **indigenous** *Naturally occurring.* |
| indigestione | **indigestion** *Inadequate digestion for various reasons.* |
| indispensabile | **mandatory** *Obligatory.* |
| indolore; torpido | **indolent** *1. Causing little pain. 2. Slow healing ulcer.* |
| indurimento | **induration** *An area that is abnormally hard.* |
| indurre | **induce, to** *Facilitated. When referring to labor, it means medication was given to assist in delivery of the fetus.* |
| inefficiente | **ineffective** *Unsuccessful or inefficient.* |
| inerzia | **inertia** *The tendency to remain unchanged.* |
| inevitabile | **inevitable** *Not preventable.* |
| infantile | **infantile** *Referring to babies or young children.* |
| infanzia | **infancy** *Early childhood.* |
| infarto | **infarct** *Referring to dead tissue.* |
| infarto | **infarction** *Dead tissue, for example, myocardial infarction.* |
| infarto bianco o ischemia | **transient ischemic attack** *Cerebral ischemic changes resulting from transitory hypoperfusion.* |
| infarto lacunare | **lacunar infarction** *Small non-cortical cerebral infarcts.* |
| infarto miocardico | **myocardial infarction** *The death of myocardial tissue as a result of an interruption in flow to the region supplied by a coronary vessel.* |
| infarto rosso o ictus cerebrale | **cerebrovascular accident (stroke)** *A decrease in level of consciousness and paralysis caused by a cerebrovascular thrombosis, hemorrhage or vasospasm.* |
| infecundo 2) asettico | **sterile** *1. Infertile 2. Refers to equipment that is free of contamination.* |
| inferiore | **inferior** *The lower aspect.* |
| infermiera | **nurse** *A person trained to care for the sick.* |
| infermiera professionista | **nurse practitioner** *A person with advanced training capable of acting as a patient's primary care provider.* |

| Italian | English |
|---|---|
| infermità; malattia | **sickness** *Illness or a state of disease.* |
| infestazione | **infestation** *The presence of large numbers, as in lice infestation.* |
| infestazione da vermi del genere Enterobius | **enterobiasis** *An infection caused by worms from the genus Enterobius.* |
| infettato da Chlamydia | **chlamydiosis** *A disease caused by the species Chlamydia.* |
| infettivo | **infectious** *Contagious.* |
| infezione crociata | **cross-infection** *Transfer of infection between individuals, each with a different organism.* |
| infezione nosocomiale | **nosocomial infection** *An infection occurring after admission to a hospital.* |
| infezione orecchio | **ear infection** *General term referring to otitis media or otitis externa.* |
| infiammazione | **inflammation** *Localized redness, excessive warmth and swelling.* |
| infiammazione del tessuto cellulare | **cellulitis** *Infection characterized by diffuse, subcutaneous inflammation.* |
| infiammazione delle guaine tendinee | **tendinitis** *Inflammation of a tendon.* |
| influenza | **influenza** *Viral infection causing fever, muscle aches and catarrh.* |
| influenza aviaria | **avian flu** *A viral disease found in birds and fowl that can be transmitted to humans; it is exhibited by respiratory and gastrointestinal symptoms but can lead to encephalitis.* |
| infraspinoso | **infraspinous** *Below the scapular spine.* |
| infundibolo | **infundibulum** *The connection between the hypothalamus and the posterior pituitary gland.* |
| infusione | **infusion** *The injection of fluid into tissue or a vein.* |
| infusione intravenoso; infusione endovenoso | **intravenous infusion** *Administration of fluid into a vein.* |
| ingestione | **ingestion** *The intake of food or liquid orally.* |
| inghiottire | **swallow, to** *To cause something to pass down the esophagus.* |
| inginocchiarsi | **kneeling** *Being on one's knees as in the prayer position.* |
| ingrossamento | **enlargement** *Becoming bigger.* |
| inguinale | **inguinal** *Referring to the groin.* |
| inguinocrurale pruriginosa dei lavandai | **dhobie itch** *So called because the contact dermatitis is caused by the soap used by laundry workers in India who are called "dhobie".* |
| inibitore dell'enzima convertitore dell'angiotensina | **angiotensin converting enzyme inhibitors (ACEI)** *A class of medicines that prevent conversion of angiotensin I to angiotensin II, a potent vasoconstrictor.* |
| inibitore monoamino-ossidasi | **monoamine oxidase inhibitor (MAOI)** *A drug used to treat depression that allows accumulation of serotonin and norepinephrine.* |
| iniezione | **injection** *The act of a needle being inserted into a body.* |
| iniezione ipodermica | **hypodermic injection** *Subcutaneous injection.* |
| inizio di travaglio | **labor onset** *The time when a pregnant woman begins uterine contractions in the process of childbirth.* |
| innervazione | **innervation** *The presence of a nerve supply.* |
| innesto autogeno | **autograft** *Grafting tissue from one part of person to another part of the same person.* |
| innesto peduncolo | **pedicle** *Part of a skin/tissue graft temporarily left connected to the original site.* |
| innocuo | **harmless** *Safe or benign.* |
| innominata | **innominate** *Referring to the innominate artery.* |
| inoculazione | **inoculation** *Injection with a vaccine to provide immunity.* |
| inorganico | **inorganic** *Not coming from natural growth.* |
| insensibile | **insensible** *Unable to perceive a stimulus.* |
| inserzione | **insertion** *The act of inserting something.* |
| insezione | **cut** *An incision.* |

| Italian | English |
|---|---|
| insidioso | **insidious** *A slow, gradual and harmful advancement.* |
| insieme | **comprehension** *Understanding.* |
| insignificante | **trivial** *Of little importance or value.* |
| insonnia | **insomnia** *Sleeplessness.* |
| insorgenza | **onset** *The beginning of an event.* |
| inspessire | **inspissate, to** *To thicken or congeal.* |
| inspirazione | **inspiration** *Drawing in a breath.* |
| insufficienza aortico | **aortic insufficiency** *A dysfunction of the aortic valve allowing backflow of blood into the heart.* |
| insufficienza cardiaca congestizia | **cardiac failure** *Decreased cardiac output of the heart.* |
| insufficienza cardiaca congestizia | **congestive heart failure** *A diminished cardiac output leading to passive engorgement.* |
| insufficienza renale | **renal failure** *Diminution of kidney function.* |
| insulina | **insulin** *A hormone produced by the pancreas and synthetically to control blood glucose levels.* |
| insulinoma | **insulinoma** *An islet cell tumor that causes abnormally high insulin secretion and thus hypoglycemia.* |
| intensivo | **intensive** *Very thorough or vigorous.* |
| interarticolare | **interarticular** *Between the articular surfaces of a joint.* |
| intercellulare | **intercellular** *Between cells.* |
| intergrigine | **intertrigo** *Irritation present because adjacent surfaces rub together.* |
| intermittente | **intermittent** *Occurring at irregular intervals.* |
| interno | **inside** *Inner part, center.* |
| interno | **internal** *Situated on the inside.* |
| interstiziale | **interstitial** *Referring to the interstices of tissue.* |
| intertrocanterico | **intertrochanteric** *Referring to the space within the trochanter.* |
| intervallo | **interval** *An intervening time.* |
| intervallo di dosaggio | **dosing interval** *The number of times per unit a medication is given.* |
| interventricolare | **interventricular** *Between the ventricles.* |
| intestinale | **intestinal** *Referring to the intestines.* |
| intestino | **intestine** *A general term used for the section of bowel from the stomach to the anus.* |
| intorno | **around** *On every side of.* |
| intorpidimento | **numbness** *Decreased sensation to tactile stimuli.* |
| intossicazione alimentare | **food poisoning** *Poisoning where the active agent is in the food.* |
| intra-articolare | **intraarticular** *Within a joint space.* |
| intracellulare | **intracellular** *Within a cell.* |
| intracerebrale | **intracerebral** *Within the cerebrum.* |
| intracranico | **intracranial** *Within the cranial vault.* |
| intradermico | **intradermal** *Within the dermis.* |
| intradurale | **intradural** *Within the dural space.* |
| intramidollare | **intramedullary** *1. Within the medulla oblongata. 2. Within the bone marrow.* |
| intramuscolare | **intramuscular** *Within a muscle.* |
| intraosseo | **intraosseous** *Within a bone.* |
| intraperitoneale | **intraperitoneal** *Within the peritoneal cavity.* |
| intratecale | **intrathecal** *Technically means within a sheath but this term is used when medication is instilled in the dura mater spinalis.* |
| intrauterino | **intrauterine** *Within the uterus.* |
| intravenoso; endovenoso | **intravenous** *Within a vein.* |

| Italian | English |
|---|---|
| intubazione | **intubation** *Placement of a tube; commonly used to refer to endotracheal intubation.* |
| intussuscezione | **intussusception** *The inversion of one portion of the bowel into another.* |
| inulina | **inulin** *A polysaccharide used in the testing of renal function.* |
| invalido | **cripple** *A person with a physical disability; not used in polite society.* |
| invecchiamento | **aging** *Becoming older.* |
| involucro | **involucrum** *A wrap or covering (referring to a sequestrum).* |
| involutivo | **involutional** *The shrinkage of an organ when it is not in use, as in the uterus after childbirth.* |
| involuto | **involved** *Difficult to comprehend.* |
| iodio | **iodine** *A chemical used as an antiseptic and a deficiency of it can lead to goiter.* |
| iodismo | **iodism** *A condition caused by excessive iodine intake resulting in diarrhea, weakness, and convulsions.* |
| iontano da | **away from** *Separated from.* |
| iper-reflessia | **hyperreflexia** *Abnormally brisk and vigorous reflex.* |
| iperacidità | **hyperacidity** *An abnormally high acid level.* |
| iperalgesia | **hyperalgesia** *Greater than normal sensitivity to pain.* |
| iperattività | **hyperactivity** *Abnormal increase in activity.* |
| iperberico | **hyperbaric** *Use of gas at a higher than normal pressure.* |
| iperbilirubinemia | **hyperbilirubinemia** *Higher than normal level of bilirubin in the blood.* |
| ipercalcemia | **hypercalcemia** *Higher than normal level of calcium in the blood.* |
| ipercapnia | **hypercapnia** *Higher than normal level of carbon dioxide in the blood stream.* |
| ipercheratosi | **hyperkeratosis** *Excessive thickening of the outer layer of skin.* |
| ipercinesia | **hyperkinesis** *Excessive activity and inability to concentrate.* |
| ipercolesterolemia | **hypercholesterolemia** *Higher than normal level of cholesterol in the blood.* |
| ipercromia | **hyperchromia** *An excessive level of hemoglobin in erythrocytes.* |
| iperdosaggio | **overdose** *An above normal dose of a medication.* |
| iperemia | **hyperemia** *An increase in blood for the area of concern.* |
| iperestensione | **hyperextension** *Extension of an articulation beyond the normal range.* |
| iperestesia | **hyperesthesia** *Higher than normal skin sensitivity.* |
| iperfagia | **hyperphagia** *Excessive food ingestion.* |
| iperflessione | **hyperflexion** *Flexion of an articulation beyond the normal range.* |
| iperforia | **hyperphoria** *Upward deviation of the visual axis of the eye.* |
| iperglicemia | **hyperglycemia** *Higher than normal level of glucose in the blood.* |
| ipergonadismo | **hypergonadism** *A condition of excessive gonadal activity and subsequently precocious sexual development.* |
| iperidrosi | **hyperhidrosis** *Excessive perspiration.* |
| iperkaliemia | **hyperkalemia** *Higher than normal level of potassium in the blood stream.* |
| iperlipemia | **hyperlipidemia** *Higher than normal level of lipids in the blood stream.* |
| iperlipemia | **lipemia** *Abnormally high fat content in the blood.* |
| ipermetrope | **longsighted** *Synonym of hyperopia.* |
| ipermetropia | **hypermetropia** *Farsightedness.* |
| ipermnesia | **hypermnesia** *Unusually good memory.* |
| ipernatremia | **hypernatremia** *Elevated level of sodium in the blood.* |
| ipernefroma | **hypernephroma** *A renal tumor that mimic adrenal cortical tissue.* |
| iperonichia | **hyperonychia** *Hypertrophic nails.* |

| Italian | English |
|---|---|
| iperopia | **hyperopia** *Farsightedness.* |
| iperosmia | **hyperosmia** *Increased sense of smell.* |
| iperparatiroidismo | **hyperparathyroidism** *Excessive level of parathyroid hormones in the blood stream causing weak bones and hypocalcemia.* |
| iperpiressia | **hyperpyrexia** *Fever.* |
| iperpituitarismo | **hyperpituitarism** *Excessive eosinophilic hormone resulting in acromegaly or excessive basophilic hormone resulting in pituitary compression and ultimately hypopituitarism.* |
| iperplasia | **hyperplasia** *Excessive growth of normal cells.* |
| iperpnea | **hyperpnea** *Abnormal increase in rate and depth of respiration.* |
| ipersensibilità | **hypersensitivity** *Abnormal increase in sensitivity.* |
| ipersplenismo | **hypersplenism** *Excessive splenic activity resulting in decreased peripheral blood elements and sometimes splenomegaly.* |
| ipertensione arteriosa | **hypertension** *Higher than normal blood pressure.* |
| ipertensione arteriosa maligno | **malignant hypertension** *Sudden, severe hypertension associated with neuroretinitis.* |
| ipertensione portale | **portal hypertension** *Hypertension in the portal system of the liver as seen in conditions causing obstruction to the portal vein.* |
| ipertermia | **hyperthermia** *Fever.* |
| ipertiroidismo | **hyperthyroidism** *Increased thyroid activity resulting in exophthalmos and increased metabolic rate.* |
| ipertonia | **hypertonia** *Excessive tone or tension.* |
| ipertonia musculare | **hypermyotonia** *Excessive muscle tone.* |
| ipertonico | **hypertonic** *Increased osmotic pressure.* |
| ipertricosi | **hypertrichosis** *Excessive hair growth.* |
| ipertrofia | **hypertrophy** *Pathologic organ enlargement.* |
| iperuricemico | **hyperuricemia** *Elevated level of uric acid in the blood.* |
| iperventilazione | **hyperventilation** *Rapid and deep respirations.* |
| ipervolemia | **hypervolemia** *Abnormally large amount of fluid in the blood stream.* |
| ipnotico | **hypnotic** *Sleep inducing agent.* |
| ipocalcemia | **hypocalcemia** *Lower than normal level of calcium in the blood.* |
| ipocapnia | **hypocapnia** *A decreased level of carbon dioxide in the blood.* |
| ipocloridria | **hypochlorhydria** *A state of decreased secretion of hydrochloric acid in the stomach.* |
| ipocondriaco | **hypochondriac** *A person suffering from hypochondriasis.* |
| ipocondrio | **hypochondrium** *The upper abdomen lateral to the epigastrium.* |
| ipocondrìa | **hypochondriasis** *Abnormal increase in concern about one's own health.* |
| ipocromico | **hypochromic** *Referring to the abnormal decrease in hemoglobin content of erythrocytes.* |
| ipoestesia | **hypoesthesia** *Abnormally decreased skin sensitivity.* |
| ipofibrinogenemia | **hypofibrinogenemia** *Diminished blood fibrinogen level.* |
| ipofisectomia | **hypophysectomy** *Surgical removal of the pituitary gland.* |
| ipofisi | **hypophysis** *Pituitary gland.* |
| ipofisi | **pituitary gland** *A gland at the base of the hypothalamus.* |
| ipoforia | **hypophoria** *Downward deviation of the visual axis of the eye.* |
| ipofosfatasia | **hypophosphatasia** *A genetic defect of diminished alkaline phosphatase in the cells leading to bone demineralization.* |
| ipogastrico | **hypogastric** *Referring to the hypogastrium.* |
| ipogastrio | **hypogastrium** *The area of the central abdomen located below the stomach.* |
| ipoglicemia | **hypoglycemia** *Abnormally low blood sugar.* |

| Italian | English |
|---|---|
| ipogonadismo | **hypogonadism** *Abnormal decrease in gonadal function with associated diminished growth and sexual development.* |
| ipokaliemia | **hypokalemia** *Diminished level of potassium in the blood stream.* |
| ipomania | **hypomania** *A moderate form of mania.* |
| iponatriemia | **hyponatremia** *Diminished level of sodium in the blood stream.* |
| ipoparatiroidismo | **hypoparathyroidism** *Abnormal decrease in parathyroid function.* |
| ipopion | **hypopyon** *The presence of purulent fluid in the anterior chamber of the eye.* |
| ipopituitarismo | **hypopituitarism** *Diminished pituitary activity exhibited by obesity and persistence of adolescent characteristics.* |
| ipoplasia | **hypoplasia** *Incomplete development.* |
| iposalivazione | **hyposalivation** *Secretion of saliva below the normal rate.* |
| ipospadia | **hypospadias** *Congenital condition exhibited by development of the urethral meatus on the inferior aspect of the penis.* |
| ipossia | **hypoxia** *Diminished oxygen content.* |
| ipostasi | **hypostasis** *The formation of a deposit.* |
| ipotalamo | **hypothalamus** *Located inferior to the thalamus it controls visceral activities, water balance, temperature and sleep.* |
| ipotensione posturale | **postural hypotension** *A significant drop in blood pressure when going from the supine or sitting position to standing.* |
| ipotermia | **hypothermia** *Lower than normal temperature.* |
| ipotiroidismo | **hypothyroidism** *Reduced functioning of the thyroid.* |
| ipotonia | **hypotonia** *Reduced tone or activity.* |
| ippocampo | **hippocampus** *The area at the base of the cerebral ventricles thought to be the center of memory and emotion.* |
| ippocratismo digitale | **clubbing** *Increase in the mass of the soft tissue of the terminal phalanges.* |
| iride | **iris** *The colored membrane posterior to the cornea.* |
| iridectomia | **iridectomy** *Surgical removal of part of the iris.* |
| iridociclite | **iridocyclitis** *Inflammation of the ciliary body and the iris.* |
| iridoplegia | **iridoplegia** *Paralysis of part of the iris with subsequent lack of contraction or dilation of the pupil.* |
| iridotomia | **iridotomy** *A surgical opening of the iris.* |
| irradiazione | **irradiation** *The process of being irradiated.* |
| irsutismo | **hirsutism** *Abnormal growth on hair on a person's face and body.* |
| ischemia | **ischemia** *Inadequate blood supply to a part of the body.* |
| ischio | **ischium** *The inferoposterior portion of the pelvis.* |
| isoanticorpo | **isoantibody** *A situation in which an antibody of person A reacts with an antigen of person B.* |
| isola | **islet** *Tissue that is structurally separate from adjacent tissues.* |
| isolamento | **isolation** *To be kept separate or apart.* |
| isotopo radioattivo | **radioactive isotope** *An isotope with an unstable nucleus that is used in diagnostic imaging.* |
| istamina | **histamine** *A chemical responsible for the reaction exhibited when a person has an allergic reaction.* |
| isterectomia | **hysterectomy** *Surgical removal of the uterus.* |
| isteria | **hysteria** *A psychological condition exhibited by uncontrolled emotion or exaggerated manifestations.* |
| isterografia | **hysterography** *1. Recording of uterine contractions. 2. Roentgenography of the uterus after administration of contrast media.* |
| isteromiomectomia | **hysteromyomectomy** *Surgical removal of a uterine myoma.* |
| isteropessi | **hysteropexy** *Surgical fixation of the uterus by shortening of the round ligaments or by other means.* |

| Italian | English |
|---|---|
| isterosalpingografia | **hysterosalpingography** *Roentgenography of the uterus and fallopian tubes after instillation of contrast media.* |
| isterotomia | **hysterotomy** *Surgical opening of the uterus.* |
| istidina | **histidine** *An amino acid precursor to histamine.* |
| istiocito | **histiocyte** *A phagocytic cell found in connective tissue.* |
| istiocitochimica | **histochemistry** *Study of intracellular distribution of chemicals, reaction sites and enzymes.* |
| istmo | **isthmus** *A narrow piece of tissue connecting two larger body parts.* |
| istologia | **histology** *The study of the structure and composition of minute structures.* |
| istoplasmosi | **histoplasmosis** *A fungal pulmonary infection from bat and bird excrement.* |
| itterizia neonatale | **jaundice of the newborn** *A form of jaundice seen in newborns in the first two weeks of life; also called icterus neonatorum.* |
| ittero | **icterus** *Yellowing of the skin and sclerae because of excess bilirubin.* |
| ittero | **jaundice** *Yellowing of the sclerae and skin because of excessive bilirubin in the blood.* |
| ittero nucleare | **kernicterus** *A condition associated with high bilirubin levels that causes yellow staining of cerebral tissues and subsequent neurologic dysfunction.* |
| ittiosi | **ichthyosis** *A congenital anomaly exhibited by excessively dry, thick skin.* |
| juxta-articolare; giusta-articolare | **juxta-articular** *Positioned near a joint.* |
| kala-azar | **kala-azar** *A disease caused by Leishmania donovani that is exhibited by weight loss, fever, anemia and hepatosplenomegaly.* |
| Klinefelter, sindrome di | **Klinefelter's syndrome** *Presence of an extra X chromosome, it is exhibited by longer legs, narrow shoulders, small testicles and gynecomastia.* |
| kopofobia | **kopophobia** *A morbid fear of fatigue.* |
| kwashiorkor | **kwashiorkor** *A form of malnutrition from inadequate protein intake.* |
| labbra meno | **labium minus (plural=labia minora)** *The folds of skin posterior to the labia majora.* |
| labbro | **labium** *Referring to any lip shaped structure.* |
| labbro dell'acetabolo | **labrum** *An edge or lip. The labrum acetabular is the fibrocartilagous rim attached to the acetabulum.* |
| labbro inferiore | **lip, lower** *Labium inferius oris.* |
| labbro leporino | **cleft lip** *A congenital abnormal opening of the lip.* |
| labbro superiore | **lip, upper** *Labium superius oris.* |
| labiale | **labial** *Referring to the lip.* |
| labile | **labile** *Easily altered; emotionally unstable.* |
| labirintite | **labyrinthitis** *Inflammation of the labyrinth.* |
| labirinto | **labyrinth** *Inner ear structure concerned with balance.* |
| laboratorio | **laboratory** *A room equipped to run blood, tissue and fluid samples.* |
| lacerazione | **laceration** *An injury that produced a cut in the skin or tissue such as a tear during childbirth.* |
| lacerazione perineale | **perineal laceration** *Tearing of the tissue adjacent to the vaginal that can occur during childbirth.* |
| lacrima | **tear** *As in, to shed a tear.* |
| lacrimale | **lacrimal** *Referring to the secretion of tears.* |
| lacrimare | **weep, to** *To shed tears.* |
| lacrimazione | **lacrimation** *The secretion of tears.* |
| lacuna | **lacuna** *A small cavity or depression.* |

| Italian | English |
|---|---|
| lagoftalmo | **lagophthalmos** *Characterized by the inability to close the eyelid completely over the eye.* |
| lalochezia | **lalochezia** *Relief of stress by uttering obscenities.* |
| lalofobia | **laliophobia** *Abnormal fear of speaking or stuttering.* |
| lambdoideo | **lambdoid** *The suture connecting the parietal bones with the occipital bone.* |
| lamella | **lamella** *A thin layer of bone.* |
| lamento | **complaint** *Grievance.* |
| laminectomia | **laminectomy** *The surgical removal of part of a vertebrae.* |
| lancetta; bisturi | **lancet** *A small sharp instrument used to obtain a drop of blood for testing.* |
| lanugine | **down** *In a lower position.* |
| laparoscopia | **laparoscopy** *A procedure utilizing a laparoscope.* |
| laparoscopio | **laparoscope** *A fiber-optic instrument used to visualize the peritoneal contents.* |
| laparotomia | **laparotomy** *A surgical incision of the abdomen.* |
| laparotomie explorative | **exploratory laparotomy** *Abdominal surgery with the intent of examining the abdominal contents.* |
| larghezza | **width** *Side to side measurement.* |
| laringe | **larynx** *A hollow muscular structure that contains the vocal cords.* |
| laringectomia | **laryngectomy** *Surgical removal of the larynx.* |
| laringeo | **laryngeal** *Referring to the larynx.* |
| laringismo stridulo | **laryngismus stridulus** *Sudden, severe laryngeal spasm.* |
| laringite | **laryngitis** *Inflammation of the larynx.* |
| laringofaringe | **laryngopharynx** *The pharyngeal space between the superior aspect of the glottis and the opening of the larynx.* |
| laringologia | **laryngology** *The study of the larynx and related diseases.* |
| laringospasmo | **laryngospasm** *Sudden, involuntary muscle contraction of the larynx.* |
| laringostenosi | **laryngostenosis** *Abnormal narrowing of the larynx.* |
| laringotomia | **laryngotomy** *Surgical creation of an opening in the larynx.* |
| laterale | **lateral** *Referring to the side of the body.* |
| laterale | **side** *A position medial or lateral to center.* |
| laterdeviazione | **laterodeviation** *Pushed to the lateral aspect.* |
| latirismo | **lathyrism** *A disease characterized by tremors, spastic paralysis and paresthesias caused by Lathyrus sativus.* |
| lattalbumina | **lactalbumin** *Proteins found in milk.* |
| lattasi | **lactase** *An enzyme that facilitates the breakdown of lactose to glucose and galactose.* |
| lattazione | **lactation** *The secretion of milk from mammary glands.* |
| latte di mucca | **cow's milk** |
| lattico | **lactic** *Referring to milk.* |
| lattosio | **lactose** *A disaccharide present in milk.* |
| lavaggio | **flush, to** *Term used to describe an irrigation procedure, as in flushing an NG tube.* |
| lavaggio gastrico | **gastric lavage** *Instillation and removal of large quantities of saline into the stomach in order to treat poisoning.* |
| lebbra | **leprosy** *A contagious disease caused by Mycobacterium leprae that causes insensate papules and disfiguration.* |
| lecitina | **lecithin** *A compound widely used by tissues, derived from egg yolks and it consists of phospholipids linked to choline.* |
| lecocitosi | **leukocytosis** *An increase in the number of leukocytes.* |
| legamento | **ligament** *A band of fibrous connective tissue that connects two bones or cartilage.* |

| Italian | English |
|---|---|
| legamento biforcuto | **bifurcate ligament** *A ligament on the dorsum of the foot that includes the calcaneonavicular and calcaneocuboid ligaments.* |
| legamento largo dell'utero | **broad ligament of uterus** *Supports the uterus on both sides.* |
| legamento pettineo | **pectineal ligament** *A continuation of the lacunar ligament along the pectineal line in the pubis.* |
| legatura | **ligature** *A thread used to tie a vessel.* |
| leggero | **light** Not heavy. |
| leishmaniosi | **leishmaniasis** *A condition caused by a flagellate protozoan parasite that is exhibited by visceral or dermatologic manifestations.* |
| lembo | **limbus** *The margin of a structure, for example, of the cornea and sclera.* |
| lembo (lembo da braccio a braccio) | **flap** *A term used to describe a piece of tissue partially excised and placed over an adjacent surface. (cross arm flap)* |
| lembo di cuticola ungueale | **hangnail** *A loose piece of skin attached near the medial or lateral nail fold.* |
| lenitivo | **demulcent** *Something that relieves irritation or inflammation.* |
| lente | **lens** *The transparent chamber between the posterior chamber and the vitreous body.* |
| lenti a contatto | **contact lens** *A lens that fits over the cornea to correct refractive errors.* |
| lenti da vista | **eyeglasses** *Eye wear used for cosmetic or prescription purposes.* |
| lenticolare | **lenticular** *Referring to the lens of the eye.* |
| lentiggine | **lentigo** *A benign condition exhibited by flat brown patches on the skin.* |
| lentiggine | **macula solaris** *Formal medical term describing a freckle.* |
| lento | **slow** *Unhurried.* |
| leontiasi ossea | **leontiasis ossea** *Bilateral hypertrophy of the bones of the face and cranium.* |
| leproma | **leproma** *A superficial granulatomous papule that is seen in leprosy.* |
| leptomeningite | **leptomeningitis** *A general term used to describe meningitis of the pia and arachnoid of the brain.* |
| leptospirosi itteroemorragica | **leptospirosis** *A zoonosis caused by the spirochete Leptospira interrogans transmitted by rats and contaminated water.* |
| lesbico | **lesbian** *A woman with same gender preference.* |
| lesione alla testa | **head trauma** *Any injury to the brain.* |
| lesione alla testa chiusa | **injury, closed head** *Brain trauma not associated with damage to the dura or skull.* |
| lesione cutanea | **skin lesion** *An abnormal but not necessarily cancerous lesion.* |
| lesione da scoppio | **blast injury** *Trauma from a wave of air pressure.* |
| lesione iperestensione-iperflessione | **injury, hyperextension-hyperflexion** *An injury, usually to the cervical spine, that involves rapid deceleration, causing pronounced extension and flexion.* |
| lesione scapsulamento | **injury, degloving** *Trauma that involves the ripping of skin and subcutaneous tissue from the underlying tissue.* |
| lesione; ingiuria | **injury** *A wound, abrasion or contusion.* |
| lesioni del ago-bastone | **needle-stick injury** *The inadvertent self-puncture with a needle that had been used previously to inject a patient.* |
| letale | **lethal** *Deadly.* |
| letargia | **lethargy** *Absence of energy.* |
| lettiga | **stretcher** *A device used to carry a patient in the supine position.* |
| letto | **bed** *A mattress resting on a frame.* |
| letto ungueale | **nail bed** *The area just beneath a finger or toenail. Also called matrix unguis.* |

| Italian | English |
|---|---|
| leucemia | **leukemia** *A malignant disease causing an increase in the number of abnormal and immature leukocytes.* |
| leucemia linfocito | **lymphocytic leukemia** *Chronic accumulation of functionally incompetent lymphocytes.* |
| leucina | **leukine (or leucine)** *An amino acid obtained from hydrolysis of some proteins.* |
| leucinosi | **leucinosis; maple syrup urine disease** *A condition characterized by an enzyme defect causing an increase in leucine in the urine.* |
| leucocitemia | **leukocythemia** *Synonym of leukemia.* |
| leucocito | **leukocyte** *A white blood cell.* |
| leucocitolisi | **leukocytolysis** *Destruction of white blood cells.* |
| leucoderma | **leukodermia** *A localized loss of skin pigment.* |
| leuconichia | **leukonychia** *A whitish discoloration of the fingernails and toenails.* |
| leucopenia | **leukopenia** *A decreased number of leukocytes in the blood.* |
| leucopoiesi | **leukopoiesis** *Production of white blood cells.* |
| leucorrea | **discharge, vaginal** *Vaginal secretions.* |
| leucorrea | **leukorrhea** *Thick white vaginal discharge.* |
| levulosio | **levulose** *Synonym for fructose.* |
| libero | **free** *Lacking or absent.* |
| libero da | **free from** *Without or clear of.* |
| libido | **libido** *Sexual desire.* |
| lichen | **lichen** *A term used to describe a variety of papular skin diseases. Lichen planus is a shiny, flat, violaceous eruption of the mucous membranes, skin and genitalia.* |
| lieve | **slight** *Minor or small.* |
| lievito | **yeast** *A unicellular fungus.* |
| ligamentum teres uteri | **round ligament of the uterus** *The supporting structure of the uterus.* |
| liipasi | **lipase** *A pancreatic enzyme that facilitates the breakdown of fats.* |
| linea alba | **linea alba** *The tendinous portion of the anterior abdomen between the two rectus muscles.* |
| linea mediana | **midline** *A median line of bilateral separation.* |
| linfa | **lymph** *A transparent and sometimes opalescent fluid that flows in the lymph channels.* |
| linfadenite | **lymphadenitis** *Inflammation of a lymph node.* |
| linfangectasia | **lymphangiectasis** *Distention of the lymph channels.* |
| linfangioma | **lymphangioma** *A mass composed of newly formed lymph tissue.* |
| linfangite | **lymphangitis** *Inflammation of the lymph vessels.* |
| linfatico | **lymphatic** *Referring to the lymph system.* |
| linfocito | **lymphocyte** *A white blood cell produced by the lymph tissue.* |
| linfocitopenia | **lymphocytopenia** *Decrease in the usual number of lymphocytes in the blood.* |
| linfocitosi | **lymphocythemia** *Abnormally high number of lymphocytes in the blood.* |
| linfocitosi | **lymphocytosis** *The organization of cysts containing lymph.* |
| linfoide | **lymphoid** *Similar to lymph.* |
| linfoma | **lymphoma** *A malignant disease of the lymph system, Hodgkin's lymphoma for example.* |
| linfosarcoma | **lymphosarcoma** *A malignant disease of the lymph system that does not include Hodgkin's lymphoma.* |
| lingua | **tongue** *The fleshy muscular organ of the mouth.* |
| lingua fragola | **strawberry tongue** *A characteristic discoloration of the tongue seen in an early phase of scarlet fever.* |

| Italian | English |
|---|---|
| lingua nigra | **lingua nigra** *A condition characterized by a dark fur-like covering on the dorsum of the tongue.* |
| linguaggio | **speech** *Oral articulation.* |
| linguale | **glossal** *Referring to the tongue.* |
| linguetta pelosa | **hairy tongue** *Lingua villosa, a benign condition associated with antibiotic used caused by candida albicans infection.* |
| lipide | **lipid** *A compound that is a fatty acid which is insoluble in water but soluble in organic solvents.* |
| lipidi abbassamento farmaco | **lipid-lowering agent** *A medication used to treat hyperlipidemia.* |
| lipoatrofia | **lipoatrophy** *Fatty tissue atrophy.* |
| lipocito | **lipocyte** *A fat cell.* |
| lipocondrodistrofia | **lipochondrodystrophy** *A congenital condition exhibited by short stature, kyphosis, mental deficiency and short fingers.* |
| lipodistrofia | **lipodystrophy** *Abnormal fat metabolism.* |
| lipoideo | **lipoid** *Referring to fat.* |
| lipoidosi | **lipoidosis** *Abnormal lipid metabolism.* |
| lipoma | **lipoma** *A benign tumor consisting of fat cells.* |
| lipoproteina | **lipoprotein** *A soluble protein used to transport fat or lipids.* |
| lipotimia momentanea da brusca | **blackout** *Common term for loss of consciousness.* |
| liquido amniotico | **amniotic fluid** *The fluid surrounding the fetus.* |
| liquido cerebrospinale | **CSF** *Abbreviation for cerebrospinal fluid.* |
| liquido sinoviale | **synovial fluid** *The fluid that surrounds, for example, the knee within a capsule.* |
| liquor cerebrale | **cerebrospinal fluid (CSF)** *The fluid between the pia mater and arachnoid membrane.* |
| lisi | **lysis** *The rupture of a cell wall or membrane.* |
| lisina | **lysine** *An amino acid found in most proteins.* |
| lisosomi | **lysosome** *An organelle contained in the cytoplasm of eukaryotic cells.* |
| lisozima | **lysozyme** *An enzyme in tears that facilitates destruction of certain bacterial cell walls.* |
| listeriosi | **listeriosis** *A disease caused by Listeria monocytogenes that occurs in the pregnant and immunocompromised.* |
| litagogo | **lithagogue** *A treatment of a calculus.* |
| litico | **lytic** *Referring to lysis.* |
| litolapassi | **litholapaxy** *The crushing and then removal of a calculus.* |
| litotomia | **lithotomy** *Surgical removal of a calculus.* |
| litotribo | **lithotriptor** *An instrument used to crush a calculus.* |
| livello di alcol nel sangue | **blood alcohol level** *A quantitative measurement of the amount of alcohol in the blood.* |
| lividezza postmortem | **post-mortem lividity** *The purplish discoloration occurring 30-120 minutes after death in dependent body parts.* |
| Loa loa, infestazione de | **loiasis** *A disease caused by the filarial nematode Loa loa.* |
| lobare | **lobar** *Referring to a lobe.* |
| lobectomia | **lobectomy** *Surgical removal of a lobe (generally lung or liver).* |
| lobo | **lobe** *A body part divided by a fissure.* |
| lobo dell'orecchio | **earlobe** *The soft, fleshy inferior portion of the pinna.* |
| lobotomia | **lobotomy** *Surgical incision into the prefrontal lobe; historically a treatment of mental illness.* |
| lobulo | **lobule** *A small lobe.* |
| localizzato | **localized** *Toward one point or area.* |
| localizzazione | **localization** *Establishment of a site of a disease process.* |

| Italian | English |
|---|---|
| lochiazione | **lochia** *Vaginal secretions noted within two weeks of childbirth.* |
| loculato | **loculated** *Divided into small cavities.* |
| logopedista | **speech therapist** *A person trained to assist people with speech and language disorders.* |
| lombaggine | **lumbago** *Pain in the region of the lumbar spine.* |
| lombare | **lumbar** *Referring to the spinal region inferior to the thoracic spine.* |
| longevità | **longevity** *Long life.* |
| lordosi | **lordosis** *An abnormal depth of the inward curvature of the spine.* |
| lottare | **cope, to** *To deal with a difficult situation.* |
| lubrificante | **lubricant** *Emollient.* |
| lucido | **clear** *Lucid.* |
| lume | **lumen** *A hollow cavity.* |
| luminoso | **light** *Illumination, bright.* |
| lunga durata d'azione | **long-acting** *Referring to a drug with long lasting effects.* |
| lunghezza | **length** *The end to end measurement.* |
| lunula | **lunula** *The pale area at the base of a fingernail.* |
| lupus eritematoso sistemico | **lupus erythematosus** *An autoimmune inflammatory disease exhibited by a butterfly shaped rash on the face along with visceral and connective tissue abnormalities.* |
| lussazione | **dislocation** *The displacement of a bone when referring to an articulation.* |
| luteotropo | **luteotropic** *Synonym of prolactin.* |
| lutto | **bereavement** *The sorrow one feels with the loss of a loved one.* |
| l'essere lamentoso | **querulousness** *Whining or complaining.* |
| macchia | **blemish** *A small mark on one's skin.* |
| macchia; chiazza | **macula** *1. The area of the eye of greatest visual acuity that surrounds the fovea. 2. A small flat discoloration of the skin (synonym for macule).* |
| macchie di Koplik | **Koplik's spots** *Red buccal macules with a blue center; seen in measles.* |
| macchina cuore -polmoni | **heart lung machine** *Device used during cardiac surgery to replace the function of the heart and lungs while surgery is performed.* |
| macrocheilia | **macrocheilia** *Abnormally large lips.* |
| macrocito | **macrocyte** *A large red blood cell.* |
| macrocitosi | **macrocytosis** *Referring to the status of an increased number of large erythrocytes as seen in Vitamin B12 deficiency.* |
| macrodattilia | **macrodactyly** *Abnormally large digits.* |
| macroencefalia | **macroencephaly** *Having an abnormally large head.* |
| macrofago | **macrophage** *A phagocytic cell that originates in the tissues.* |
| macroglia | **astroglia** *The neurologic tissue which is composed of astrocytes.* |
| macroglobulinemia | **macroglobulinemia** *A condition exhibited by an increase number of macroglobulins in the blood.* |
| macroglossia | **macroglossia** *Abnormally large tongue.* |
| macromastia | **macromastia** *Abnormally large breasts.* |
| macromelia | **macromelia** *Abnormally large head or extremity.* |
| macrostomia | **macrostomia** *Abnormal increase in the width of the mouth.* |
| maculopapula | **maculopapule** *A skin lesion that is similar to both a macule and a papule.* |
| madido | **moist** *Damp or humid.* |
| maggiore del normale | **greater than normal** *Above normal.* |
| magnetico | **magnetic** *Having the properties of a magnet.* |
| magro | **thin** *Lean or slender.* |
| mal di gola | **sore throat** *Common term for pharyngitis.* |

| Italian | English |
|---|---|
| mal di lombi; coxalgia | **coxalgia** *Pain in the hip.* |
| mal di schiena | **low back pain** *Pain in the lumbar region.* |
| malacia | **malacia** *The abnormal softening of a body part or tissue.* |
| malallineamento | **malalignment (dental)** *Displacement of the teeth from their normal position.* |
| malaria | **malaria** *A condition caused by a protozoan of the genus Plasmodium. It is transmitted by mosquitos and is exhibited by fever, chills, headache. In the severe form it can lead to convulsions, increased ICP and death.* |
| malaria cerebrale | **cerebral malaria** *A severe form of malaria manifested by seizures and a decreased level of consciousness.* |
| malatti di Crohn | **Crohn's disease** *An inflammatory bowel disease.* |
| malatti di memielinizzazione | **demyelinating disease** *A condition characterized by the loss of myelin.* |
| malattia da graffio di gatto | **cat scratch fever** *An infectious disease characterized by local inflammation a the site of the scratch, local lymph adenopathy and fever.* |
| malattia da reflusso gastroesofageo | **GERD gastroesophageal reflux disease** *A condition characterized by gastric contents being regurgitated into the esophagus or mouth.* |
| malattia dei capelli riorti | **kinky-hair syndrome** *Inborn error of copper metabolism, noted in the first few weeks of life. Exhibited by sparse kinky hair, failure to thrive and seizures. Also called Menke's syndrome or trichopoliodystrophy.* |
| malattia dei cassoni | **caisson disease** *Decompression sickness.* |
| malattia del legionario | **legionnaires' disease** *The name was derived after an outbreak at a convention of the American Legion; it is manifested by fever, chills, dyspnea, and cough.* |
| malattia del sonno; tripanosomiasi | **sleeping sickness** *Also called Trypanosomiasis, this disease is caused by a parasitic protozoa and transmitted by the tsetse fly.* |
| malattia delle Azzorre | **Azorean disease** *A form of hereditary ataxia found in peoples of Azorean descent. Also called Machado-Joseph disease or Portuguese-Azorean disease.* |
| malattia dell'urina a sciroppo diacero | **maple syrup urine disease** *A condition characterized by an enzyme defect causing an increase in leucine in the urine.* |
| malattia di Adams-Stokes | **Adams-Stokes Syndrome** *Characterized by bradycardia, syncope and convulsions.* |
| malattia di altitudine | **altitude sickness** *A general term used for an illness that occurs at high altitude.* |
| malattia di Alzheimer | **Alzheimer's disease** *A dementia of unknown cause or pathogenesis.* |
| malattia di cuore congenito | **congenital heart disease** *A cardiac disorder present prior to birth.* |
| malattia di De Quervain | **De Quervain tenosynovitis** *Inflammation of the tendons of the wrist including the abductor pollicis longus and extensor pollicis brevis.* |
| malattia di foresta Kyasanur | **Kyasanur Forest disease** *A viral fever noted in Mysore, India transmitted by Haemaphysalis spinigera. It is characterized by fever, headache, generalized pains, diarrhea, and intestinal bleeding.* |
| malattia di Hansen; lebbra | **Hansen's disease** *Leprosy* |
| malattia di Köhler | **Köhler's disease** *A genetic disease characterized by osteonecrosis and subsequent collapse of the tarsal navicular bone.* |
| malattia di Lobo | **Lobo's disease** *A condition exhibited by small, red, hard papules in the sacral region caused by Lacazia loboi.* |
| malattia di Strümpell | **Strümpell's disease** *Also known as spondylitis deformans, it is characterized by arthritis and osteitis deformans of the spinal cord with a rounded kyphosis and rigidity.* |

| Italian | English |
|---|---|
| malattia infiammatoria pelvica | **pelvic inflammatory disease** *Generally a bacterial infection affecting a woman with potential involvement of the uterus, fallopian tubes, ovaries and cervix.* |
| malattia mentale | **behavior disorder** *An abnormal mental state.* |
| malattia periodontale | **periodontal disease** *Present around to a tooth.* |
| malattia trasmessa sessualmente | **sexually transmitted disease (STD)** *A condition one obtains from another during sexual relations.* |
| malattia, infermità | **disease** *Malady or disorder.* |
| maleducato | **rude** *Ill-mannered.* |
| malessere | **malaise** *A vague feeling of discomfort or unease.* |
| malformazione arterovenoso | **arteriovenous malformation** *A sac like structure created by the abnormal communication of an adjacent artery and vein.* |
| malgrado | **despite** *Notwithstanding.* |
| maligno | **malignant** *Tendency of a tumor to invade normal tissue.* |
| malleolo | **malleolus** *A bony protrusion on medial and lateral aspect of each ankle.* |
| malleolo esterno | **malleolus, lateral** *The lateral aspect of the distal fibula.* |
| malleolo tibiale interno | **malleolus, medial** *The medial aspect of the distal portion of the tibia.* |
| malnutrizione | **malnutrition** *Lack of appropriate nutrition.* |
| maltosio | **maltose** *A disaccharide hydrolyzed by amylase.* |
| malunione | **malunion** *The union of a fracture in a faulty position.* |
| mammario | **mammary** *Referring to the breast.* |
| mammillare | **mammillary** *Referring to a nipple.* |
| mammografia | **mammography** *Roentgenography of the breasts, used as a screening test for cancer.* |
| mammoplastica | **mammaplasty** *Plastic surgery of the breast.* |
| mancanza | **absence of** |
| mancanza | **deficiency** *Insufficiency or deficit.* |
| mancanza di peristalsi | **aperistalsis** *Lack of intestinal peristalsis.* |
| mancino | **left-handed** *The preference of using the left hand for common tasks.* |
| mandibola | **jaw** *Mandible.* |
| mandibola | **mandible** *The lower jaw.* |
| mandorla | **amygdala** *Any almond shaped structure such as the tonsil* |
| mangiare | **eat, to** *To consume food.* |
| mania | **mania** *A mental disorder exhibited by hyperexcitability, delusions and euphoria.* |
| mano | **hand** *The upper extremity distal to the wrist.* |
| mano ad artiglio | **clawhand** *A hand deformity caused by ulnar nerve palsy exhibited by the hyperextension of the metacarpophalangeal joints and flexion of the interphalangeal articulations.* |
| mano di scimmia | **monkey-paw** *An appearance due to median nerve palsy causing atrophy of the thenar eminence with adduction and elevation of the thumb, resembling that of a simian.* |
| manometro | **manometer** *Device used for pressure monitoring.* |
| manovra di Adson | **Adson maneuver** *A test used to screen for thoracic outlet syndrome.* |
| manovra di Bill | **Bill maneuver** *During childbirth, use of forceps at midpelvis to help extract the head.* |
| manovra di Bracht | **Bracht maneuver** *Delivery of a fetus in a breech position.* |
| manovra di Buzzard | **Buzzard maneuver** *Testing of the patellar reflex while the client firmly touches the floor with their toes in a sitting position.* |
| manovra di Hampton | **Hampton maneuver** *Rolling a patient during gastrointestinal fluoroscopy in order to obtain an air contrast of the antrum and duodenum.* |

| Italian | English |
|---|---|
| manovra di Heimlich | **Heimlich maneuver** *A forceful upward thrust to the diaphragm to dislodge an airway obstruction.* |
| manovra di Hillis-Müller | **Hillis-Müller maneuver** *A procedure to determine the descent of the head during active labor.* |
| manovra di Hueter | **Hueter's maneuver** *The application of downward and forward pressure on the tongue while passing an gastric tube.* |
| manovra di Jendrassik | **Jendrassik's maneuver** *A method of distracting a patient while checking the patellar reflex.* |
| manovra di Leopold | **Leopold's maneuver** *Used to determine fetal position.* |
| manovra di Mcdonald | **Mcdonald's maneuver** *A measurement of the uterus in centimeters that corresponds to gestational age in weeks.* |
| manovra di Ritgen | **Ritgen's maneuver** *A procedure that controls the rate of delivery of the infant's head during childbirth.* |
| manovra di Valsalva | **Valsalva's maneuver** *A technique in which one attempts to exhale with the mouth and nose closed; this equalizes pressure in the ears.* |
| manubrio dello sterno | **manubrium sterni** *The superior segment of the sternum which articulates with the clavicle and first rib.* |
| marasma | **marasmus** *Progressive weight loss and emaciation.* |
| marihuana | **marijuana** *Cannabis.* |
| marsupializzazione | **marsupialization** *Creation of a surgical pouch.* |
| martello | **malleus** *Small bone in the inner ear that articulates with the incus.* |
| mascella | **maxilla** *The upper jaw that also forms the inferior portion of the orbit and part of the nose.* |
| maschera a ossigeno a circuito aperto | **non-rebreather mask** *A type of oxygen mask used to deliver a higher oxygen concentration.* |
| mastectomia | **mastectomy** *Surgical resection of one or both breasts.* |
| masticare | **chew, to** *Masticate.* |
| masticazione | **mastication** *Chewing.* |
| mastite | **mastitis** *Inflammation of the breast.* |
| mastodinia | **mastodynia** *Breast pain.* |
| mastoide | **mastoid** *Referring to the mastoid process.* |
| mastoidectomia | **mastoidectomy** *Surgical removal of the mastoid.* |
| mastoidite | **mastoiditis** *Inflammation of the mastoid process.* |
| mastzellen | **mast cell** *A cell containing basophilic granules that releases histamine and other substances during allergic reactions.* |
| materasso | **mattress** *A fabric case filled with material, used for sleeping.* |
| materia grigia | **gray matter** *The section of the brain and spinal cord composed of branching dendrites and nerve cell bodies.* |
| maxillo-facciale | **maxillofacial** *Referring to the maxilla and the face.* |
| mazamorra | **mazamorra** *Dermatitis caused by hookworm larvae indigenous to Puerto Rico.* |
| meato | **meatus** *Opening to the body, such as urethral meatus.* |
| meconio | **meconium** *The first newborn feces which are green.* |
| mediale | **medial** *Situated toward the midline.* |
| mediastino | **mediastinum** *The thoracic area between the lungs.* |
| mediastinoscopia | **medianstinoscopy** *Visual inspection of the mediastinum with a scope.* |
| medicazione | **medication** *A substance used for medical treatment.* |
| medicazione (medicazione a secco) | **dressing** *The gauze applied to a wound. (dry dressing)* |
| medicazione compressiva | **pressure dressing** *A dressing used for compression to reduce bleeding.* |
| medicina 2) medicamento | **medicine** *A substance used for medical treatment or 2) the art and science of healing patients.* |

| Italian | English |
|---|---|
| medicina mucleare | **nuclear medicine** *The branch of medicine associated with the use of radioactive material in the evaluation and treatment of disease.* |
| medico | **physician** *Medical practitioner.* |
| medico dentista | **dentist** *A professional capable of treating diseases of the teeth and gums.* |
| medicochirurgico | **medicosurgical** *Referring to medicine and surgery.* |
| medulloblastoma | **medulloblastoma** *A malignant tumor of the cerebellum found mostly in children.* |
| megacariocito | **megakaryocyte** *A cell found in the bone marrow that is a source of platelet production.* |
| megacolon | **megacolon** *Abnormal enlargement and dilatation of the colon.* |
| megaloblasto | **megaloblast** *A large red blood cell noted primarily in pernicious anemia.* |
| megalocefalia | **megacephaly** *Having a larger than normal cranial capacity.* |
| megalomania | **megalomania** *A mental disorder characterized by abnormal feelings of self-importance.* |
| meiosi | **meiosis** *Cell division creating two daughter cells each with half the number of cells as the parent cell.* |
| melancolia | **melancholia** *Profound sadness.* |
| melanina | **melanin** *A dark pigment found on the skin, hair or iris.* |
| melanoma | **melanoma** *Malignant cancer, typically found in the skin.* |
| melena | **melena** *The passage of black, tarry stools indicative of upper gastrointestinal bleeding.* |
| melissofobia | **melissophobia** *Also called apiphobia, a fear of bees.* |
| melite | **melitis** *Inflammation of the cheek.* |
| membrana cellulare | **cell membrane** *The semipermeable structure surrounding the cytoplasm of a cell.* |
| membrana del timpano | **ear-drum** *Common term for tympanic membrane.* |
| membrana timpanica | **tympanic membrane** *The membrane between the external and middle ear.* |
| membro | **limb** *An extremity or branch.* |
| membro | **member** *Referring to an extremity (arm or leg).* |
| memoria | **memory** *Ability to remember.* |
| memoria | **recollection** *Memory.* |
| menarca | **menarche** *The time of the initial menstrual period.* |
| meningeo | **meningeal** *Referring to the dura mater, arachnoid and the pia mater.* |
| meningioma | **meningioma** *A tumor of the meningeal tissue; generally benign.* |
| meningismo | **meningism** *Signs and symptoms of meningitis without infection of the meninges.* |
| meningite | **meningitis** *Inflammation of the meninges exhibited by fever, photophobia, nuchal rigidity and in severe cases coma and convulsions.* |
| meningite criptococcica | **cryptococcal meningitis** *A meningeal infection associated with AIDS.* |
| meningocele | **meningocele** *A congenital defect exhibited by protrusion of the meninges through a defect in the spinal column.* |
| meningococcemia | **meningococcemia** *Presence of N. meningitidis in the blood.* |
| menisco | **meniscus** *A thin cartilage between joint surfaces.* |
| menisectomia | **meniscectomy** *Surgical excision of a meniscus.* |
| menopausa | **menopause** *The time when menstruation ceases.* |
| menorragia | **menorrhagia** *Abnormally large amount of menstrual blood.* |
| mentale | **mental** *Cognitive or psychological.* |
| mento | **chin** *Mentum; the anterior projection of the lower jaw.* |
| menzionare | **mention, to** *Refer to or allude to.* |

| Italian | English |
|---|---|
| merluzzo | **cod** *A large marine fish, also called codfish.* |
| mesarterite | **mesarteritis** *Inflammation of the middle layer of an artery.* |
| mesencefali tetto | **tectum mesencephali** *The posterior portion of the mesencephalon including the sup. and inf. colliculi and tectal lamina.* |
| mesencefalo | **mesencephalon** *Midbrain.* |
| mesencefalo | **midbrain** *The portion of the brainstem superior to the pons.* |
| mesenchima | **mesenchyme** *Organized mesodermal cells that produce connective tissue, lymphatics and bone.* |
| mesentere | **mesentery** *The fold of peritoneum that connects the small bowel, pancreas and spleen to the posterior portion of the abdominal wall.* |
| mesoappendice | **mesoappendix** *The portion of the mesentery vermiform appendix.* |
| mesocolon | **mesocolon** *The mesentery connecting the colon to the posterior abdominal wall.* |
| mesoderma | **mesoderm** *The middle germ layer in an embryo that is the source of bone, muscle and skin.* |
| mesonefroma | **mesonephroma** *Usually a tumor of the female genital tract that is thought to stem from the mesonephros.* |
| mesosalpinge | **mesosalpinx** *A portion of the broad ligament supporting the fallopian tubes.* |
| mesotelioma | **mesothelioma** *A tumor that stems from mesothelial tissue; a known cause is asbestos exposure.* |
| mesovario | **mesovarium** *The portion of the mesentery connecting the ovary with the abdominal wall.* |
| mestruazioni | **menses** *The blood and other material expelled from the uterus during menstruation.* |
| mestruazioni | **menstruation** *Synonym of menses.* |
| metabolico | **metabolic** *Referring to the physical and chemical reactions involved with keeping an organism functioning.* |
| metacarpale | **metacarpal** *The name for any of the five hand bones.* |
| metacarpofalangeo | **metacarpophalangeal** *Referring to the metacarpus and the phalanges.* |
| metaemoglobina | **methemoglobin** *A substance formed with the oxidation of hemoglobin.* |
| metafisi | **metaphysis** *The region between the diaphysis and the epiphysis.* |
| metaplasia | **metaplasia** *Abnormal change in the nature or character of tissue.* |
| metatarsale | **metatarsal** *Any of the bones of the foot.* |
| metatarsalgia | **metatarsalgia** *Foot pain.* |
| metencefalo | **hindbrain** *The brainstem which includes the pons, medulla oblongata and cerebellum.* |
| metionina | **methionine** *A sulfur-containing amino acid used in the biosynthesis of cysteine.* |
| metodo di Crede | **Credé's maneuver** *Manual pressure over the bladder to assist in expression of urine in an atonic bladder.* |
| metro | **meter** *Unit if measurement. (instrument for measurement)* |
| metro a nastro | **tape measure** *A long length of tape, marked at intervals for measuring.* |
| metrorragia | **metrorrhagia** *Uterine bleeding in normal amounts but at irregular intervals.* |
| mezzo | **half** *Divided in two.* |
| mezzogiorno | **noon** *The 12 o'clock mid-day hour.* |
| mialgia | **myalgia** *Muscle pain.* |
| miastenia gravis | **myasthenia gravis** *An autoimmune disease characterized by fluctuating weakness of the ocular, limb and respiratory muscles.* |
| micetoma | **mycetoma** *Persistent inflammation of the tissues caused by an infection.* |
| micosi | **mycosis** *A disease caused by a fungal infection.* |

| Italian | English |
|---|---|
| micotossina | **mycotoxin** *A substance toxic to fungus.* |
| microbiologia | **microbiology** *The study of microorganisms.* |
| microbo | **microbe** *A microorganism.* |
| microcefalico | **microcephalic** *A congenital deformity exhibited by an abnormally small head.* |
| microcito | **microcyte** *An unusually small erythrocyte associated with anemias, such as iron deficiency anemia.* |
| microftalmo | **microphthalmos** *A congenital condition characterized by smallness of the eyes.* |
| micrognazia | **micrognathia** *Abnormally small maxilla or mandible.* |
| microgrammo | **microgram** *One millionth of one gram.* |
| micrometro | **micrometer** *One millionth of one meter.* |
| microorganismo | **microorganism** *An organism only seen with a microscope.* |
| microscopio | **microscope** *A instrument used to magnify and view small objects.* |
| microscopio elettrone | **electron microscope** *A device that uses electron beams and lenses to give high magnification.* |
| midollare | **medullary** *1. The inner part of an organ. 2. Referring to the medulla oblongata.* |
| midollare del surrene | **adrenal medulla** *The innermost part of the adrenal gland.* |
| midollo allungato | **medulla oblongata** *The inferior portion of the brainstem.* |
| midollo osseo | **bone marrow** *The soft material filling the cavity of bones.* |
| midollo spinale | **spinal cord** *The bundle of nerves that with the brain comprise the central nervous system.* |
| midriasi | **mydriasis** *Pupillary dilation.* |
| mielina | **myelin** *The substance that forms a sheath around some nerve fibers.* |
| mielite | **myelitis** *Inflammation of the spinal cord.* |
| mielocele | **myelocele** *Protrusion of the spinal cord through a defect in the bony structure.* |
| mielogramma | **myelogram** *CT scan or roentgenography of the spinal canal after injection of contrast media.* |
| mieloide | **myeloid** *Referring to the bone marrow or spinal cord.* |
| mieloma | **myeloma** *Malignant tumor of the bone marrow.* |
| mielomatosi | **myelomatosis** *A leukemic disease in which there is an abnormally high amount of myeloblasts in the blood.* |
| mielomeningocele | **myelomeningocele** *A protrusion of the spinal cord and its meninges through a defect in the vertebral canal.* |
| mielopatia | **myelopathy** *A condition of the spinal cord.* |
| migliorare | **ameliorate** *To make something better or to improve.* |
| migliore | **best** *Optimal or ideal.* |
| miliare | **miliary** *Referring to a disease that is exhibited by small seed-like lesions (millet), such as miliary tuberculosis.* |
| miliaria rubra | **prickly heat** *A rash with small vesicles that is pruritic and associated with a warm moist environment.* |
| milligrammo | **milligram** *A unit of weight, 1/1000 of a gram.* |
| millilitro | **milliliter** *A unit of volume, 1/1000 of a liter.* |
| millimetro | **millimeter** *A unit of measurement, 1/1000 of a meter.* |
| milza | **spleen** *The visceral organ that is involved with production and removal of blood cells.* |
| minore | **less** *A smaller amount.* |
| minuscolo | **minute** *Something very small.* |
| minuto | **minute** *A unit of time.* |
| minzione | **micturition** *Synonym of urination.* |
| miocardico | **myocardial** *Referring to the muscular tissue of the heart.* |

| Italian | English |
|---|---|
| miocardio | **myocardium** *The middle layer of the heart wall.* |
| miocardiopatia | **cardiomyopathy** *Chronic cardiac muscle disease.* |
| miocardite | **myocarditis** *An inflammation of the heart.* |
| mioclonio | **myoclonus** *Contraction or spasm of a group of muscles.* |
| mioglobina | **myoglobin** *A protein within muscle that carries and stores oxygen.* |
| mioma | **myoma** *A benign neoplasm of muscular tissue.* |
| miomatectomia | **myomectomy** *Surgical resection of a myoma.* |
| miometrio | **myometrium** *The smooth muscle layer of the uterus.* |
| miopatia | **myopathy** *Muscle disease.* |
| miopia | **myopia** *Nearsightedness.* |
| mioscaroma | **myosarcoma** *A mass with myoma and sarcoma characteristics.* |
| miosina | **myosin** *A protein that when coupled with actin form the contractile complex of a muscle cells.* |
| miosite | **myositis** *Inflammation of muscle tissue.* |
| miosite ossificante | **myositis ossificans** *Inflammation of muscle tissue with presence of bony deposits.* |
| miotomia | **myotomy** *The surgical removal of muscle tissue.* |
| miotonia distrofica | **myotonia dystrophica; Steinert's disease** *A condition exhibited initially by hypertonic muscles followed by atrophy of the facial and neck muscles.* |
| miringite | **myringitis** *Inflammation of the tympanic membrane.* |
| miringoplastica | **myringoplasty** *Surgical repair of tympanic membrane defects.* |
| miringotomia | **myringotomy** *Surgical opening of the tympanic membrane.* |
| miryachit | **miryachit** *A disease of Siberia characterized by an exaggerated startle response; also referred to as jumping disease.* |
| misantropia | **misanthropy** *A severe dislike of homo sapiens.* |
| misofobia | **mysophobia** *Severe fear of dirt or contamination from common objects.* |
| mite | **mild** *Slight, nominal.* |
| mitocondrio | **mitochondria** *Organelle found in cells responsible for energy production.* |
| mitosi | **mitosis** *Cell division in which two daughter cells are formed that have the same number of chromosomes as the parent cell.* |
| mitrale | **mitral** *Referring to the mitral valve.* |
| mixedema | **myxedema** *Diffuse edema with a wax-like appearance of the skin; this condition is associated with hypothyroidism.* |
| mixoma | **myxoma** *A tumor composed of mucous tissue.* |
| mixosarcoma | **myxosarcoma** *A sarcoma that also has mucous tissue.* |
| modello in gesso | **plaster cast** *Use of gypsum impregnated gauze to immobilize fractured extremities.* |
| modifica | **adjustment** *A modification of a plan.* |
| modifica | **alteration** *The process of change or modification.* |
| modiolo | **modiolus** *A column located in the cochlea.* |
| modulo di domanda | **application** *The forms one fills out to obtain a grant.* |
| molalità | **molality** *The number of moles of a solution per kilogram of pure solvent.* |
| molecola | **molecule** *A combination of at least two atoms.* |
| mollezza | **laxity** *A description of a joint that is loose.* |
| mollusco | **shellfish** *An aquatic shelled crustacean or mollusk.* |
| molti | **lots of** *An abundance of.* |
| molto caldo | **hot** *Very warm.* |
| moncone di arto amputato | **stump** *Term used to designate what remains of an amputated extremity.* |

| Italian | English |
|---|---|
| mondiplopia | **monodiplopia** *Double vision in only one eye.* |
| monitoraggio ambulatoriale electrocardiografico | **ambulatory electrocardiographic monitoring** *A continuous recording of the electrocardiogram used to detect occult dysrhythmias.* |
| monitoraggio cardiaco fetale | **fetal cardiac monitor** *Device used to monitor fetal heart rate and rhythm.* |
| mono-ovulare | **uniovolar** *Referring to one fertilized ovum.* |
| monocito | **monocyte** *A leukocyte with an oval nucleus and grey cytoplasm.* |
| monocitosi | **monocytosis** *An abnormal increase in the number of monocytes in the blood.* |
| monoclonale | **monoclonal** *Asexual formation of a clone from a single cell.* |
| monolaterale | **unilateral** *One side only.* |
| monomania | **monomania** *A psychotic obsession about a single subject.* |
| mononervite | **mononeuritis** *Inflammation of a single nerve.* |
| mononeuropatia craniale III | **cranial mononeuropathy III** *Dysfunction of the third cranial nerve causes double vision and eyelid drooping.* |
| mononeuropatia craniale VI | **cranial mononeuropathy VI** *A disorder of the sixth cranial nerve causes double vision.* |
| mononucleato | **mononuclear** *A cell having only one nucleus.* |
| mononucleosi | **mononucleosis** *An infectious disease exhibited by malaise and lymphadenopathy.* |
| monoplegia | **monoplegia** *Paralysis of a single limb.* |
| monte del pube | **mons pubis** *The fleshy protuberance over the symphysis pubis.* |
| morbillo | **measles** *A childhood viral, infectious disease exhibited by rash and fever.* |
| morbillo | **Rubeola** *Another term for measles, an acute exanthematous disease.* |
| morbo di Addison | **Addison's disease** *A disease of the adrenal gland exhibited by anemia, hypotension and a bronze tone to the skin.* |
| morbo di Cushing | **Cushing's syndrome** *Characterized by truncal obesity, moon face, acne, abdominal striae, hypertension, decreased carbohydrate tolerance, protein catabolism, psychiatric disturbances, and osteoporosis.* |
| morbo di Dupuytren | **Dupuytren's contracture** *A disease of the palmar fascia causing a flexion contracture of the fourth and fifth fingers.* |
| morbo di Grave | **Graves' disease** *A form of hyperthyroidism exhibited by a goiter and exophthalmos.* |
| morbo di Hodgkin | **Hodgkin's disease** *Also called Hodgkin's lymphoma, it is a cancer that begins in the lymphocytes.* |
| morbo di Milroy | **Milroy's disease** *Hereditary disease exhibited by leg edema.* |
| morbo di Parkinson | **paralysis agitans** *Synonym of Parkinson's disease (obsolete phrase).* |
| morbo di Parkinson | **Parkinson's disease** *A progressive neuromuscular disease exhibited by masklike facial expression, resting tremor, cogwheel rigidity and abnormal gait.* |
| morbo di Peyronie | **Peyronie's disease** *Curvature of the penis during an erection to to plaque.* |
| morbo di Pott; spondilite tubercolare | **Pott's disease** *Also referred to as tuberculous spondylitis it is caused by a spinal deformity caused by a tuberculosis infection of the spine.* |
| morbo di Werner-His | **quintan fever** *Also known as trench fever as it was first noted during trench warfare in WW I. It is a rickettsial fever caused by Bartonella quintana and transmitted by a louse; signs and symptoms are myalgia, headache, malaise, fever and chills.* |
| morbo itai-itai | **ouch-ouch disease** *Common term for Itai-Itai disease that is derived from "it hurts, it hurts" said by patients suffering from cadmium poisoning.* |

| Italian | English |
|---|---|
| morbo terminale | **terminal illness** *A disease with no viable treatment with death being inevitable.* |
| morbo tsutsugamushi | **tsutsugamushi disease** *An acute febrile infectious disease caused by Rickettsia tsutsugamushi. It is characterized by fever, pain lymphadenopathy, small black lesions on the genitals, neck or axilla.* |
| morbo venereo | **venereal disease** *A condition transmitted via sexual intercourse.* |
| morbosità | **morbidity** *The state of disease.* |
| morboso | **morbid** *Indicative of disease.* |
| morfea | **morphea** *A condition exhibited by an elevated or depressed patch of pink skin with a purple border.* |
| morfina | **morphine** *An opioid analgesic.* |
| morfologia | **morphology** *The study of living organisms and the correlation between their structure.* |
| moribondo | **moribund** *Near death.* |
| morire | **die, to** *To stop living, to expire.* |
| mortale | **fatal** *Lethal.* |
| morte | **death** *The action of dying.* |
| morte cerebrale | **brain death** *Cessation of cerebral functioning.* |
| morte per annegamento | **drowning** *The process of dying from submerging in and inhaling water.* |
| morto | **dead** *Deceased.* |
| morula | **morula** *A solid mass created by the splitting of an ovum.* |
| mosca nera | **black fly** *From the family Simuliidae, a gnat that can cause disease in humans; also called buffalo fly.* |
| mosca tse-tse | **tsetse fly** *An insect that transmits the protozoa trypanosoma and can cause sleeping sickness.* |
| motore | **motor** *Referring to muscles.* |
| movimenti oculari rapidi | **Rapid Eye Movement** *The movement of a person's eyes during this period of sleep.* |
| movimenti oculari rapidi | **REM (rapid eye movement) sleep** *This period of sleep is associated with irregular respirations and heart rate, involuntary movements and dreaming.* |
| movimento fetale intrauterina | **fetal movements** *Sensations by the mother of fetal activity.* |
| mucca pazza; encefalopatia spongiforme bovina | **mad cow disease** *Bovine spongiform encephalopathy, a disease that cause cerebral degeneration exhibited by ataxia.* |
| mucillagine | **mucilage** *1. A viscous bodily fluid. 2. A polysaccharide used in medicines and glue.* |
| mucina | **mucin** *A glycoprotein that is the primary constituent in mucous.* |
| muco | **sputum** *A mixture of respiratory tract secretions and saliva.* |
| muco | **mucus** *A substance secreted by mucous membranes.* |
| mucocele | **mucocele** *An accumulation of mucous in a dilated cavity.* |

| Italian | English |
|---|---|
| mucoide | **mucoid** *Referring to mucous.* |
| mucolitico | **mucolytic** *A substance that breaks down mucous.* |
| mucopolisaccaridosi tipo I | **mucopolysaccharidosis type I** *Also referred to as Hurler syndrome, persons cannot make lysosomal alpha-L-iduronidase which breaks down glycosaminoglycans.* |
| mucopolisaccaridosi tipo II | **mucopolysaccharidosis type II** *Also referred to as Hunter syndrome, persons with this inherited condition cannot produce iduronate sulfatase. There are mild to severe forms but all forms have deafness, coarse facial features, hypertrichosis and macrocephaly.* |
| mucopolisaccaridosi tipo III | **mucopolysaccharidosis type III** *Also referred to as Sanfilippo syndrome, persons cannot catabolize the heparan sulfate sugar chain. Symptoms include stiff joints, thick eyebrows, coarse facial features and developmental delays.* |
| mucopolisaccaridosi tipo Is | **mucopolysaccharidosis type Is** *Also referred to as Scheie syndrome, persons cannot produce lysosomal alpha-L-iduronidase. Symptoms include cloudy cornea, hirsutism, prognathism and stiff joints.* |
| mucopolisaccaridosi tipo IV | **mucopolysaccharidosis type IV** *Also referred to as Morquio syndrome, persons do not produce galactosamine-6-sulfatase or in some cases beta-galactosidase. Symptoms include hypermobile joints, macrocephaly, short stature and wide spaced teeth.* |
| mucopolisaccaridosi tipo VI | **mucopolysaccharidosis type VI** *Also referred to as Maroteaux-Lamy syndrome. It is characterized by hydrocephalus, macroglossia and coarse facial features but normal intelligence.* |
| mucopurulento | **mucopurulent** *That which contains both mucous and pus.* |
| mucosa | **mucosa** *A mucous membrane like the buccal mucosa.* |
| mughetto | **thrush** *Candida albicans* |
| multigravida | **multigravida** *A woman who has been pregnant more than once.* |
| multiloculare | **multilocular** *The presence of more than one cell within a cavity.* |
| multipara | **multipara** *A woman with more than one live births.* |
| muscolare | **muscular** *Referring to muscles.* |
| muscolo | **muscle** *A band if fibrous tissue that can contract.* |
| muscolo bicipite | **biceps** *A muscle with two heads usually referring to the biceps brachii which is used for forearm flexion.* |
| muscolo buccinatore | **buccinator muscle** *Pulls the mouth posteriorly.* |
| muscolo flessore | **flexor** *A muscle that bends an extremity or part of an extremity.* |
| muscolo gastrocnemio | **gastrocnemius** *A large muscle in the lower leg, responsible for ankle plantar flexion, that is attached to the distal femur and achilles tendon.* |
| muscolo gluteo | **gluteal or gluteus muscle** *A paired set of three muscles, the gluteus maximus, medius and minimus, that all have origins in the ilium and insertions in the femur. (buttocks)* |
| muscolo interosseo | **interosseous muscles** *Referring to the interosseous muscles of the hand.* |
| muscolo occipitofrontale | **occipitofrontal muscle** *Raises the eyebrows.* |
| muscolo pubovescicale | **detrusor urinae** *Smooth muscle fibers that extend from the urinary bladder to the pubis.* |
| muscolo retto dell'addome | **rectus abdominis muscle** *The pair of long, flat muscles that connect the sternum with the pubis.* |
| muscolo sartorio | **sartorius muscle** *The thigh muscle that runs from the pelvis to the proximal, medial aspect of the tibia.* |

| Italian | English |
|---|---|
| muscolo stapedio | **stapedius muscle** *Located in the tympanic interior, it reduces stapedial movement.* |
| muscolo trapezio | **trapezius muscle** *The muscle with an origin of occipital bone and seventh cervical vertebra, insertion of clavicle and scapula, and it draws the scapula backward.* |
| muscolo tricipite | **triceps** *Referring to something having three heads like the triceps muscle.* |
| mutazione | **mutation** *A gene alteration that can be passed to the next generation.* |
| mutismo | **mutism** *Inability to speak.* |
| muto | **mute** *Refraining from or being speechless.* |
| narcisismo | **narcissism** *Abnormally excessive self-interest.* |
| narcolepsia | **narcolepsy** *A condition exhibited by a strong desire to sleep and by sudden onset of sleep at increased intervals.* |
| narcosi | **narcosis** *A reversible medication-induced condition of excessive drowsiness or unconsciousness.* |
| narcotico | **narcotic** *A medication that produces narcosis.* |
| narice | **nostril** *One of two openings in the nose used for air passage.* |
| nasale | **nasal** *Referring to the nose.* |
| nascita | **birth** *The process of bearing offspring from the uterus.* |
| naso | **nose** *The midface protuberance used for smelling and breathing.* |
| nasofaringe | **nasopharynx** *The part of the pharynx which lies superior to the soft palate.* |
| nasofaringeo | **nasopharyngeal** *Referring to the nose and pharynx.* |
| nasolacrimale | **nasolacrimal** *Referring to the nose and tear apparatus.* |
| nastro adesivo | **adhesive tape** *Tape used to secure dressings or intravenous lines to the body.* |
| natiche (natica) | **buttocks (buttock)** *The bilateral region covering the gluteal muscles.* |
| nato morto | **stillborn** *Refers to a newborn that died in utero.* |
| nausea | **nausea** *A feeling that one wants to vomit.* |
| nausea gravidica | **morning sickness** *Nausea associated with pregnancy.* |
| navicolare | **navicular** *1. boat shaped 2. Referring to the navicular bone of the hand or foot.* |
| nebbiolina | **nebula** *An opaque spot on the cornea causing impaired vision.* |
| nebulizzatore | **nebulizer** *A device used for transforming a liquid into a fine mist for inhalation as in nebulized albuterol for an acute exacerbation of asthma.* |
| necropsia | **necropsy** *Synonym of autopsy.* |
| necrosi | **necrosis** *The death of most of the cells of the affected part.* |
| necrosi avascolare | **avascular necrosis** *Bone death caused by poor blood supply.* |
| necrotico | **necrotic** *Referring to necrosis.* |
| nefrectomia | **nephrectomy** *Surgical removal of a kidney.* |
| nefrite | **nephritis** *A general term meaning inflammation of a kidney that is further categorized depending on the associated pathology.* |
| nefroblastoma; tumore di Wilms | **nephroblastoma** *Congenital tumor of the kidney, also called Wilms' tumor.* |
| nefrocalcinosi | **nephrocalcinosis** *A condition exhibited by calcium phosphate deposition in the renal tubules; a cause of renal insufficiency.* |
| nefrolitiasi | **nephrolithiasis** *A calculus in the kidney.* |
| nefrolitotomia | **nephrolithotomy** *Surgical removal of a renal calculus.* |
| nefroma | **nephroma** *A renal tumor.* |
| nefrone | **nephron** *A functional unit of the kidney that consists of the glomerulus, the proximal and distal convoluted tubules, the loop of Henle and the collecting tubule.* |
| nefropatia | **nephropathy** *Renal disease.* |

| Italian | English |
|---|---|
| nefropessi | **nephropexy** *The surgical fixation of a kidney that was previously floating.* |
| nefroptosi | **nephroptosis** *Inferior displacement of the kidney.* |
| nefrosclerosi | **nephrosclerosis** *Hardening of the kidney.* |
| nefrosi | **nephrosis** *A kidney disease exhibited by edema and proteinuria; also called nephrotic syndrome.* |
| nefrosico | **nephrotic** *Referring to nephrosis.* |
| nefrostomia | **nephrostomy** *Surgical creation of an opening between the renal pelvis and an opening in the skin.* |
| nefrotomia | **nephrotomy** *Surgical incision of the kidney.* |
| negare | **deny, to** *To reject or repudiate.* |
| negativo | **negative** *Contrary or opposing.* |
| nematode | **nematode** *An endoparasite belonging to the class of the Nemathelminthes including roundworms and threadworms.* |
| neonatale | **neonatal** *Referring to the first four weeks after birth.* |
| neonato | **baby** *A newborn.* |
| neonato | **infant** *Newborn.* |
| neonato | **neonate** *The term for a newborn infant for the first four weeks.* |
| neonato a termine | **infant, term** *A neonate born at expected date.* |
| neonato postmaturo | **infant, post-term** *A neonate born after the normal gestation.* |
| neonato prematuro | **infant, pre-term** *A neonate born prior to normal gestation.* |
| neoplasma | **neoplasm** *A new and abnormal growth.* |
| nero | **black** *Referring to the color, as in the color of coal.* |
| nervastenico | **neurasthenia** *A psychoneurosis exhibited by severe fatigue.* |
| nervi splancnico | **splanchnic nerves** *The nerves supplying the abdominal viscera and blood vessels.* |
| nervo | **nerve** *A fibrous band made up of axons and dendrites that connects the nervous systems with other organs.* |
| nervo abducente | **abducens nerve** *A motor nerve (6th cranial nerve) that controls the lateral rectus muscle of the eye.)* |
| nervo accessorio | **accessory nerve (XI)** *Supplies motor innervation to the sternocleidomastoid and trapezius.* |
| nervo circonflesso | **circumflex nerve** *The axillary nerve that has an origin in the posterior branch of the brachial plexus.* |
| nervo facciale | **facial nerve** *Cranial nerve VII that supplies the face and tongue.* |
| nervo femorale | **femoral nerve** *Supplies the motor function of the quadriceps and the sensation over the anterior and medial thigh.* |
| nervo ipoglosso | **hypoglossal nerve** *Twelfth cranial nerve pair.* |
| nervo oculomotore; III nervo cranico | **oculomotor nerve** *Referring to cranial nerve III which is one of the nerves responsible for extraocular movements.* |
| nervo sensitivo | **sensory nerve** *A nerve that receives input from various receptors.* |
| nervo spinale | **spinal nerve** *The term for each of the thirty pairs of nerves that originate in the spine and traverse between the vertebrae. There are eight cervical, twelve thoracic, five lumbar, five sacral and one coccygeal nerve pairs.* |
| nervo trigemino | **trigeminal nerve** *The fifth cranial nerve which supplies the motor function of mastication and has three sensory branches, the ophthalmic, maxillary and mandibular.* |
| nervo trocleare | **trochlear nerve** *The fourth cranial nerve that supplies the superior oblique muscle of the eyeball.* |
| nervo ulnare | **ulnar nerve** *Arises from the C8-T1 nerves and supplies the hand. (Injury to the ulnar nerve causes loss of flexion of the metacarpophalangeal joints and extension at the interphalangeal joints, thus the common term, claw hand.)* |

| Italian | English |
|---|---|
| nervo vago | **vagus nerve** *The tenth cranial nerve that supplies the heart, lungs visceral organs; its function is tested by assessment of elevation of the uvula.* |
| nervosa anoressia | **anorexia nervosa** *A mental disorder characterized by the desire to avoid eating and to lose weight.* |
| nervrectomia | **neurectomy** *Excision of a section of a nerve.* |
| neurale | **neural** *Referring to a nerve or nerve impulse.* |
| neuralgia | **neuralgia** *Severe pain along the course of a nerve.* |
| neuralgia genicolato | **geniculate neuralgia** *Severe intermittent pain in the external ear and deep in the ear.* |
| neuralgia trigeminale | **trigeminal neuralgia** *Pain in the region of one or more branches of the fifth cranial nerve sensory branches.* |
| neuraprassia | **neurapraxia** *Paralysis from nerve injury but no degeneration of the nerve.* |
| neurilemma | **neurilemma** *The membrane covering a myelinated nerve fiber or the axon of an unmyelinated nerve fiber.* |
| neurinoma dell'acustico | **acoustic neuroma** *A nonmalignant tumor that can cause deafness, tinnitus and vertigo.* |
| neurite retrobulbare oculare | **retrobulbar optic neuritis** *An inflammatory, demyelinating condition in the retrobulbar region.* |
| neuroblastoma | **neuroblastoma** *A nervous system malignant tumor composed of neuroblasts.* |
| neurochirurgia | **neurosurgery** *Surgery of the brain or spinal cord.* |
| neurodermatite | **neurodermatitis** *A pruritic, thickened eruption in the axillary and inguinal thought to be exacerbated by emotions.* |
| neuroepitelio | **neuroepithelium** *Cells specialized to serve as sensory cells such as cells of the cochlea and tongue.* |
| neurofibroma | **neurofibroma** *A tumor formed by excessive growth of perineurium and endoneurium.* |
| neurofibromatosi | **neurofibromatosis** *A hereditary condition exhibited by formation of multiple soft tumors scattered throughout the skin surface. Also known as von Recklinghausen disease.* |
| neurolettico | **neuroleptic** *A drug that causes neurologic symptoms.* |
| neurolog | **neurologist** *A physician who specializes in the study of the nervous system.* |
| neurologia | **neurology** *The study of the nervous system.* |
| neuroma | **neuroma** *A mass composed of nerve cells and fibers.* |
| neuromielite ottica di Devic | **devic disease** *Also known as neuromyelitis optica; it is a demyelinating disorder associated with a transverse myelopathy and optic neuritis.* |
| neurone | **neuron** *A nerve cell.* |
| neuropatia | **neuropathy** *Structural of pathologic changes of the peripheral nervous system.* |
| neuropatia bulbo di cipolla; neuropatia ipertrofica interstiziale | **onion bulb neuropathy** *Also known as hypertrophic interstitial neuropathy which is a sensorimotor polyneuropathy.* |
| neuropatia del plesso brachiale | **brachial plexus neuropathy** *Characterized by acute arm or shoulder pain followed by focal muscle weakness.* |
| neuropatia di carenz di vitamina B12 | **vitamin B12 neuropathy** *Abnormal sensation related to a chronic deficiency of cyanocobalamin; also called subacute combined degeneration of the spinal cord or Putnam-Dana syndrome.* |
| neuropatia diabetico | **diabetic neuropathy** *Pain and burning initially in the feet, associated with diabetes mellitus.* |
| neuropatia intrappolamento | **entrapment neuropathy** *Weakness or numbness caused by compression of a peripheral nerve.* |

| Italian | English |
|---|---|
| neuropatia ottica ischemica | **ischemic optic neuropathy** *A general category of a cause of blindness with several subcategories.* |
| neuropatico | **neuropathic** *Referring to neuropathy.* |
| neurosi | **neurosis** *A mental disorder.* |
| neurosi d'ansia | **anxiety neurosis** *Abnormal presence of anxiety.* |
| neurosifilide | **neurosyphilis** *Infection of the central nervous system with Treponema pallidum.* |
| neurotmesi | **neurotmesis** *The severing of a nerve.* |
| neurotomia | **neurotomy** *Surgical incision into a nerve.* |
| neurotrasmettitore | **neurotransmitter** *A substance released at the end of a nerve fiber that facilitates transmission of an impulse.* |
| neutrofilo | **neutrophil** *A polymorphonuclear leukocyte.* |
| neutropenia | **neutropenia** *Diminished number of neutrophils in the blood.* |
| nevo | **nevus** *A benign, well-circumscribed growth of tissue of congenital origin.* |
| nevo capillare | **capillary nevus** *A growth of skin that involves the capillaries.* |
| nevo flammeus | **port-wine mark** *Also called nevus flammeus, it is a vascular anomaly characterized by purplish skin discoloration.* |
| nevo ragno | **spider nevus** *A papule with telangiectases radiating from the center.* |
| nevralgia del trigemino | **tic douloureux** *Also referred to as trigeminal neuralgia.* |
| nevrite | **neuritis** *Inflammation of a nerve.* |
| nevroglia | **neuroglia** *A type of connective tissue of the nervous system.* |
| nistagmo | **nystagmus** *Rapid involuntary movement of the eyes; it can be horizontal, vertical or rotary.* |
| nistagmo ondulatorio | **oscillating nystagmus** *Abnormal movement of the eyes in a wave-like pattern.* |
| nittalopia | **night blindness** *Common term for nyctalopia, it refers to low vision with reduced illumination, often seen with Vitamin A deficiency.* |
| nocca | **knuckle** *A metacarpophalagngeal joint or a finger joint when the fist is closed.* |
| nocca scoppiettante | **crack one's knuckles** *Moving the fingers side to side or with flexion in such a manner to cause a popping or crackling sound.* |
| nocivo | **noxious** *Harmful or poisonous.* |
| nocturia | **nocturia** *Urination at night.* |
| nodo | **node** *A swelling or prominence.* |
| nodo chirurgico | **knot** *A fastening made by tying a suture, for instance.* |
| nodo linfa | **lymph node** *An area of organized lymphatic tissue.* |
| nodo senoatriale | **sinoatrial node** *A mass of cardiac tissue that acts as the pacemaker.* |
| nodo sinciziale | **syncytial knot** *Aggregation of syncytiotrophoblastic nuclei in the villi of the placenta during early pregnancy.* |
| noduli di Heberden | **Heberden's node** *Hard nodules formed at the distal interphalangeal joints in osteoarthritis.* |
| nodulo di Caplan | **Caplan nodules** *These are pulmonary nodules noted in people with rheumatoid arthritis who were exposed to coal dust.* |
| nodulo di Schmorl | **Schmorl's nodule** *Protrusion of the nucleus pulposus through the vertebral body endplate into the adjacent vertebra.* |
| nodulo di Suor Maria Giuseppa | **Sister Mary Joseph nodule** *A nodule at the umbilicus associated with metastatic abdominal cancer.* |
| nodulo; nodo | **nodule** *A small node in the skin of up to 1cm and in the lung up to 3cm.* |
| nome | **name** *A word by which a person is known.* |
| nome da ragazza | **maiden name** *The surname a woman uses prior to being married.* |

| Italian | English |
|---|---|
| non conserva fossetta dopo compressione digitale | **nonpitting edema** *Subcutaneous swelling that cannot be indented with compression.* |
| non più in uso | **outdated** *Something that has passed the expiration date.* |
| non rianimare | **DNR Do not resuscitate.** *The term used to indicate a person should not have life sustaining measures taken if they were to have cardiopulmonary arrest.* |
| non vascolare | **avascular** *An area with no blood supply.* |
| nonostante tutto di | **regardless of** *Without consideration of.* |
| norepinefrina | **norepinephrine** *A hormone secreted by the adrenal medulla and a synthetic drug used as a pressor agent.* |
| normoblasto | **normoblast** *A precursor cell for erythrocytes.* |
| normocito | **normocyte** *A normal erythrocyte.* |
| nosofobia | **nosophobia** *Unwarranted, excessive fear of any disease.* |
| nosologia | **nosology** *The medical science of disease classification.* |
| notturna | **nocturnal** *Referring to events that happen at night.* |
| nucleare | **nuclear** *Referring to a nucleus.* |
| nucleo arcuato | **arcuate nucleus** *Small masses of gray matter found on the medulla oblongata.* |
| nucleo dentato | **dentatum** *Also referred to as dentate nucleus of cerebellum.* |
| nucleo rosso | **red nucleus** *A collection of gray matter near the subthalamus that receives data from the superior cerebellar peduncle.* |
| nucleoproteina | **nucleoprotein** *A substance composed of a nucleic acid and a protein.* |
| nulligravida | **nulligravida** *A woman who has never been pregnant.* |
| nullipara | **nullipara** *A woman who has never given birth.* |
| nummulazione | **nummulation** *Formed as round, flat discs.* |
| nutazione | **nutation** *Referring to nodding of the head.* |
| nutriente | **nutrient** *A substance that provides essential nourishment.* |
| nutrimento | **food** *Nutrition.* |
| nutrizione | **nutrition** *The process of supplying food needed for growth.* |
| obesità | **obesity** *Having a body mass index over 30kilograms/meters squared.* |
| obitorio | **morgue** *A room where deceased patients are housed until sent to a funeral home.* |
| obsoleto | **obsolete** *No longer in use; antiquated.* |
| occhiali di protezione | **goggles** *Close fitting, protective eyeglasses.* |
| occhiata | **glance** *A brief look at something.* |
| occhio rosa; congiuntivite acuta | **pink eye** *Common term for acute contagious conjunctivitis.* |
| occipitale | **occipital** *Referring to the back part of the head.* |
| occlusione | **occlusion** *A pathway that is blocked or obstructed.* |
| occlusione coronarica | **coronary occlusion** *A blockage in a coronary artery.* |
| oculare | **ocular** *Referring to the eye.* |
| oculogiro | **oculogyric** *Referring to movement of the eye around the anteroposterior axis.* |
| odinofagia | **odynophagia** *Pain associated with swallowing.* |
| odinofobia | **odynophonia** *Pain associated with speaking.* |
| odontalgia | **odontalgia** *Tooth pain.* |
| odontalgia; mal di dente | **toothache** *Dental pain.* |
| odontoide | **odontoid** *A prominence on the second cervical vertebra on which the first cervical vertebra pivots.* |
| odontologia | **odontology** *Synonym of dentistry.* |
| odore | **odor** *A smell that is given off someone or something.* |
| odorifero | **odiferous** *Having an unpleasant or distinctive smell.* |

| Italian | English |
|---|---|
| oftalmia | **ophthalmia** *Profound inflammation of the eye or its structures.* |
| oftalmia blenorragica | **gonorrheal ophthalmia** *An acute purulent conjunctivitis that can occur in neonates within 2-5 days of birth.* |
| oftalmico | **ophthalmic** *Referring to the eye.* |
| oftalmologia | **ophthalmology** *The study of diseases of the eye.* |
| oftalmologo | **ophthalmologist** *A physician specializing in diseases of the eye.* |
| oftalmoplegia | **ophthalmoplegia** *Paralysis of the eye muscles.* |
| oftalmoplegia sovranucleare | **supranuclear ophthalmoplegia** *A disorder that effects the extraocular movements especially limiting the upward movement of the eyes.* |
| oftalmoscopio | **ophthalmoscope** *A device used to visually inspect the interior eye.* |
| ogni | **every** *Each or all possible.* |
| ogni altro giorno | **every other day** *On alternate days.* |
| ogni giorno | **every day** *Each day.* |
| olecrano | **olecranon** *The bony protrusion at the proximal ulna at the elbow.* |
| olfattivo | **olfactory** *Referring to the sense of smell.* |
| oligodattilia | **oligodactyly** *Presence of fewer than 5 digits on a hand or foot.* |
| oligodendrociti | **oligodendroglia** *The ectodermal cells forming part of the central nervous system.* |
| oligofrenico | **feeble-minded** *Antiquated term used to describe a person unable to make seemingly simple decisions because of a cognitive impairment.* |
| oligoidramnios | **oligohydramnios** *Inadequate amount of amniotic fluid.* |
| oligomenorrea | **oligomenorrhea** *Infrequent menstruation or low volume menstrual flow.* |
| oligoptialismo | **oligoptyalism** *Insufficient secretion of saliva; also oligosialia.* |
| oligospermia | **oligospermia** *Abnormally low sperm count.* |
| oligotrofia | **oligotrophia or hypotrichosis** *Less than normal amount of head/body hair.* |
| oliguria | **oliguria** *Abnormally low urine output.* |
| oltre | **above** |
| oltre | **beyond** *On the farther side.* |
| ombelicato | **umbilicated** *Referring to depressed areas that resemble the umbilicus.* |
| ombelico | **navel** *Umbilicus.* |
| ombelico | **umbilicus** *The scar that denotes the end of the umbilical cord.* |
| ombrofobia | **ombrophobia** *An abnormal fear of rain.* |
| omento | **omentum** *A fold of peritoneum fastening the stomach to other organs in the viscera.* |
| omentocele | **omentocele** *A herniated protrusion of omentum.* |
| omentopessia | **omentopexy** *Surgically fastening the omentum to an adjacent tissue it was not previously attached to.* |
| omeopatia | **homeopathy** *A treatment of disease by use of minute doses of toxic substances that would normally be harmful.* |
| omeostasi | **homeostasis** *The tendency of an organism to maintain a stable and uniform state.* |
| omero | **humerus** *The long bone in the upper arm.* |
| omicida | **homicide** *When one person kills another.* |
| omolaterale | **homolateral** *Ipsilateral.* |
| omolaterale | **ipsilateral** *On the same side.* |
| omologo | **homologous** *Referring to something derived from the same species but different genotype.* |
| omosessuale | **homosexual** *A person sexually attracted to someone of the same gender.* |
| omotrapianto | **homograft** *A graft of tissue from the same species as the recipient.* |
| omozigotico | **homozygous** *Having identical alleles for a particular trait.* |

| Italian | English |
|---|---|
| oncologia | **oncology** *The study of cancer.* |
| oncologista | **oncologist** *A physician specializing in the treatment of cancer.* |
| onda Alfa | **alpha wave** *Electroencephalographic waves with a frequency of 8-13 per second.* |
| onfalite | **omphalitis** *Inflammation of the umbilicus.* |
| onfalocele | **omphalocele** *A large congenital, umbilical hernia with only a thin membranous covering.* |
| onichia | **onychia** *Inflammation of the toenail or fingernail matrix.* |
| onichia fragile | **onychia sicca** *Brittle fingernails or toenails.* |
| onicocriptosi | **onychocryptosis** *Ingrown toenail.* |
| onicofagia | **onychophagia** *Habitually chewing on one's fingernails.* |
| onicogrifosi | **onychogryphosis** *A deformed nail that is incurved or hooked.* |
| onycomicosi | **onychomycosis** *Fungal disease of the toenails or fingernails.* |
| oocito | **oocyte** *An ovarian cell that needs to undergo meiotic division to become an ovum.* |
| ooforectomia | **oophorectomy** *Surgical removal of an ovary.* |
| ooforite | **oophoritis** *Inflammation of an ovary.* |
| ooforosalpingectomia | **oophorosalpingectomy** *Surgical removal of an ovary and fallopian tube.* |
| oogenesi | **oogenesis** *The initiation and development of an ovum.* |
| operazione | **operation** *A surgical procedure.* |
| operazione chirurgica | **surgery** *The incision of a body part using sterile technique in order to treat disease or injury.* |
| opistotono | **opisthotonos** *A profound spasm in which the head/neck is hyperextended, the feet are touching the bed and with the patient supine the body arched upward.* |
| oppiato | **opiate** *Referring to opium.* |
| oppio | **opium** *An addictive drug derived from opium poppy; synthetic versions are used as analgesics.* |
| oppioide | **opioid** *A substance similar to opium that binds to at least one of the opium receptors in the body.* |
| opponente | **opponens** *Synonym for opponent muscle.* |
| opsonina | **opsonin** *An antibody used to facilitate phagocytosis of a bacterium.* |
| optometria | **optometry** *The profession of examination of the eyes for disease (not a medical doctor).* |
| optometrista | **optometrist** *A person who practices optometry.* |
| orale | **oral** *Relating to the mouth.* |
| oralmente | **orally** *By mouth.* |
| orbicolare; circolare | **orbicular** *Rounded or circular.* |
| orbita | **orbit** *The bony structure enclosing the eyeball.* |
| orbitario | **orbital** *Referring to the orbit.* |
| orchialgia | **orchialgia** *Testicular pain.* |
| orchiectomia | **orchidectomy** *Synonym of orchiectomy; removal of one or both testes.* |
| orchiepididimite | **epididymo-orchitis** *Inflammation of the epididymis and the testis.* |
| orchiepididimite | **orchiepididymitis** *Inflammation of the testis and epididymis.* |
| orchipessia | **orchidopexy** *Surgical repair of an undescended testis.* |
| orchite | **orchitis** *Inflammation of one or both testes.* |
| orecchio | **ear** *The organ of hearing and balance.* |
| orecchio esterno | **ear, external** *Auris externa.* |
| orecchio interno | **ear, inner** *Auris interna.* |
| orecchio medio | **ear, middle** *Auris media.* |
| orecchio medio | **middle ear** *The portion of the ear containing the stapes, incus and malleus.* |

| Italian | English |
|---|---|
| Orecchio, naso, gola | **ENT** *Abbreviation for ears, nose and throat.* |
| orecchioni | **mumps** *A contagious viral disease that is exhibited by parotid swelling and puts males at risk for sterility. Also called epidemic parotitis.* |
| Organizzazione Mondiale della Sanità | **World Health Organization (WHO)** |
| organo | **organ** *A part of the body that is self contained and serves a vital function.* |
| organomegalia | **organomegaly** *Enlargement of an organ, typically referring to an intraabdominal organ.* |
| orifizio | **orifice** *Synonym of foramen.* |
| orinale | **urinal** *Device used by men to void while in bed or sitting.* |
| ormone | **hormone** *A substance produced in the body that effects a specific organ.* |
| ormone adrenocorticotropo | **adrenocorticotrophic hormone (ACTH)** *A hormone that influences the cortex of the adrenal glands.* |
| ormone antidiuretico | **antidiuretic hormone** *Vasopressin.* |
| ormone luteinizzante | **luteinizing hormone (LH)** *A pituitary hormone that stimulates ovulation in females and androgen in males.* |
| ormone tireotropo | **thyroid stimulating hormone (TSH)** *A thyroid secreted by the pituitary that regulates the thyroid.* |
| ormoni liberatori | **releasing hormone** *Hormones that come from one gland such as the thalamus that cause release of hormones from another gland such as the pituitary.* |
| ornitosi | **ornithosis** *A viral infection transmitted by birds that is manifested by chills, headache, photophobia, fever, nausea and vomiting.* |
| oro | **gold** *Precious metal with atomic number of 79.* |
| orofaringe | **oropharynx** *The portion of the pharynx between the soft palate and the superior aspect of the epiglottis.* |
| ortesi | **orthosis** *Straightening of a malaligned part with the use of braces and other supportive devices.* |
| orticaria | **urticaria** *A diffuse pruritic macular rash, caused by an allergy.* |
| ortodonzia | **orthodontics** *A subspecialty of dentistry concerned with treatment of dental irregularities and malocclusion, including the use of braces.* |
| ortopedia | **orthopedics** *A surgical specialty concerned with treatment of skeletal problems.* |
| ortopnea | **orthopnea** *The inability to breath comfortably except in the upright position.* |
| ortostatico | **orthostatic** *Referring to the standing position. Orthostatic hypotension is low blood pressure in the standing position.* |
| orzaiolo | **hordeolum** *Inflammation of the sebaceous gland of the eye.* |
| orzaiolo | **sty** *Also called hordeolum externum, it is inflammation of the sebaceous gland of an eyelash.* |
| osmolalità | **osmolality** *The concentration expressed in total number of solute particles per kilogram.* |
| osmole | **osmole** *The recognized unit of osmotic pressure.* |
| osmosi | **osmosis** *The movement of a solvent from a solution of greater concentration to one of lower concentration through a semi-permeable membrane until the two solutions have equal concentration.* |
| osmotico | **osmotic** *Referring to osmosis.* |
| ospedale | **hospital** *Acute care medical/surgical facility.* |
| ossa dell carpo | **trapezium** *The lateral bone in the distal row of carpal bones.* |
| ossaluria | **oxaluria** *Existence of oxalates in the urine.* |
| osseo | **osseous** *Possessing the quality of bone.* |
| osservazione | **comment** *A remark providing an opinion.* |

| Italian | English |
|---|---|
| ossessione | **obsession** *A pathologic preoccupation.* |
| ossicino | **ossicle** *A small bone. (auditory ossicle)* |
| ossidazione | **oxidation** *The process of a chemical combining with oxygen.* |
| ossido di azoto | **nitrous oxide** *An inhalant gas used as an anesthetic agent.* |
| ossiemoglobina | **oxyhemoglobin** *The combination of oxygen and hemoglobin using a covalent bond.* |
| ossificazione | **ossification** *The formation of bone.* |
| ossigenazione | **oxygenation** *Saturated with oxygen.* |
| ossigeno | **oxygen** *A colorless, odorless gas with atomic number 8.* |
| ossimetro | **oximeter** *A medical device used to measure the percent of oxygen that is saturated in the blood (oxygen saturation).* |
| ossitocico | **oxytocic** *Referring to rapid parturition.* |
| ossitocina | **oxytocin** *A natural hormone released by the pituitary or a synthetic hormone that facilitates uterine contraction.* |
| osso | **bone** *Skeletal tissue formed by osteoblasts.* |
| osso capitato del carpo | **capitate bone** *The bone at the base of the palm that articulates with the third metacarpal.* |
| osso del carpo (situato fra trapezio e capitato) | **trapezoid bone** *A bone that articulates with the second metacarpal, trapezium, capitate and scaphoid.* |
| osso del pube | **pubis** *The anterior inferior part of the hip bone on each side that articulates at the pubic symphysis.* |
| osso etmoide | **ethmoid bone** *A bone at the root of the nose which has perforations for the olfactory nerves to transit.* |
| osso iliaco | **ilium** *The large bone at the superior aspect of the pelvis which is present bilaterally.* |
| osso ioide | **hyoid bone** *A horseshoe shaped bone located between the chin and thyroid cartilage.* |
| osso naviculare | **navicular bone** *The most lateral bone in the proximal row of carpal bones.* |
| osso sacro | **sacrum** *The bone formed by five fused vertebrae that is situated between the two hip bones.* |
| osso scafoide | **scaphoid bone** *The most lateral of the carpal bones; it articulates with the radius.* |
| osso semilunare del carpo | **lunate bone; os lunatum** *A carpal bone that articulates with the wrist.* |
| osso turbinato | **turbinate bones** *The three curved shelves in the nasal cavity.* |
| osso uncinato | **hamate bone; uncinate bone** *The medial bone in the distal row of carpal bones adjacent to the fifth metacarpal.* |
| osso uncinato del carpo | **unciforme bone** *Hamate bone. The bone on the ulnar side of the distal row of the carpus. It articulates withe the 4th and 5th metacarpal, triquetral, lunate and capitate.* |
| osso zigomatico | **zygomatic bone** *The triangular cheek bone.* |
| osteite | **osteitis** *Inflammation of the bone.* |
| osteoartrite | **osteoarthritis** *A long term, progressive degenerative joint disease.* |
| osteoartrosi | **osteoarthrosis** *Arthritis without inflammation.* |
| osteoblasto | **osteoblast** *A cell that matures from a fibroblast and produces bone.* |
| osteocito | **osteocyte** *An osteoblast within the bone matrix.* |
| osteoclasia | **osteoclasis** *The surgical fracture of a bone usually in order to restore proper alignment.* |
| osteoclasto | **osteoclast** *A large bone cell that is associated with bone reabsorption and removal.* |
| osteoclastoma | **osteoclastoma** *A tumor composed of giant cells or osteoclasts.* |
| osteocondrale | **osteochondral** *Referring to bone and cartilage.* |
| osteocondrite | **osteochondritis** *Inflammation of bone and cartilage.* |

| Italian | English |
|---|---|
| osteocondroma | **osteochondroma** *A tumor with bony and cartilaginous characteristics.* |
| osteodistrofia | **osteodystrophy** *Abnormal bone formation.* |
| osteofito | **osteophyte** *Abnormal growth of a bone protuberance.* |
| osteofonia | **osteophony** *The sound conduction of bone.* |
| osteogenesi | **osteogenesis** *Development of new bones.* |
| osteogenesi imperfetta | **fragilitas ossium** *A condition exhibited by excessively brittle bones. Also called osteogenesis imperfecta.* |
| osteogenesi imperfetta | **osteogenesis imperfecta** *A connective tissue disorder characterized by bone fragility, skeletal deformity, blue sclerae, ligament laxity, and hearing loss.* |
| osteolitico | **osteolytic** *Referring to the removal or loss of calcium from the bone.* |
| osteomalacia | **osteomalacia** *Softening of the bones because of a deficiency of vitamin D, calcium or phosphorus.* |
| osteomielite | **osteomyelitis** *Inflammation of the bone or bone marrow because of a microorganism.* |
| osteopatia | **osteopathy** *1. Any disease of the bone. 2. Medical practice concerning treatment of disease by manipulation and massage of bones, joints, and muscles.* |
| osteopetrosi | **osteopetrosis** *Increased bone density with no change in modeling.* |
| osteoporosi | **osteoporosis** *Loss of bone substance because the osteoblasts fail to produce bone matrix.* |
| osteosarcoma | **osteosarcoma** *A tumor composed of a sarcoma and osseous material.* |
| osteosclerosi | **osteosclerosis** *Abnormal hardening of bone.* |
| osteotomia | **osteotomy** *Creation of a surgical opening in bone.* |
| ostetrica; levatrice | **midwife** *A person trained to assist in childbirth.* |
| ostetricia | **midwifery** *The occupation of assisting in childbirth.* |
| ostetrico | **obstetric** *Referring to The management of pregnancy, labor and the peuperium.* |
| ostetrico | **obstetrician** *A physician who specializes in the management of pregnancy, labor and the peuperium.* |
| ostio | **ostium** *A vessel or body cavity opening.* |
| ostruzione intestinale | **intestinal obstruction** *Blockage of the intestine by mass or volvulus.* |
| otalgia | **otalgia** *Ear pain.* |
| otalgia; dolore all'orecchio | **earache** *Pain associated with the ear.* |
| otite | **otitis** *Inflammation of the ear. (otitis media or otitis externa)* |
| otite interna | **inner ear** *Made up of the cochlea and semicircular canals.* |
| otolaringologo | **otolaryngologist** *Surgical specialist concerned with organs of the ears, nose and throat.* |
| otolito | **otolith** *A calcium based calculus in the inner ear.* |
| otologia | **otology** *Study of conditions and anatomy of the ear.* |
| otomicosi | **otomycosis** *Fungal infection of the ear.* |
| otosclerosi | **otosclerosis** *A hereditary condition exhibited by progressive hearing loss because of bone overgrowth in the inner ear.* |
| otoscopio | **otoscope** *A device used for inspection of the tympanic membrane.* |
| ototossico | **ototoxic** *A substance harmful to the ear or its nerve supply.* |
| ottico | **optic** *Referring to the eye.* |
| ottico diplomato | **optician** *A person who makes eyeglasses.* |
| otturatore | **obturator** *A device used to close an artificial or natural opening.* |
| ottuso | **blunt** *Having a flat or rounded end.* |
| ottuso | **obtuse** *Rather insensitive or hard to understand.* |
| ovario | **oophoron** *Synonym for ovary.* |
| ovarite | **ovaritis** *Synonym for oophoritis.* |

| Italian | English |
|---|---|
| ovidotto | **oviduct** *The channel which an ovum passes from the ovary.* |
| ovulazione | **ovulation** *The release of an ova from the ovary.* |
| ovulo | **ovule** *An immature ovum.* |
| oxicefalia | **oxycephaly** *The deformation of the skull so that it appears pointed.* |
| ozena | **ozena** *Various nasal conditions, all of which include fetid discharge.* |
| ozono | **ozone** *A toxic chemical that has profound oxidizing properties. It has three atoms in its molecule compared with oxygen which has two.* |
| pacemaker | **pacemaker** *An electrical device used to stimulate the heart used for bradyarrhythmias.* |
| pachidermia | **pachydermia** *An abnormally thick skin.* |
| pachimeningite | **pachymeningitis** *Inflammation of the dura mater.* |
| padella da letto | **bedpan** *A metal or plastic vestibule one sits on while in bed to defecate.* |
| pagofagia | **pagophagia** *Compulsive need to eat ice which is usually associated with iron deficiency anemia.* |
| palato | **palate** *The roof of the mouth.* |
| palatoplegia | **palatoplegia** *Paralysis of the palate.* |
| palliativo | **palliative** *A treatment used to reduce pain when cure is not possible.* |
| palliectomia | **pallidectomy** *Surgical resection of all or part of the palate.* |
| pallore | **pallor** *Unusually pale appearance.* |
| palmare | **palmar** *Referring to the palm.* |
| palmo della mano | **palm** *The anterior aspect of the hand.* |
| palpazione | **palpation** *The assessment of the body with the use of one's hands.* |
| palpebra | **eyelid** *Palpebra.* |
| palpebra | **palpebra, palpebrae** *Eyelid, eyelids.* |
| palpitazioni | **palpitation** *Sensation of a forceful, rapid, irregular heartbeat present after exercise or with anxiety.* |
| paludismo; malaria | **paludism** *Synonym of malaria.* |
| panartrite | **panarthritis** *Inflammation of the joints.* |
| pancardite | **pancarditis** *Inflammation of pericardium, myocardium and endocardium.* |
| pancreas | **pancreas** *A gland that secretes digestive enzymes into the duodenum and insulin and glucagon into the blood.* |
| pancreatectomia | **pancreatectomy** *Surgical excision of part or all of the pancreas.* |
| pancreatite | **pancreatitis** *Inflammation of the pancreas.* |
| pancreozimina | **pancreozymin** *A duodenal mucosal enzyme that facilitates the secretion of amylase and other enzymes from the pancreas.* |
| pandemico | **pandemic** *When a disease is present over an entire region.* |
| panipopituitarismo | **panhypopituitarism** *Insufficiency of the anterior pituitary.* |
| pannicolite | **panniculitis** *Inflammation of a section of subcutaneous tissue containing large amounts of fat.* |
| pannolino assorbente | **diaper** *Undergarment worn to absorb urine in incontinent persons.* |
| panoftalmite | **panophthalmia** *Inflammation of the eye and all its structures.* |
| panotite | **panotitis** *Inflammation of each part of a bone.* |
| papilledema | **papilledema** *Swelling of the optic disc.* |
| papillite | **papillitis** *Swelling of a papilla.* |
| papilloma | **papilloma** *A benign, lobulated tumor coming from epithelium.* |
| papula | **papule** *A small, well-circumscribed elevation of the skin.* |
| paracentesi | **nyxis** *Paracentesis or a puncture.* |
| paracentesi | **paracentesis** *A procedure involving aspiration of fluid from the abdominal cavity.* |
| paracusia | **paracusia** *Any abnormality in the sense of hearing.* |

| Italian | English |
|---|---|
| parafimose | **paraphimosis** *A condition in which the foreskin is retracted but cannot be replace because of a restricted foreskin.* |
| paralisi | **palsy** *Paralysis that is usually associated with tremors.* |
| paralisi bulbare | **bulbar palsy** *Paralysis due to changes in the motor center of the medulla oblongata.* |
| paralisi cerebrale | **cerebral palsy** *A condition exhibited by motor incoordination and speech changes that is the result of brain injury occurring ante-, intra- or post- partum.* |
| paralisi di Bell | **Bell's palsy** *Unilateral facial paralysis related to dysfunction of the seventh cranial nerve.* |
| paralisi facciale | **facial paralysis** *Lack of movement or sensation in the distribution of the facial nerve.* |
| paralisi oculare | **ocular paralysis.** *Paralysis of intraocular and extraocular muscles.* |
| paralisi periodica ipokaliemica | **hypokalemic periodic paralysis** *An inherited disorder that leads to muscle weakness related to a low serum potassium level.* |
| paralisi periodico | **periodic paralysis** *A familial muscle disorder exhibited by recurrent episodes flaccid paralysis without change in level of consciousness.* |
| paralisi pseudobulbare | **pseudobulbar palsy** *Sudden outbursts of laughter or tearfulness sometimes seen in amyotrophic lateral sclerosis.* |
| paralitico | **paralytic** *1. Referring to paralysis. 2. A person who is paralyzed.* |
| paramediano | **paramedian** *Situated toward the middle of the body.* |
| paramedico | **paramedical** *Hospital support staff excluding physicians.* |
| parametrio | **parametrium** *The connective tissue and smooth muscle between the broad ligament serous layers.* |
| parametrite | **parametritis** *Inflammation of the parametrium.* |
| paramnesia | **paramnesia** *A condition exhibited by a person's belief they have memory for an event that never happened.* |
| paranasali | **paranasal** *Situated adjacent to the nose.* |
| paranoia | **paranoia** *A mental condition exhibited by delusions of persecution.* |
| paranoideo | **paranoid** *Having the symptom of paranoia.* |
| paraplegia | **paraplegia** *Paralysis of the lower extremities.* |
| paraprassia | **parapraxis** *1. Unable to perform purposeful movements. 1. Irrational behavior.* |
| pararettale | **pararectal** *Adjacent to the rectum.* |
| parasimpatico | **parasympathetic** *Part of the autonomic nervous system that opposes sympathetic stimulation.* |
| parassita | **parasite** *An organism that lives on or within another organism without benefit to the latter.* |
| paratiroideo | **parathyroid** *Positioned adjacent to the thyroid.* |
| paratormone | **parathormone** *Synonym for parathyroid hormone.* |
| paravertebrale | **paravertebral** *Positioned adjacent to the vertebra.* |
| parenchima | **parenchyma** *The functional elements of an organ.* |
| parenterale | **parenteral** *Other than the alimentary canal.* |
| paresi | **paresis** *Incomplete paralysis.* |
| parestesia | **paresthesia** *An abnormal sensation usually described as pins and needles.* |
| parete cellulare | **cell wall** *The peripheral border of the cell.* |
| parete toracica | **chest wall** *Thoracic wall.* |
| parete toracica flaccida (respiro paradosso) | **flail chest** *The term used when one has multiple rib fractures causing a segment of the chest wall to move incongruently with the rest of the chest wall.* |
| parietale | **parietal** *Referring to the wall of a part or cavity.* |
| paronichia | **paronychia** *Inflammation of the tissue bordering a fingernail* |
| paronichia | **whitlow** *An abscess occurring on the palmar surface of the fingertips.* |

| Italian | English |
|---|---|
| parosmia | **parosmia** *An alteration in the sense of smell.* |
| parossismo | **attack** *A fit or paroxysm.* |
| parossistico | **paroxysmal** *Occurring in sudden attacks.* |
| parotico | **parotid** *A gland near the ear.* |
| parotite | **parotiditis** *Inflammation of the parotid gland.* |
| parte centrale | **core** *Central part of a structure.* |
| parte dorsale dell'arco del piede | **instep** *The medial aspect of the foot between the ankle and the ball of the foot.* |
| partenogenesi | **parthenogenesis** *Reproduction that occurs without an egg being fertilized by sperm.* |
| parto | **delivery** *The process of giving birth.* |
| parto | **childbirth** *Parturition; the process of labor and delivery of an infant.* |
| parto podalico | **breech birth** *Delivery with the feet or buttocks coming first.* |
| passare appena | **squeeze, to** *To apply pressure.* |
| passeggio | **ambulation** *Relating to walking.* |
| passivo | **passive** *Not achieved through active effort.* |
| passo | **pace** *Consistent and continuous movement.* |
| pasta | **paste** *A thick, soft moist substance usually with medicine mixed in.* |
| patella, rotula | **patella** *The bone situated in the anterior portion of the knee.* |
| patellectomia | **patellectomy** *Surgical excision of the patella.* |
| patogenesi | **pathogenesis** *The course of a disease.* |
| patogeno | **pathogenic** *Referring to an organism that can cause disease.* |
| patognomonico | **pathognomonic** *Characteristic of something.* |
| patologia | **pathology** *1. The branch of medicine dealing with the study of tissues and the forensic application. 2. Referring to a condition that is abnormal.* |
| patologico | **pathological** *Referring to pathology.* |
| paura | **fear** *Fright or trepidation.* |
| pavor nocturnus | **night terror** *Sensation of profound fear upon wakening.* |
| pediatra | **pediatrician** *Physician who is a specialist in pediatrics.* |
| pediatria | **pediatrics** *Medical specialty concerned with the treatment and prevention of childhood disease.* |
| pediculosi | **pediculosis** *Lice infestation.* |
| peduncolato | **pediculate** *Referring to pedicle.* |
| peduncolo | **peduncle** *1. A stalk-like protrusion. 2. A bundle of nerve fibers connecting two parts of the brain.* |
| peduncolo crebellare superiore | **brachium cerebelli** *Synonym of pedunculus cerebellaris superior (upper portion the cerebellum).* |
| peggioramento | **impairment** *A specific disability.* |
| peli del pube | **pubic hair** *Hair present in the perineal area.* |
| pellagra | **pellagra** *A deficiency in nicotinic acid exhibited by diarrhea and dermatitis.* |
| pelle | **skin** *Flesh.* |
| pelle d'oca; cutis anserina | **goose bumps** *Cutis anserina.* |
| peloso | **hairy** *A profuse amount of hair.* |
| pelvi | **pelvis** *The bony structure at the base of the spine.* |
| pelvi maschile | **android pelvis** *A pelvis shaped like a man's.* |
| pelvi renale | **renal pelvis** *The kidney collecting system.* |
| pelvico | **pelvic** *Referring to the pelvis.* |
| pelvimetria | **pelvimetry** *Measurement of the dimensions of the pelvis to determine whether a patient is capable of natural childbirth.* |

| Italian | English |
|---|---|
| pemfigoide bolloso | **bullous pemphigoid** *A benign disease of the aged characterized by large bullae forming on the torso and extremities.* |
| pena | **sorrow** *A feeling of deep despair.* |
| pene | **penis** *Male genital organ used for the transfer of sperm and elimination of urine.* |
| penetrazione | **penetration** *The process of making a way through something.* |
| penfigo | **pemphigus** *A skin disorder with large bullous lesions.* |
| penicillina | **penicillin** *A synthetic antibiotic originally produced from blue mold.* |
| pentosuria | **pentosuria** *The presence of pentose in the urine (a monosaccharide with five carbon atoms in the molecule).* |
| pepsina | **pepsin** *A proteolytic gastric enzyme.* |
| peptico | **peptic** *Referring to pepsin or concerning digestion.* |
| peptide | **peptide** *A compound with low molecular weight and containing two or more amino acids.* |
| per sentirsi meglio | **feel better, to** *To have improved health symptomatically.* |
| percuotere leggermente | **tap** *A puncture with the intent of draining fluid as in spinal tap.* |
| percussione | **percussion** *A manual procedure involving tapping a body part to determine the size or density (liquid or air) of a part.* |
| perdita di coscienza | **loss of consciousness** *Unresponsive to verbal and tactile stimuli.* |
| perdita di funzione | **loss of function** *Inability to complete routine activities.* |
| perdita di successivo | **lost to follow-up** *This describes a situation in which a patient has a chronic medical problem but has not been seen regularly.* |
| perforazione | **perforation** *Presence of a hole.* |
| periarterite nodosa | **polyarteritis nodosa** *A systemic necrotizing vasculitis that effects medium sized arteries.* |
| periartrite | **periarthritis** *Inflammation of the tissues around a joint.* |
| pericardico | **pericardial** *Referring to around the heart.* |
| pericardio | **pericardium** *The structure enclosing the heart which contains a fibrous outer layer and serous inner layer.* |
| pericardite | **pericarditis** *Inflammation of the pericardium.* |
| pericolite | **pericolitis** *Inflammation of the membrane covering the colon.* |
| pericolo di vita | **life-threatening** *Potentially fatal.* |
| pericondrio | **perichondrium** *The membrane that encloses a cartilage.* |
| pericondrite | **perichondritis** *Inflammation of the perichondrium.* |
| periferico | **peripheral** *Referring to an outward part or surface.* |
| perilinfa | **perilymph** *The fluid separating the membranous and osseous labyrinth.* |
| perinataligo | **perinatology** *The study of disease in the period just before and right after birth.* |
| perineale | **perineal** *Referring to the perineum.* |
| perineo | **perineum** *The area between the anus and scrotum or anus and vulva.* |
| perineorrafia | **perineorrhaphy** *Surgical repair of the perineum.* |
| periosteo | **periosteal** *Referring to the periosteum.* |
| periosteo | **periosteum** *A layer of connective tissue covering the bones.* |
| periostite | **periostitis** *Inflammation of the periosteum.* |
| periproctite | **periproctitis** *Inflammation of the tissue encircling the anus and rectum.* |
| perirenale | **perinephric** *Around the kidney.* |
| peristalsi | **peristalsis** *The contraction of the longitudinal and circular muscle fibers of the alimentary canal so food is propelled.* |
| peritomia | **peritomy** *Surgically creating an opening of the periosteum.* |
| peritoneale | **peritoneal** *Referring to the peritoneum.* |

| Italian | English |
|---|---|
| peritoneo | **peritoneum** *The serous membrane covering the abdominal organs and lining the abdominal walls.* |
| peritonite | **peritonitis** *Inflammation of the peritoneum.* |
| peritonsillare | **peritonsillar** *Surrounding the tonsils.* |
| periuretrale | **periurethral** *Surrounding the urethra.* |
| pernicioso, 2) anemia perniciosa | **pernicious** *1. Having a detrimental effect. 2. Pernicious anemia is a reduced red blood cell count due to Vitamin B12 deficiency.* |
| peroneale | **peroneal** *Referring to the fibula or the outer part of the leg.* |
| persona che controlla | **monitor** *A person that observes a process or a monitoring device.* |
| persona che ha subito un infortunio | **casualty** *A person who is killed or seriously injured.* |
| personalità | **personality** *Qualities that form a person's unique character.* |
| pertosse | **pertussis** *Synonym for whooping cough.* |
| pertosse | **whooping cough** *Pertussis* |
| pesante | **heavy** *Possessing great weight.* |
| pesce | **fish** *A cold-blooded vertebrate with gills and fins.* |
| peso corporeo | **body weight** *Relative mass as measured in kilograms or pounds.* |
| pessario | **pessary** *A supportive device placed in the rectum or vagina.* |
| peste bubbonica | **bubonic plague** *A form of plague exhibited by the formation of buboes.* |
| petecchia | **petechia** *A small red or purple macule on the skin caused by bleeding.* |
| petroso | **petrous** *Possessing a density of a stone.* |
| petto | **breast** *Mammary tissue including the areola.* |
| pettorale | **pectoral** *Referring to the pectoral muscle.* |
| pettoriloquia | **pectoriloquy** *The examiner's voice is clearly audible when the patient speaks as when the examiner listens to an area of consolidation in the lungs of the speaker.* |
| pettoriloquia bisbigliata | **whispered pectoriloquy** *The sound heard through the stethoscope when listening to a person's lungs. The sound resonates as it would when listening over a bronchus if there is an area of consolidation.* |
| peurperio | **puerperium** *The six week period after childbirth.* |
| phthirus pubis | **crab louse** *Phthirus pubis is formal name for a louse that infests pubic hair and causes intense itching.* |
| pia madre | **pia mater** *The first layer of three covering the brain and spinal cord.* |
| piaga da decubito | **decubitus ulcer** *A wound caused by laying in one position for too long; also referred to as a pressure ulcer.* |
| piaga da decubito; ulcera da compressione | **pressure ulcer** *Loss in skin integrity due to a portion of the body being in the same position for too long and possibly other factors.* |
| piaga orientali | **oriental sore** *A stigmata of cutaneous leishmaniasis caused by a bite from a sand fly.* |
| pianta del piede | **sole of foot** *Common term for plantar aspect of the foot.* |
| piastrina | **platelet** *An oval cell without a nucleus used in coagulation; also called a thrombocyte.* |
| piatto | **flat** *Level or even; without bulges.* |
| picacismo | **pica** *A desire for unusual substances as occurs in pregnancy and some psychological conditions.* |
| piccola compressa | **pledget** *A small plug of cotton or other synthetic material inserted into a wound.* |
| picnico | **pyknic** *Possessing a short, stocky physique.* |
| picnosi | **pyknosis** *The degeneration of a cell with the nucleus shrinking.* |
| picollo insetto | **bug** *Insect.* |
| pidocchio | **lice** *Plural for louse, a small parasite that lives on the skin. Pediculus humanus capitis is a head louse.* |
| piede | **foot** *The lower extremity distal to the ankle.* |

| Italian | English |
|---|---|
| piede cadente | **drop foot** *The symptom in a person with a nerve injury causing impaired ankle dorsiflexion.* |
| piede cadente | **foot drop** *Caused by palsy of the nerve controlling foot dorsiflexion.* |
| piede cavo | **pes cavus** *Excessive height of the longitudinal arch of the foot.* |
| piede d'atleta | **athlete's foot** *Common term for tinea pedis.* |
| piede piatto | **flatfoot** *Common term for pes planus.* |
| piede piatto | **pes planus** *Medical term for flat foot.* |
| piede valgo | **pes valgus** *Abnormal longitudinal arch- it is flat.* |
| piega della pelle | **skin fold** *An overlapping of skin formed by subcutaneous tissue.* |
| piega glutea | **gluteal fold** *The horizontal crease between the buttock and upper thigh.* |
| pielite | **pyelitis** *Renal pelvis inflammation.* |
| pielografia | **pyelography** *Use of a contrast agent to radiologically study the kidney, ureters and bladder.* |
| pielolitotomia | **pyelolithotomy** *Surgical excision of a calculus from the renal pelvis.* |
| pielonefrite | **pyelonephritis** *Inflammation of the renal parenchyma usually due to bacterial infection.* |
| pielonefrosi | **pyelonephrosis** *Term, rarely used anymore, used to describe disease of the renal pelvis.* |
| piemia | **pyemia** *Sepsis characterized by the presence of secondary abscesses.* |
| pietra miliare | **milestone** *An event indicative of a certain stage of development.* |
| pigmenti biliari | **bile pigments** *The golden brown or green-yellow color associated with bile.* |
| pillola | **pill** *A medicated tablet or capsule.* |
| pillola rivestimento | **coated tablet** *A pill covered with a substance to slow absorption or reduce gastric irritation.* |
| pilorico | **pyloric** *Referring to the pylorus.* |
| piloro | **pylorus** *The opening at the distal stomach that opens into the duodenum.* |
| piloroplastica | **pyloroplasty** *Surgical enlargement of a pylorus that previously was stenotic.* |
| pinguecola | **pinguecula** *The yellow tissue on the bulbar conjunctiva adjacent to the sclerocorneal junction.* |
| pinocitosi | **pinocytosis** *The absorption of fluid into a cell by the formation of vesicles on the cell membrane.* |
| pinza per aghi; porta aghi | **needle holder** *A surgical instrument used to grasp a needle during suturing.* |
| piochilocitosi | **poikilocytosis** *The presence of abnormally shaped erythrocytes.* |
| piodermite | **pyoderma** *A purulent skin infection.* |
| piogeno | **pyogenic** *Referring to the formation of pus.* |
| piombo | **lead** *An element with an atomic number of 82.* |
| pionefrosi | **pyonephrosis** *Injury to the renal parenchyma due to pus.* |
| piorrea | **pyorrhea** *Emission of pus.* |
| piosalpinge | **pyosalpinx** *Purulent material in the oviduct.* |
| pipetta | **pipet** *A slender tube with a bulb used for transferring liquids.* |
| piramidale | **pyramidal** *A term that is used to describe various spinal tracts that originate in the cerebral cortex.* |
| piressia | **pyrexia** *Fever.* |
| piridossina; vitamina B6 | **pyridoxine** *Synonym for vitamin B6.* |
| pirogeno | **pyrogen** *A fever producing substance released by bacteria.* |
| pirosi | **pyrosis** *Synonym for heartburn.* |
| pirosi esofagea | **heartburn** *Synonym of pyrosis.* |
| pisolino | **nap** *A brief sleep or catnap.* |

| Italian | English |
|---|---|
| pitiriasi rosea | **pityriasis rosea** *A skin disease characterized by dry pink oval papulosquamous eruptions.* |
| piuria | **pyuria** *Presence of purulent material in the urine.* |
| placca neuromuscolare motore | **motor end plate** *The expansions on a motor nerve where the branches terminate on muscle fiber.* |
| placenta | **placenta** *The vascular tissue that nourishes a fetus through an umbilical cord.* |
| placenta (espulsa dopo il parto) | **afterbirth** *The tissue expelled after the birth of a child that includes the placenta and allied membranes.* |
| placenta previa | **placenta praevia** *A condition in which the placenta covers the cervical os.* |
| placentare | **placental** *Referring to the placenta.* |
| plagiocefalia | **plagiocephaly** *A condition characterized by an asymmetric skull because the cranial sutures do not close normally.* |
| plantare | **plantar** *Referring to the bottom of the foot.* |
| plasmacitosi | **plasmacytosis** *The existence of plasma cells in the blood.* |
| plasmaferesi | **plasmapheresis** *A method of removing blood and reinfusing it after the elimination of antibodies.* |
| pleomorfismo | **pleomorphism** *The ability of an organism or substance to attain distinct forms.* |
| plesso brachiale | **brachial plexus** *A cluster of nerves coming off the last four cervical and first thoracic spinal nerves form the nerve supply the the chest and arms.* |
| plesso solare | **solar plexus** *A cluster of ganglia and nerves, located at the base of the sternum, that surround the celiac trunk.* |
| pletismografo | **plethysmograph** *A device used to measure the amount of blood flowing through a body part; impedance plethysmography is used to check for deep venous thrombosis.* |
| pletora | **plethora** *An excess of something.* |
| pleura | **pleura** *The serous membrane lining each lung.* |
| pleura cervicale | **cervical pleura** *The dome-like cap of the pleura.* |
| pleurite | **pleurisy** *Inflammation of the pleura.* |
| plica | **plica** *A fold, as in a fold in the peritoneum.* |
| pneumatocele | **pneumatocele** *1. A hernia-like protrusion of lung tissue. 2. A collection of gas in a sac such as the scrotum.* |
| pneumaturia | **pneumaturia** *Presence of air or gas in the urine.* |
| pneumococco | **pneumococcus** *A bacterium causing pneumonia and meningitis. A common type is Streptococcus pneumoniae.* |
| pneumoconiosi | **anthracosis** *Pneumoconiosis caused by coal dust.* |
| pneumoconiosi | **pneumoconiosis** *Fibrosis of the lung due to dust inhalation.* |
| pneumonectomia | **pneumonectomy** *Surgical excision of all or part of a lung.* |
| pneumopatia granluomatosa interstiziale | **farmer's lung** *Coined because farmers are susceptible to this disease by inhaling fungi from hay; also called Aspergillosis.* |
| pneumoperitoneo | **pneumoperitoneum** *Abnormal or induced presence of air or gas in the peritoneum.* |
| pneumotorace | **pneumothorax** *Abnormal presence of air between the lung and chest wall.* |
| podiatra | **chiropodist** *A doctor trained in the treatment of feet.* |
| poichilotermia | **poikilothermy** *A condition of cold-blooded animals in which their temperature varies based on the ambient temperature.* |
| poliambulatorio; centro sanitario | **health center** *A physical location where patients are treated.* |
| policistico | **polycystic** *Possessing more than one cyst.* |
| policitemia | **polycythemia** *Excess in the number of erythrocytes in the blood.* |

| Italian | English |
|---|---|
| policitemia vera | **polycythemia vera** *Condition characterized by increase in erythrocytes, thrombocytes and leukocytes, as well as, splenomegaly.* |
| policondrite | **polychondritis** *Inflammation of the cartilage at more than one site.* |
| polidattilia | **polydactyly** *Congenital anomaly exhibited by more than 5 digits on the hands and/or feet.* |
| polidipsia | **polydipsia** *Profound thirst.* |
| polimenorrea | **polymenorrhea** *Increase in the frequency of menstruation.* |
| polimiosite | **polymyositis** *Inflammation of several muscle groups at once.* |
| polineuropatia | **polyneuropathy** *A condition involving more than one nerve.* |
| polinevrite | **polyneuritis** *Inflammation of more than one nerve.* |
| polioencefalite | **polioencephalitis** *Polio infection of the brain.* |
| poliomielite | **poliomyelitis** *An infectious viral disease exhibited by constitutional symptoms that can lead to quadriplegia.* |
| poliopia | **polyopia** *A condition in which one object is seen abnormally as two or more.* |
| poliposi | **polyposis** *The formation of multiple polyps.* |
| poliposo | **polypus** *Synonym of polyp (a prominent growth from a mucous membrane).* |
| polisaccaride | **polysaccharide** *A carbohydrate that upon hydrolysis forms more than ten monosaccharides.* |
| polisialia | **polysialia** *Abnormal increase in saliva.* |
| politraumatismo | **polytrauma** *A condition exhibited by multiple injuries from blunt or penetrating trauma.* |
| poliuria | **polyuria** *Abnormal increase in volume of urine excreted.* |
| pollice | **thumb** *The first digit of each hand.* |
| polluzione notturna | **nocturnal emission** *Involuntary emission of semen at night.* |
| polmonare | **pulmonary** *Referring to the lungs.* |
| polmone | **lung** *One of a pair of respiratory organs.* |
| polmonite | **pneumonia** *Inflammation of the lung due to an infection caused by a virus or bacterium.* |
| polmonite aspirazione | **aspiration pneumonia** *Taking air or matter into the lungs.* |
| polmonite pneumocisti jiroveci | **pneumocystis jiroveci pneumonia.** *A pulmonary infection associated with AIDS. Formerly called pneumocystis carinii pneumonia* |
| polpa | **pulp** *The tissue filling the root canals of a tooth.* |
| polpaccio | **calf** *Muscles of the posterior portion of the lower leg.* |
| polpastrello | **fingertip** *Distal aspect of a finger.* |
| polso | **pulse** *The rhythmic throbbing of arteries felt at major vessels.* |
| polso | **wrist** *The articulation of the hand and radius/ulna.* |
| polso alternanza | **pulsus alternans** *A regular alternation of weak and strong beats of the pulse.* |
| polvere | **dust** *Dry earthen particles found on the ground and surfaces.* |
| polvere | **powder** *Fine dry particles.* |
| pomo d'Adamo | **Adam's apple** *A prominence on the anterior neck caused by the thyroid cartilage of the larynx.* |
| ponfolice | **pompholyx** *A condition exhibited by interdigital vesicles of the hands and feet.* |
| ponte | **pons** *The part of the brainstem that connects the medulla oblongata with the thalamus.* |
| pontino | **pontine** *Referring to the pons.* |
| popliteo | **popliteal** *Referring to the posterior aspect of the knee.* |
| popora di Henoch | **Henoch purpura** *Exhibited by vomiting, diarrhea, abdominal pain and hematuria; a non-thrombocytopenic purpura.* |

| Italian | English |
|---|---|
| porfiria | **porphyria** *A hereditary condition currently classified based on the specific enzyme deficiency. The most common form is porphyria cutanea tarda that causes blistering lesions.* |
| porfirina | **porphyrin** *A class of pigments that contain a flat ring of four heterocyclic groups.* |
| porpora | **purpura** *The presence of patches of ecchymosis or petechiae.* |
| portale | **portal** *Referring to an entrance such as porta hepatis.* |
| portare | **bring, to** *To carry or transport something.* |
| positivo | **positive** *Indicating the presence of something.* |
| posizione fetale | **fetal position** *Refers to how the fetus lies within the uterus.* |
| posizione genu-cubitale | **knee elbow position** *Knees and elbows are on the table and the chest is in the air.* |
| posizione litotomia | **lithotomy position** *Buttocks positioned at the end of the OR table, the hips and knees flexed and the feet strapped in. Dorsosacral position.* |
| posizione varo | **varus position** *Refers to a joint being abnormally angulated toward the midline of the body.* |
| posporre | **postpone, to** *To delay.* |
| post-carico | **after-load** *Referring to the amount of pressure the heart needs to pump against. If one has left heart failure it is beneficial to reduce after-load.* |
| post-termine nascita | **post-term birth** *An infant born after the normal length of pregnancy.* |
| postaccessuale | **postictal** *The period of time after a seizure.* |
| posteriore | **posterior** *Further back in position; opposite of anterior.* |
| postmaturità | **postmaturity** *Generally referring to a pregnancy that goes beyond the due date.* |
| posturale | **postural** *Referring to position or posture.* |
| potassio | **potassium** *A chemical of the alkali metal group.* |
| potenza | **potency** *Strength or power.* |
| potenziale d'azione | **action potential** *The alteration in electrical potential associated with the movement along a nerve cell.* |
| potenziali evocati | **evoked potential** *Electrical impulses that can be noted after stimulation of sensory organs.* |
| pre-eclampsia | **pre-eclampsia** *Hypertension with proteinuria and/or edema in the setting of pregnancy.* |
| preauricolare | **preauricular** *Anterior to the ear.* |
| precanceroso | **precancerous** *Referring to an early stage in cancer development.* |
| preciptina | **precipitin** *An antibody-antigen reaction producing a precipitate.* |
| precordialgia | **precordialgia** *Pain in the precordium.* |
| precordio | **precordium** *The area occupying the epigastrium and lower sternum.* |
| prematuro | **beforehand** *In advance or previously.* |
| prematuro | **premature** *Occurring earlier than expected.* |
| premesturale | **premenstrual** *Occurring prior to the onset of menstruation.* |
| premolare | **premolar** *The teeth anterior to the molars.* |
| prenatale | **prenatal** *Referring to the time prior to birth.* |
| prendersi un raffreddore | **catch a cold** *To come down with a viral upper respiratory tract infection.* |
| preoccupare | **worry, to** *To fret or have unease.* |
| preparato anatomico ottenuto per dissezione | **dissection** *Autopsy or postmortem exam.* |
| prepuzio | **foreskin** *Also called prepuce, the skin that naturally covers the glans but can be rolled back.* |
| presbiacusia | **presbyacusia** *An age related, progressive hearing loss.* |
| presbiopia | **presbyopia** *Farsightedness associated with aging.* |

| Italian | English |
|---|---|
| presentazione del cordone ombelicale | **cord presentation** *The presence of the umbilical cord at the cervix during active labor.* |
| presentazione di faccia | **face presentation** *Referring to the part of the body coming out of the cervix first during childbirth.* |
| presentazione di fronte | **brow presentation** *The term used to describe which part of the body (forehead) is being delivered first in childbirth.* |
| presentazione di podice | **breech presentation** *Position of the feet or buttocks near the cervix.* |
| preservativi | **condom** *A covering for the penis or the vagina (female condom) used during sexual intercourse that is meant to reduce the chance of pregnancy or infection.* |
| presistole | **presystolic** *The time just before systole.* |
| pressione, tensione | **stress** *Strain or pressure.* |
| prevedere | **expect, to** *To suppose or presume.* |
| prevenire | **prevent, to** *To stave off or hinder.* |
| previo | **former** *Prior.* |
| priapismo | **priapism** *A painful and abnormally prolonged erection.* |
| prima della morte | **antemortem** *Refers to: before death.* |
| primi movimento del feto nell'utero precepiti dalla madre | **quickening** *Signs of life noted by a mother as the fetus moves.* |
| primipara | **primipara** *A woman giving birth for the first time.* |
| probabilità | **likelihood** *The probability or feasibility.* |
| problema; difficoltà | **problem** *Difficulty or complaint.* |
| processo mastoideo | **mastoid process** *The posterior part of the temporal bone bordered by the parietal bone superiorly and the occipital bone posteriorly.* |
| processo xifoideo dello sterno | **xiphoid process** *The inferior segment of the sternum.* |
| proctalgia | **proctalgia** *A chronic high, dull rectal pain worse with sitting position.* |
| proctectomia | **proctectomy** *Surgical excision of the rectum.* |
| proctite | **proctitis** *Inflammation of the rectum.* |
| proctocele | **proctocele** *A hernia-type protrusion of the rectum into the vagina.* |
| proctoscopia | **proctoscopy** *Inspection of the rectum with a scope.* |
| profilassi | **prophylaxis** *That which is done to prevent disease.* |
| profondo | **deep** *Having significant depth.* |
| profondo | **wise** *Possessing much knowledge.* |
| progenie | **offspring** *One's children.* |
| progeria | **progeria** *A childhood disorder exhibited by signs of aging including gray hair, wrinkled skin and short height.* |
| progestogeno | **progesterone** *A steroid hormone that prepares the uterus for pregnancy.* |
| prognatismo | **prognathism** *Protrusion of the mandible which can cause malocclusion.* |
| prognosi | **prognosis** *The likely course of a disease.* |
| programmazione della famiglia | **family planning** *Birth control.* |
| progressivo | **progressive** *Developing gradually.* |
| prolasso | **prolapse** *The slipping downward of a body part, such as rectal prolapse.* |
| prolasso uterino | **prolapse of the uterus** *Eversion of the uterus through the vagina.* |
| prolasso uterino | **uterine prolapse** *Protrusion of the uterus out the vagina.* |
| prolattina | **prolactin** *A pituitary hormone that facilitates milk production.* |
| promonocito | **promonocyte** *An intermediate cell stage between monocyte and monoblast.* |

| Italian | English |
|---|---|
| promontorio | **promontory** *A protruding eminence.* |
| pronazione | **pronation** *Turning posteriorly. When the hand is pronated, it is turned medially until the palm is facing posteriorly (when the body was initially in the anatomic position).* |
| prono | **prone** *Lying with the abdomen and face downward.* |
| pronto soccorso | **first aid** *The initial treatment after an injury.* |
| propriocettore | **proprioceptor** *A receptor that responds to sensory input including position sense.* |
| prosencefalo | **forebrain** *The part of the brain that includes the thalamus, hypothalamus and cerebral hemispheres.* |
| prossimale | **proximal** *Situated closer to the center of the body (opposed to that which is farther away, as in distal).* |
| prossimo | **next** *The following or upcoming.* |
| prostaciclina | **prostacyclin** *A prostaglandin that functions as an anticoagulant and vasodilator.* |
| prostaglandine | **prostaglandin** *A compound first found in semen (thus "prosta" in the name from prostate) with many effects including uterine contraction.* |
| prostata | **prostate** *A gland found in men that surrounds the neck of the urethra and bladder.* |
| prostatectomia | **prostatectomy** *Surgical excision of the prostate.* |
| prostrazione | **prostration** *Profound exhaustion.* |
| proteina | **protein** *A class of nitrogenous organic compound.* |
| proteinuria | **proteinuria** *The presence of protein in the urine.* |
| proteolisi | **proteolysis** *Enzyme action on proteins to form amino acids.* |
| protesi | **prosthesis** *An artificial body part. (above the knee) [below the knee]* |
| protesi per palatoschisi | **cleft palate** *A congenital abnormal opening in the palate.* |
| protoplasma | **protoplasm** *The cytoplasm, organelles and nucleus of a living cell.* |
| Protozoi | **Protozoa** *A single celled microscopic organism including amoebas among others.* |
| protrombina | **prothrombin** *A compound converted to thrombin during coagulation of blood.* |
| protuberanza | **lump** *A protuberance.* |
| prova crociata di compatibilità | **cross-matching (blood)** *Evaluation of blood to determine compatibility between the donor and recipient prior to transfusion.* |
| prova di Finkelstein | **Finkelstein test** *Pain elicited with thumb flexion and wrist flexion is indicative of De Quervain tenosynovitis.* |
| prova di fissazione del complemento | **complement fixation test** *A laboratory test for the presence of an antibody in the serum that involves inactivation of the complement in the serum.* |
| prova di fragilità capillare | **capillary fragility test** *Application of a blood pressure cuff high enough to restrict venous return and after five minutes count the number or petechiae produced.* |
| prova di intradermoreazione di Casoni | **Casoni's test** *Hydatid fluid is injected intradermally; subsequent formation of a larger papule indicates hydatid disease.* |
| prova sussurro | **whisper test** *The examiner whispers into one ear while blocking the other ear to see if the patient can hear in the ear whispered into.* |
| prove calcagno-ginocchio | **heel-shin test (heel to knee to toe test)** *A test of position sense and coordination; one moves the heel of one foot from the knee on the other foot down to the foot.* |
| prove indice-naso | **finger nose test** *A test for dysmetria in which a person reaches out to touch their own nose with an extended finger with their eyes closed.* |
| provetta | **test tube** *A glass or plastic tube used to hold a medical specimen.* |
| provocare | **provoke, to** *To evoke or elicit.* |
| provvedere | **endow, to** *To supply or provide for.* |

| Italian | English |
|---|---|
| provviste | **supplies** *Stock or reserves.* |
| prurigine | **prurigo** *A chronic, pruritic papular skin eruption.* |
| prurito | **pruritus** *A general term for conditions exhibited by itching.* |
| prurito aestivalis | **summer itch** *Pruritus noted upon exposure to hot weather, also known as pruritus aestivalis.* |
| prurito avicoltore | **poultryman's itch** *Pruritus associated with the mite Dermanyssus gallinae.* |
| prurito azo | **azo itch** *A pruritus noted in people who use azo dyes.* |
| prurito copra | **copra itch** *A pruritus noted in people working with copra (dried kernel from a coconut).* |
| prurito da freddo | **frost itch** *A pruritus noted when exposed to cold weather.* |
| prurito del nuotatore | **swimmer's itch** *Pruritus caused by exposure to schistosomes.* |
| prurito di Malabar | **Malabar itch.** *Pruritus associated with tinea imbricata which is characterized by overlapping rings of papulosquamous patches. It is also known as oriental ringworm.* |
| prurito di Saint Ignatius; pellagra | **Saint Ignatius' itch** *Pruritus noted with a cluster of symptoms related to niacin deficiency. Generally referred to as pellagra.* |
| prurito Norway | **Norway itch** *A severe pruritus caused by scabies and is associated with immune disorders such as AIDS.* |
| pseudoartrite | **pseudarthrosis** *Deossification of weight bearing long bones.* |
| pseudomnesia | **pseudomnesia** *Sensing the memory of an event that has never happened.* |
| psicastenia | **psychasthenia** *Essentially any non-hysterical neuroses.* |
| psichiatria | **psychiatry** *A branch of medicine specializing in the treatment of mental disorders.* |
| psicologia | **psychology** *The study of the human mind and emotions.* |
| psicologo | **psychologist** *A professional specializing in psychology.* |
| psiconevrosi | **psychoneurosis** *A mental disorder that could include depression or anxiety but does not include hallucinations.* |
| psicopatologia | **psychopathology** *Scientific examination of mental disease.* |
| psicosi | **psychosis** *A profound mental disorder that can include delusions and hallucinations.* |
| psicosi affettivo | **affective disorders** *Manic-depressive psychosis.* |
| psicosi maniaco-depressiva | **manic-depressive psychosis** *A mental disorder exhibited by alternating periods of depression and mania.* |
| psicosi postpartum | **postpartum psychosis** *A episode of abnormal thought or hallucinations following delivery.* |
| psicosomatico | **psychosomatic** *Physical ailments arising from mental disease.* |
| psicoterapia | **psychotherapy** *Treatment of mental disease with cognitive-behavioral approaches.* |
| psittacosi | **psittacosis** *A chlamydial pneumonia that is transmitted by birds.* |
| psoriasi | **psoriasis** *A chronic papulosquamous dermatosis characterized by silver plaques.* |
| pterigio | **pterygium** *A membrane in the interpalpebral fissure present from the conjunctiva to the cornea.* |
| ptialina | **ptyalin** *An enzyme found in saliva.* |
| ptosi (della palpebra superiore) | **ptosis** *Drooping of the upper eyelid usually due to paralysis of the third cranial nerve.* |
| pubertà | **puberty** *The time when adolescents become capable of sexual reproduction.* |
| pudendo | **pudendal** *Referring to the female genitalia* |
| pudendo | **pudendum** *The mons, pubis, labia majora, labia minora and the vagina.* |
| puerpera | **puerpera** *A woman who just gave birth.* |

| Italian | English |
|---|---|
| pugno | **fist** *When a person has their fingers clenched tightly to the palm.* |
| pulce | **flea** *A small wingless insect that feeds on blood of mammals.* |
| pulpite | **pulpitis** *Dental pulp inflammation.* |
| pulsatile | **pulsatile** *Relating to pulsation.* |
| pulsazione | **pulsation** *The action of expanding and contracting.* |
| pungiglione | **sting** *A small puncture as in a bee sting.* |
| punteggiatura | **stippling** *Having numerous small specks or spots.* |
| Punteggio di Apgar | **Apgar score** *A scoring system for newborns that utilizes heart rate, respiratory effort, muscle tone, responsiveness and skin color.* |
| punto cieco | **blind spot** *An area of insensitivity to light located at the point of entry of the optic nerve on the retina.* |
| punto estremo | **end point** *The last stage of a process.* |
| puntura cisterna | **cisternal puncture** *A trans-occipitoatlantoid ligament puncture of the cisterna magna so CSF can be obtained.* |
| puntura di api | **bee sting** *A piercing from a bee.* |
| puntura di zecca | **tick bite** |
| puntura lombare | **lumbar puncture** *Insertion of a needle into the spinal canal in the region of L3-4 to obtain a sample of CSF.* |
| pupilla | **pupil** *The opening at the center of the iris.* |
| pupilla amaurotico | **amaurotic pupil** *A pupil that will not respond to light when directly exposed but will respond when the other eye is exposed to light.* |
| pupilla di Adie | **Adie's pupil** *Characterized by a weak light reaction and a strong but slow near response.* |
| pupilla di Bumke | **Bumke's pupil** *Dilation of the pupil in response to anxiety.* |
| pupilla di Hutchinson | **Hutchinson's pupil** *Dilation of a pupil related to third nerve palsy on the side of the lesion as seen in herniation.* |
| pupilla paradossale | **paradoxical pupil** *Constriction of the pupil when exposed to darkness.* |
| purulento | **purulent** *Referring to pus.* |
| pus | **pus** *Thick yellow or green opaque liquid as seen with infection.* |
| putrefazione | **putrefaction** *The rotting or decaying of organic matter.* |
| quadricipite | **quadriceps** *The anterior thigh muscle composed of four muscles.* |
| quadriplegia | **quadriplegia** *Paralysis of all four extremities.* |
| qualificato | **qualify** *To become eligible by fulfilling a necessary standard.* |
| quantità | **amount** *The total or the aggregate.* |
| quarantena | **quarantine** *A place of isolation for infectious persons until it can be certain it is safe to let them mingle.* |
| quiescenza | **quiescent** *A time of inactivity.* |
| quieto | **quiet** *Making little or no noise.* |
| quinta malattia | **Fifth disease** *Erythema infectiosum is a viral disease caused by parovirus B19.* |
| quoziente dell'intelligenza | **intelligence quotient (IQ)** *A number representing a person's ability to problem solve compared to a matched-control.* |
| rabbia | **rabies** *An infectious viral disease transmitted through the bite of a mammal. Symptoms include hydrophobia, pharyngeal spasms and hyperactivity.* |
| rabbia | **rage** *Uncontrollable anger.* |
| rabdomiolisi | **rhabdomyolysis** *A acute destruction of muscle documented by myoglobinemia and myoglobinuria.* |
| racemoso | **racemose** *A gland having the form of a cluster.* |
| rachitismo | **rickets** *A condition exhibited by softening and bowing of the long bones; caused by Vitamin D deficiency.* |
| radiale | **radial** *Referring to the radius.* |

| Italian | English |
|---|---|
| radiazione | **radiation** *1. The emission of energy in the form of electromagnetic waves. 2. Divergence from a common point.* |
| radiazioni ionizzanti | **ionizing radiation** *High energy radiation that produces ion pairs in matter.* |
| radice | **root** *An embedded part of an organ or structure.* |
| radice dorsale | **dorsal root** *A description of the site of ganglion found on the dorsal root of each spinal nerve.* |
| radice quadrata | **square root** *The result noted when a number is multiplied by itself.* |
| radioattivo | **radioactive** *Referring to the emission of ionizing particles or radiation.* |
| radiobiologia | **radiobiology** *The study of the effects of radiation on organisms.* |
| radiocolite | **radiculitis** *Inflammation of a spinal nerve root.* |
| radiodermatite | **radioepithelitis** *The injury to epithelial cells due to effects of radiation.* |
| radiografia | **radiography** *The department where images are produced on sensitive film by x-rays.* |
| radiologia | **radiology** *The branch of medicine concerned with roentgenography and other high-energy radiation.* |
| radiologo | **radiologist** *A physician specializing in radiology.* |
| radionuclide | **radionuclide** *A radioactive nuclide.* |
| radioscopia | **fluoroscopy** *The continuous viewing of roentgenographic images with a fluorescent screen.* |
| radiosensibilità | **radiosensitivity** *The susceptibility of the skin to radiation.* |
| radioterapia | **radiotherapy** *Treatment of cancer with radiation.* |
| raffreddare | **cool** *Chilly or cold.* |
| raffreddore comune | **cold** *Viral upper respiratory tract infection.* |
| ragadi | **rhagade** *Fissures in the skin, particularly adjacent to body orifices.* |
| raggi gamma | **gamma ray** *A type of electromagnetic radiation.* |
| raggi ultravioletti | **ultraviolet rays** *Electromagnetic radiation with wavelength longer than x rays.* |
| raggi x | **x-ray** |
| raggio X di torace | **chest x-ray** *Roentography of the thorax.* |
| rame | **copper** *A chemical element with atomic number of 29.* |
| ramo | **ramus** *A branch; a term used to describe a smaller vessel branching off from a larger one.* |
| rana | **frog** *A tailless amphibian that is short with long hind legs for jumping.* |
| rantoli crepitanti | **crackles or rales** *A crackling noised noted while auscultating the lungs.* |
| rantolo | **rale** *An abnormal lung sound noted during auscultation.* |
| ranula | **ranula** *A retention cyst formed because of obstruction of a salivary gland in the floor of the mouth.* |
| rapporto sessuale | **sexual intercourse** *The act of copulation.* |
| raschiaperiostio | **rugine** *A surgical instrument that resembles a rasp.* |
| raschiatura | **scrape** *An injury caused by having a body part rubbed against a rough surface.* |
| rauco | **hoarse** *A rough, harsh sounding voice.* |
| reattivo | **reactive** *A response to a stimulus.* |
| reazione | **reaction** *A response to an action.* |
| reazione conversione | **conversion reaction** *When referring to a psychiatric condition it is the exhibition of physical symptoms as a manifestation of mental disease.* |
| reazione della droga | **drug reaction** *Typically refers to an adverse effect of medication.* |
| reazione di risveglio | **arousal reaction** *The change in brain wave patterns upon awakening.* |

| Italian | English |
|---|---|
| reazione dopa | **dopa reaction** *A dopa-oxidase reaction, changing dopa into melanin.* |
| recessivo | **recessive** *This refers to genetic controlled traits that are only inherited when code from both parents is the same.* |
| recidiva | **relapse** *The return to a prior state of ill health.* |
| regione inguinale | **groin** *The genital region.* |
| relazione | **relation** *1. A person who has a blood or marriage connection.* |
| remissione | **remission** *A decrease in severity or a temporary resolution.* |
| renale | **renal** *Referring to the kidney.* |
| rene | **kidney** *One of two glandular organs that form urine.* |
| rene a ferro di cavallo | **horseshoe kidney** *Anomalous renal development.* |
| renina | **renin** *A renal enzyme that facilitates the production of angiotensin.* |
| reparto di isolamento | **isolation ward** *A ward where patients with infectious disease are housed.* |
| reparto osedaliero | **ward** *A section of a hospital where patients reside.* |
| reposo | **rest** *Relaxation or respite.* |
| resezione | **resection** *The removal of tissue.* |
| resina | **resin** *An organic substance that is insoluble in water. There are many types. Cholestyramine resin is used for hypercholesterolemia.* |
| respiratorio | **respiratory** *Referring to respiration or the organs of respiration.* |
| respiro | **breath** *One respiration.* |
| respiro boccheggiante di Kussmaul | **Kussmaul respiration** *The slow, deep breathing noted in patients with acidosis.* |
| respiro di Cheyne-Stokes | **Cheyne-Stokes respirations** *A breathing pattern characterized by alternating apnea with hyperpnea.* |
| respiro di Kussmaul | **air hunger** *The sensation of shortness of breath.* |
| responsabile | **causative** *Something that induces an effect.* |
| restringimento | **stricture** *A narrowing of a canal or duct.* |
| reticolare | **reticular** *Referring to a matrix of membranous tubules inside the cytoplasm of a eukaryotic cells.* |
| reticolo endoplasmico | **endoplasmic reticulum** *A framework of tubules within the cytoplasm of eukaryotic cells.* |
| reticolo-endoteliale | **reticulo-endothelial** *Referring to the system of phagocytes involved in the immune system.* |
| reticolocitosi | **reticulocytosis** *An abnormal increase in circulating reticulocytes.* |
| reticulocito | **reticulocyte** *A red blood cell without a nucleus.* |
| retina | **retina** *The innermost of three layers of the eyeball; it surrounds the vitreous body and is continuous with the optic nerve.* |
| retinite | **retinitis** *Inflammation of the retina.* |
| retinoblastoma | **retinoblastoma** *A tumor consisting of retinal germ cells.* |
| retinopatia | **retinopathy** *Any one of a number of retinal inflammatory conditions.* |
| retrazione | **retraction** *Being drawn back.* |
| retrofaringeo | **retropharyngeal** *Referring to the area posterior to the pharynx.* |
| retrogrado | **retrograde** *Referring to backward movement.* |
| retrogusto | **after-taste** *The sensation of a prolonged savor following eating/drinking.* |
| retroperitoneale | **retroperitoneal** *Situated or referring to the area posterior to the peritoneum.* |
| rettale | **rectal** *Referring to the rectum.* |
| rettocele | **rectocele** *A herniation of the wall between the rectum and vagina.* |
| rettoscopia | **rectoscopy** *Visualization of the rectum with a scope.* |
| rettosigmoidectomia | **rectosigmoidectomy** *Surgical resection of the rectum and sigmoid colon.* |
| reumatico | **rheumatic** *Referring to rheumatism.* |

| Italian | English |
|---|---|
| reumatismo | **rheumatism** *Any condition exhibited by inflammation and pain in the joints and muscles.* |
| rianimazione bocca a bocca | **mouth to mouth resuscitation** *A form of emergency management of respiratory failure.* |
| rianimazione cardiorespiratoria | **cardiopulmonary resuscitation** *Use of artificial means to support respiration and circulation.* |
| riboflavina; vitamina B2 | **riboflavin** *Also called vitamin B2, this essential vitamin is present in food such as eggs and is synthesized in the small bowel.* |
| ricetta | **prescription** *The action of prescribing a medication or treatment.* |
| Rickettsia | **Rickettsia** *A genus of bacteria transmitted by ticks or fleas; Rocky Mountain Spotted fever is one of many diseases caused by this bacterium.* |
| ridere | **laugh, to** |
| riduzione | **reduction** *Return of a dislocated joint or fractured bone to its proper position.* |
| riduzione aperta di una frattura | **open reduction (of fractures)** *The realignment of a fractured bone using a surgical approach.* |
| riduzione chiusa | **closed reduction** *The realignment of a fracture without use of surgery.* |
| riesacerbazione | **flare-up** *A sudden worsening one's condition.* |
| riflesso achilleo | **Achilles tendon reflex** *The normal response to tapping the achilles tendon with a reflex hammer is the plantar flexion of the foot.* |
| riflesso Bainbridge | **Bainbridge reflex** *Increase in heart rate due to increased pressure in the right atrium.* |
| riflesso Bechterew-Mendel | **Bechterew-Mendel reflex** *Plantar flexion of the toes when the examiner percusses the dorsum of the foot; seen with pyramidal lesion.* |
| riflesso Bezold-Jarisch | **Bezold-Jarisch reflex** *A reflex in the vagus, originating in the heart, resulting in sinus bradycardia, hypotension and peripheral vasodilation.* |
| riflesso bicipite | **biceps reflex** *The biceps brachii tendon is hit with a reflex hammer and results in flexion of the forearm as a normal response. This assesses the C5-C6 region.* |
| riflesso bulbocavernoso | **bulbocavernosus reflex** *Brisk contraction of the ischiocavernosus and bulbocavernosus muscles when the glans penis is compressed.* |
| riflesso bulmomimic | **facial reflex or bulbomimic reflex** *Pressure on the eyeballs causes contraction of facial muscles on the side contralateral to the side of the lesion in the patient in a coma. In coma from a metabolic problem the reflex is present bilaterally.* |
| riflesso congiuntivale | **conjunctival reflex** *Closure of the eyes in response to irritation of the conjunctiva.* |
| riflesso corneale | **corneal reflex** *Closure of the eyelids when the cornea is touched lightly with a soft material. Also called the lid reflex.* |
| riflesso cremasterico | **cremasteric reflex** *Retraction of the testicle and scrotum upon stroking of the ipsilateral inner thigh.* |
| riflesso del dito pollice | **finger-thumb reflex** *Opposition and adduction of the thumb with flexion at the MCP joint and extension at the interphalangeal joint when there is flexion of the 3rd, 4th, and 5th finger. This is present normally and absent with with pyramidal lesions.* |
| riflesso del seno carotideo | **carotid sinus reflex** *Bradycardia as a result of pressure on the carotid sinus.* |
| riflesso di Strümpell | **Strümpell reflex** *Flexion of the leg and adduction of the foot elicited by stroking of the thigh or abdomen.* |
| riflesso faringeo | **gag reflex** *Contraction of the pharynx muscles when the back of the pharynx is stimulated by touch.* |
| riflesso gastrocolico | **gastrocolic reflex** *Peristalsis of the colon produced by food entering the stomach.* |

| Italian | English |
|---|---|
| riflesso gluteale | **gluteal reflex** *After the skin of the buttocks are stimulated the gluteal muscles contract.* |
| riflesso in prensione forzata | **grasp reflex** *Flexion of the fingers or toes when stimulated.* |
| riflesso mandibola | **jaw reflex** *Contraction of the temporal muscles when a relaxed mandible is given a downward tap. Also, masseter reflex or jaw jerk.* |
| riflesso Rossolimo | **Rossolimo reflex** *Flexion of the toes when the tips of the toes are flicked. This abnormal response is present in pyramidal tract lesions.* |
| riflesso rotuleo | **knee jerk reflex** *Contraction of the quadriceps, yielding leg extension when the quadriceps tendon is tapped.* |
| riflesso rotulo; riflesso del tendine del quadricipite | **quadriceps jerk (reflex)** *Also referred to as the patellar reflex.* |
| riflesso spinale | **spinal reflex** *A reflex that has an arc passing through the spine.* |
| riflesso tendine | **tendon reflex** *A deep reflex elicited by gently tapping the tendon.* |
| riflesso tendine profondo | **deep tendon reflex** *Reflexes exhibited by the stretching of a tendon.* |
| riflesso tricipite | **triceps reflex** *A tendon reflex causing extension of the arm when the triceps tendon is gently tapped.* |
| riflusso epatogiugulare | **hepatojugular reflex** *The presence of jugular venous distension with compression of the abdomen for at least 10 seconds.* |
| rigidità a troclea dentata | **cogwheel rigidity** *As in cogwheel rigidity which is a jerky passive movement after there was increased tone.* |
| rigidità cadaverica | **rigor mortis** *The normal stiffening of the muscles and joints that occurs a few hours after death.* |
| rigidità decerebrato | **decerebrate rigidity** *Rigid extension of the arms which is an abnormal posture associated with increased intracranial pressure.* |
| rigidità nucale | **stiff-neck** *Cervical sprain with reduced range of motion.* |
| rigidità spastica | **clasp knife reflex** *An abnormal response seen in the setting of a pyramidal tract lesion in which there is a rapid decrease in resistance during passive movement of a joint.* |
| rigonfiamento esterno | **bulge** *A protuberance on a flat surface.* |
| rigonfio | **bloated** *Sensation of having an abnormally large amount of air in the viscera.* |
| rigurgito | **regurgitation** *1. Backflow of blood in the heart. 2. Movement of gastric contents into the mouth.* |
| rigurgito mitrale | **mitral regurgitation** *Backflow of blood from the left ventricle to the left atrium because of dysfunctional valve.* |
| rilassante | **relaxant** *Term generally used to refer to a muscle relaxant.* |
| rilassina | **relaxin** *A hormone secreted by the placenta which dilates the cervix.* |
| rinite | **rhinitis** *A viral infection or allergic reaction exhibited by nasal mucosal inflammation.* |
| rinoplastica | **rhinoplasty** *Plastic surgery performed on the nose.* |
| rinorrea | **rhinorrhea** *Abundant nasal mucosal drainage.* |
| rinoscopia | **rhinoscopy** *Examination of the nasal passages.* |
| riposta immunitaria | **immune response** *The body's reaction to what is perceived as a foreign substance.* |
| riposta plantare dell'estensore | **extensor plantar response** *Great toe extension indicating a positive Babinski sign.* |
| ripugnanza del cuoio capelluto | **scalp avulsion** *An injury causing the skin along with some subcutaneous tissue to be pulled from the skull.* |
| riso sardonico | **risus sardonicus** *A spasm of the facial muscles causing what appears to be a smile on one's face.* |
| risonanza magnetica nucleare | **nuclear magnetic resonance (NMR)** *A type a diagnostic body imaging utilizing electromagnetic radiation in a magnetic field.* |

| Italian | English |
|---|---|
| risultato di laboratorio | **lab result** *The data obtained from a laboratory test.* |
| risveglio | **awakening** *The state of being conscious.* |
| ritmo | **rhythm** *The pattern or cadence.* |
| ritmo circadiano | **circadian rhythm** *Naturally recurring fluctuations in a 24 hour period.* |
| ritmo di galoppo | **cantering rhythm** *Gallop rhythm.* |
| ritrattazione | **withdrawal** *The action of being without drugs or alcohol.* |
| rizotomia | **rhizotomy** *Interruption of the spinal nerve roots within the spinal canal.* |
| rodopsina | **rhodopsin** *A reddish purple light sensitive pigment in the human retina.* |
| roentgen | **Roentgen** *One unit of ionizing radiation named after the German physicist Wilhelm Conrad Röntgen.* |
| romboide | **rhomboid** *A back muscle that elevates, retracts and adducts the scapula.* |
| ronco | **rhonchus** *A coarse, dry sound heard on auscultation of the lungs.* |
| ronzio nelle orecchie; tinnito | **ringing in the ears** *Common term for tinnitus.* |
| rosolia | **German measles** *(rubella) A contagious viral infection.* |
| rosolia | **rubella** *Also called German measles, it is characterized by a rash, fever, headache.* |
| rotazione | **rotation** *Movement around an axis.* |
| rottura | **rupture** *An instance of bursting suddenly.* |
| rottura delle membrane prolungata | **prolonged rupture of the membranes** *Rupture of the membranes more than 24 hours before delivery.* |
| rotula | **kneecap** *Common term for patella.* |
| rrecettore | **receptor** *A cell or organ that accepts stimuli and transmits data to a sensory nerve.* |
| rubefacente | **rubefacient** *A substance that reddens the skin.* |
| rumore di sfegamento | **friction rub** *A noise heard during cardiac auscultation in patients with pericarditis, for example.* |
| rumore, soffio | **bruit** *An abnormal sound heard through a stethoscope indicating turbulent blood flow.* |
| rupia | **rupia** *A sign of tertiary syphilis in which there are bullae or vesicles formed on the skin that erupt and form crusts.* |
| russare | **snore, to** *To snore or grunt while breathing during sleep.* |
| sacco colostomia | **colostomy bag** *A pouch attached to the skin with a mild adhesive that collects stool emitted from a colostomy.* |
| sacrale | **sacral** *Referring to the sacrum.* |
| sacralizzazione | **sacralization** *The fusion of the fifth lumbar vertebra to the sacrum.* |
| safena | **saphena** *Referring to either of the two superficial saphenous veins.* |
| saggio biologico | **bioassay** *A laboratory test determination as compared to normal.* |
| saggio; prova | **assay** *A procedure for measuring the activity of a biological sample.* |
| sala iperbarico | **hyperbaric chamber** *A device used to treat decompression illness.* |
| sala parto | **labor room** *The hospital room used while a woman is in labor.* |
| sala postoperatoria | **recovery room** *The immediate post-operative room where patients are stabilized prior to going to a general ward.* |
| sala pronto soccorso | **emergency room** *A ward used for initial treatment of critical patients.* |
| sala; camera | **room** *A division in a building surrounded by walls.* |
| salato | **salt** *Typically referring to sodium chloride.* |

| Italian | English |
|---|---|
| salato biliari | **bile salts** *Normally occurring salts of bile acids.* |
| salino | **saline** *A solution of sodium chloride.* |
| saliva | **saliva** *The watery liquid secreted by the salivary glands.* |
| saliva | **spit** *A term used to describe saliva that is ejected from the mouth.* |
| salivazione | **salivation** *The process of secreting saliva.* |
| salpingectomia | **salpingectomy** *Surgical resection of the fallopian tubes.* |
| salpingite | **salpingitis** *Inflammation of the fallopian tubes.* |
| salpingografia | **salpingography** *Roentgenography of the fallopian tubes after administration of contrast media.* |
| salpingostomia | **salpingostomy** *A surgical procedure involving cutting the fallopian tube.* |
| salubre | **healing** *The process of becoming healthy again.* |
| saluretico | **saluretic** *An agent that promotes excretion of sodium and chloride in the urine.* |
| salute | **health** *The state of being free of illness.* |
| sangue | **blood** *Plasma containing erythrocytes, leukocytes and platelets.* |
| sangue occulto | **occult blood** *Presence of blood from an unknown source.* |
| sanguinamento uterino | **uterine bleeding** *Bleeding that emanates from the uterus.* |
| sanguisuga | **leech** *An annelid used in some tropical regions for drawing out blood; they have an anticoagulant effect locally and have been attached to digits of persons with acute peripheral ischemia.* |
| sano | **healthy** *In good health.* |
| sano | **sound** *Vibrations that travel through air and are heard when reaching the ears.* |
| sapone | **soap** *A compound made with fats/oils and an alkali; it is used for washing.* |
| saponificare | **saponify,to** *The creation of soap from oil using an alkali.* |
| saprofita | **saprophyte** *Any organism living on dead organic material.* |
| sarcoide | **sarcoid** *Referring to sarcoidosis.* |
| sarcoidosi | **sarcoidosis** *A chronic disease characterized by lymphadenopathy and widespread granulomas.* |
| sarcolemma | **sarcolemme** *The sheath that covers skeletal muscle fibers.* |
| sarcoma | **sarcoma** *A non-epithelial malignant tumor.* |
| saturazione | **saturation** *An amount, expressed in a percentage, that expresses the degree something is absorbed versus the maximal absorption possible.* |
| sbadiglio | **gaping** *Wide open.* |
| sbadiglio | **yawn** *Opening one's mouth and inhaling deeply due to sleepiness/ boredom* |
| sbagliare a scrivere | **misspelling** *Incorrect spelling of a word.* |
| sbrigliamento | **debridement** *Trimming the dead tissue adjacent to a wound.* |
| scabbia | **scabies** *A skin condition exhibited by intense pruritus and a macular rash commonly in the perineal and interdigital spaces.* |
| scadenza | **deadline** *Cutoff date.* |
| scafocefalia | **scaphocephaly** *A condition exhibited by a long narrow skull because of early closure of the sagittal sutures.* |
| scala | **scale** *A device to check a person's weight.* |
| scala di Glasgow del coma | **Glasgow coma scale** *A scale used to grade one's level of consciousness with a score of 3 being totally unresponsive and a score of 15 being normal.* |
| scalfittura | **scratch** *A long, narrow superficial wound.* |
| scalpello | **scalpel** *A knife used during surgery for incision of skin and tissue.* |
| scanner della risonanza magnetica | **magnetic resonance imaging (MRI)** *Images are produced by evaluating the response of body tissue. nuclei to radio waves in a magnetic field.* |

| Italian | English |
|---|---|
| scapola | **scapula** *Medical term for the shoulder blade.* |
| scarico dell'ospedale | **hospital discharge** *To leave the hospital.* |
| scarificazione | **scarification** *Multiple small scratches of the skin, as is sometimes used for vaccine administration.* |
| scarlattina | **scarlet fever** *A condition caused by streptococci that is exhibited by fever and a bright red (scarlet) rash.* |
| scarpa | **shoe** *Article of clothing worn on each foot.* |
| scavalcamento | **bypass** *An alternate route, typically referring to an arterial bypass.* |
| scelta | **choice** *Selection or decision.* |
| scheda paziente | **patient chart** *The file containing the client's medical record.* |
| scheggia | **splinter** *A small, thin object; usually refers to the object being imbedded in the body.* |
| scheletro | **skeleton** *Internal bony framework.* |
| schema | **scheme** *A program or plan.* |
| schermo | **shield** *A protective device, as in eye shield.* |
| schermo fluorescente | **fluorescent screen** *A screen used to view x-rays.* |
| schiarirsi la voce | **clear one's throat, to** *To cough lightly in attempt to speak more clearly.* |
| schistocito | **schistocyte** *Part of a red blood cell seen in hemolytic anemia.* |
| schistosoma | **Bilharzia** *Historical name of a genus of flukes or nematodes now known as Schistosoma.* |
| schistosomiasi | **schistosomiasis** *A condition, sometimes known as bilharzia, which involves infestation with flukes of the genus Schistosoma.* |
| schiuma | **foam** *A mass of small bubbles in a liquid.* |
| schiuma | **froth** *Covered with a mass of small bubbles.* |
| schiuma alla bocca | **froth at the mouth, to** *To have a mass of saliva with small bubbles in it coming out of the mouth.* |
| schizofrenia | **schizophrenia** *A chronic mental condition exhibited by delusions, hallucinations, and faulty perception.* |
| sciatica | **sciatica** *Pain radiating from the buttock down the back of the leg; it is caused by a compressed spinal nerve root.* |
| scibale | **scybalum** *A hard, dry formation of stool in the bowel.* |
| scintigrafia osseo | **bone scan** *Bone imaging using technetium 99m (99mTc) diphosphate.* |
| scioltezza | **looseness** *Possessing a quality of not being tight.* |
| sciolto | **loose** *Not tight.* |
| sciroppo | **syrup** *A thick sweet liquid.* |
| scirro | **scirrhus** *A cancer that is hard to palpation.* |
| sclera | **sclera** *The white outer covering of the eyeball.* |
| sclerite | **scleritis** *Inflammation of the eyeball.* |
| sclerodattilia | **sclerodactylia** *Scleroderma of the digits.* |
| sclerodermia | **scleroderma** *A systemic disease of the connective tissues.* |
| sclerosi laterale amiotrofica | **amyotrophic lateral sclerosis** *A progressive neurodegenerative disorder.* |
| sclerosi multipla | **multiple sclerosis** *A chronic neurologic disease exhibited by numbness, vision and speech problems, and motor incoordination.* |
| sclerotomia | **sclerotomy** *Surgical incision of the sclera.* |
| scolice | **scolex** *The front end of a tapeworm.* |
| scoliosi | **scoliosis** *A lateral curvature of the spine.* |
| scomparsa | **disappearance** *An instance of something/someone gone missing.* |
| scompenso | **decompensation** *The inability of an organ to respond to functional overload.* |
| sconosciuto | **unknown** *Uncertain or undisclosed.* |
| scopofilia | **scopophilia** *Sexual pleasure attained by viewing sexual organs.* |

| Italian | English |
|---|---|
| scorbuto | **scurvy** *A disease of vitamin C deficiency exhibited by bleeding gums.* |
| scoreggiare | **fart, to** *Slang term for releasing flatus.* |
| scorrettezza professionale | **malpractice** *Negligent professional activity.* |
| scotoma | **scotoma** *A blind spot within an otherwise normal visual field.* |
| scottatura | **scald** *A burn injury from extremely hot water.* |
| screziato | **mottled** *An irregular arrangement of patches of color.* |
| scrofola | **scrofula** *Cervical tuberculous lymphadenitis.* |
| scrotale | **scrotal** *Referring to the scrotum.* |
| scroto | **scrotum** *The sac which contains the testes.* |
| scuotere | **shake, to** *To tremble uncontrollably.* |
| scutulo | **scutulum** *A crust of tinea capitis.* |
| sebaceo | **sebaceous** *Referring to a sebaceous gland or what it secretes.* |
| seborrea | **seborrhea** *Abnormal amount of sebum production.* |
| secco; asciutto | **dry** *Absence of moisture.* |
| seconda vertebra cervicale | **axis** *The second cervical vertebra.* |
| secondo | **according to** |
| secretina | **secretin** *A hormone that increases secretion from the pancreas and liver.* |
| secrezione | **secretion** *The discharge of substances from cells or glands.* |
| secrezioni gastriche | **gastric secretions** *Fluids secreted from gastric mucosa.* |
| sedativo | **sedative** *A medication used to facilitate sleep or calm a person.* |
| sedia a rotelle | **wheelchair** *A wheeled device used for propulsion.* |
| sedimento urinario | **urinary sediments** *The debris that settles in a urine sample when left undisturbed.* |
| sega | **saw** *A hand or power-driven tool used for cutting.* |
| segni vitali | **vital signs** *The designation for blood pressure, pulse, respirations and temperature.* |
| segno di Argyll-Robertson | **Argyll Robertson symptom** *Presence of small pupils that do not react to light but will constrict when the person focuses on a near object.* |
| segno di Babinski | **Babinski's sign** *A reflex that occurs when the plantar surface of the foot is stimulated. The great toe turns upward- normal in infancy but when it turns upward in an adult it means there is central nervous system injury.* |
| segno di Brudzinski | **Brudzinski sign** *Involuntary flexion of the knees and hips after flexion of the neck while supine; seen in meningitis.* |
| segno di Graefe | **Graefe's sign** *Also called lid lag, a sign characterized by the upper eyelid not closing over the globe. This is seen commonly in exophthalmic goiter.* |
| segno di Oppenheim | **Oppenheim reflex** *Extension of the toes elicited by scratching of the medial leg; present when the patient has cerebral irritation.* |
| segno di scimitar | **scimitar sign** *An abnormal radiologic finding associated with anomalous pulmonary venous drainage.* |
| semi di ricino | **castor bean** *A bean that can yield the poisonous compound ricin.* |
| seminoma | **seminoma** *A malignant tumor of the testis.* |
| senescenza | **senescence** *The normal process of deterioration with age.* |
| seni paranasali | **paranasal sinuses** *Any of the sinuses (ethmoidal, frontal, maxillary or sphenoidal) that communicate with the nasal cavity.* |
| senile | **senile** *Generally referring to mental deterioration associated with aging.* |
| senilità | **senility** *The process of being senile.* |
| seno cavernoso | **cavernous sinus** *Large venous sinus located adjacent to the sphenoid bone and posterior to the petrosal sinuses.* |

| Italian | English |
|---|---|
| seno frontale | **frontal sinus** *A paranasal sinus on both sides of the lower part of the frontal bone.* |
| seno sfenoidale | **sphenoidal sinus** *Part of the sphenoid bone; it communicates with the most superior aspect of the nasal meatus.* |
| senoatriale | **sinoatrial** *Referring to the cardiac node of the same name.* |
| sensazione | **sensation** *A perception when one is touched.* |
| sensibile | **sensible** *When referring to a choice, chosen with wisdom.* |
| sensibilità | **sensibility** *Ability to feel or perceive.* |
| sensibilizzato | **sensitized** *Being abnormally sensitive to a substance.* |
| sensibilizzazione | **sensitization** *The change in an organ by a hormone so it will respond to another stimulus.* |
| senso del tatto | **touch** *Tactile stimulation.* |
| senza casa | **homeless** *Having nowhere to live.* |
| senza denti; edentato | **toothless** *Edentulous.* |
| senza senso | **meaningless** *Having no significance.* |
| separarsi | **parting** *Separating.* |
| separato, distinto | **discrete** *Separate and distinct.* |
| sepsi | **sepsis** *A condition exhibited by overwhelming inflammation due to infection.* |
| sequela | **sequela** *A medical problem related to an initial injury or disease.(late sequelae)* |
| sequestro osseo | **sequestrum** *Necrotic bone present in an injured or diseased bone.* |
| seriato | **serial** *In a series.* |
| serotonina | **serotonin** *A neurotransmitter that constricts blood vessels.* |
| serpiginoso | **serpiginous** *A skin lesion having wavy margin.* |
| sessile | **sessile** *Having a broad base with no stalk.* |
| sesso | **sex** *Gender.* |
| sete | **thirst** *The desire to drink.* |
| setticemia | **septicemia** *A systemic disease in which microorganisms or their toxins are in the blood stream.* |
| settico | **septic** *Referring to a state of sepsis.* |
| settimanale | **weekly** *That which occurs every seven days.* |
| setto | **septum** *A wall separating two chambers, the nasal septum for example.* |
| setto deviazione | **deviated septum** *Characterized by deviation of the nasal septum.* |
| setto rettovescicale | **rectovesical septum** *The wall between the rectum and the urinary bladder.* |
| severo | **severe** *Intense or very great.* |
| sezione trasversale | **cross-section** *A transverse section through a specimen or structure.* |
| sferocito | **spherocyte** *An erythrocyte without the usual central pallor; it is noted in spherocytosis and some hemolytic anemias.* |
| sferocitosi | **spherocytosis** *The presence of spherocytes in the blood.* |
| sferocitosi ereditaria | **hereditary spherocytosis** *A familial hemolytic disease exhibited by abnormally thick erythrocytes.* |
| sfigmomanometro | **sphygmomanometer** *Device for measuring blood pressure.* |
| sfintere | **sphincter** *A muscle the surrounds an orifice or duct so it closes when the muscle contracts.* |
| sfinterotomia | **sphincterotomy** *Surgical incision of the anal sphincter.* |
| sforzo | **effort** *Attempt or endeavor.* |
| sfregamento | **rub** *A sound heard at times with pericarditis called more specifically a pericardial friction sound.* |
| sgombero | **clearance** *The process of removing something.* |
| sgorbia | **gouge** *A chisel with a concave blade used in surgery.* |

| Italian | English |
|---|---|
| sguardo | **gaze** *Steady, intent look.* |
| sguardo furioso | **glare** *An angry stare.* |
| shock cardiaco | **shock** *A condition characterized by systemic hypoperfusion.* |
| shock spinale | **spinal shock** *Hypotension related to injury or intervention of the spine.* |
| sialadenitis | **sialadenitis** *Inflammation of a salivary gland.* |
| sialolito | **sialolith** *A calculus in a salivary duct.* |
| sicosi | **sycosis** *A bacterial infection affecting the hair follicles on a person's face.* |
| siderosi | **siderosis** *Discoloration of a part due to iron deposition.* |
| siero | **serum** *The fluid that isolates out when blood coagulates.* |
| sieroso | **serous** *Referring to serum or similar to serum.* |
| sifilide | **syphilis** *A infectious disease caused by Treponema pallidum that causes a painless penile ulcer in the primary stage but can lead to irreversible brain damage in the untreated tertiary stage.* |
| sifilide congenita | **congenital syphilis** *Passed to the child in utero, the child may have failure to thrive, fever and a flattened bridge of the nose.* |
| sifiloma | **chancre** *The initial ulcer that is seen with primary syphilis.* |
| sigillo | **seal** *A device or substance used to bind two things together.* |
| sigmoide | **sigmoid** *Referring to the portion of the colon that leads into the rectum.* |
| sigmoidoscopia | **sigmoidoscopy** *Visualization of the sigmoid colon with a scope.* |
| sigmoidostomia | **sigmoidostomy** *Formation of an opening in the sigmoid colon that communicates with the outside of the body.* |
| silente | **silent** *Absence of noise or no indication of something.* |
| silicosi | **silicosis** *Grinders's disease; fibrotic lung disease caused by inhalation of silica.* |
| simbiosi | **symbiosis** *The living together of two organisms.* |
| simmetria | **symmetry** *Being equally bilaterally.* |
| simpatectomia | **sympathectomy** *The surgical resection of a sympathetic nerve to reduce undesired effects.* |
| simulazione di malattia | **malingerer** *A person who feigns illness.* |
| simultaneo | **simultaneous** *Occurring at the same time.* |
| sinapsi | **synapse** *The intersection of two nerve cells.* |
| sinartrosi | **synarthrosis** *Adjacent bones connected by a joint but the joint is fixed.* |
| sincondrosi | **synchondrosis** *A joint with little motion that uses cartilage such as the vertebral bodies.* |
| sincope | **syncope** *Sudden loss of consciousness.* |
| sincope del seno carotideo | **carotid sinus syncope** *Dizziness and syncope that results from hyperactivity of the carotid sinus reflex.* |
| sindorme di trisomia 21 | **trisomy 21** *A congenital anomaly in which chromosome 21 is effected and results in Down's syndrome.* |
| sindrome di Rett | **Rett syndrome.** *A rare inherited disorder causing developmental delays and is seen mostly in girls.* |
| sindrome alcolica fetale | **fetal alcohol syndrome** *A condition caused by alcohol use by the mother during pregnancy and exhibited by poor intrauterine growth, decreased muscle tone, delayed development and widened palpebral fissures.* |
| Sindrome da immunodeficienza acquisita | **Acquired Immunodeficiency Syndrome (AIDS)** *Presence of an AIDS defining illness or having a CD4 of less than 200/mm3.* |
| sindrome da rapido svuotamento | **dumping syndrome** *Characterized by rapid bowel evacuation after eating in patients with prior gastric surgery.* |

| Italian | English |
|---|---|
| sindrome del chiavistello | **locked-in syndrome** *A neurologic condition characterized by a person being conscious of their surroundings but being unable to verbally communicate that understanding.* |
| sindrome del colon irritabile | **irritable bowel syndrome** *A condition exhibited by chronic diarrhea or constipation and abdominal pain; it is sometimes associated with a labile emotional state.* |
| sindrome del furto della succlavia | **subclavian steal syndrome** *Retrograde vertebral artery flow due to ipsilateral subclavian artery stenosis.* |
| sindrome del grido di gatto | **cat cry syndrome** *A hereditary congenital disorder exhibited by microcephaly, hypertelorism, and cognitive deficits.* |
| sindrome del pannolino blu | **blue diaper syndrome** *A disorder of tryptophan absorption. Excess tryptophan is metabolized to indicans in the bowel, excreted in the urine and oxidized in the diaper to indigo, thus the blue diaper.* |
| sindrome del tunnel carpale | **carpal tunnel syndrome** *Paresthesia that results from compression of the median nerve.* |
| sindrome del tunnel tarsale | **tarsal tunnel syndrome** *Characterized by impingement of various nerves of the ankle.* |
| sindrome della coda equina | **cauda equina syndrome** *Neurologic condition manifested by pain, paresthesia and weakness but no bowel/bladder dysfunction.* |
| sindrome della sella turcica vuota | **empty sella syndrome** *Compressed or flattened pituitary related to herniating arachnoid, surgery or radiotherapy.* |
| sindrome dell'ansa afferente | **afferent loop syndrome** *The obstruction of the duodenum or jejunum after gastrojejunostomy, resulting in duodenal distention.* |
| sindrome dell'ansa cieca | **blind loop syndrome** *A condition in which there is a non-functional section of the bowel that is thought to be responsible for malabsorption and Vitamin B12 deficiency.* |
| sindrome dell'arteria basilare | **vertebrobasilar insufficiency** *Diminished flow to the vertebral and basilar arteries causing posterior fossa symptoms.* |
| sindrome di Aicardi | **Aicardi syndrome** *A rare genetic anomaly in which the corpus callosum is absent or insufficient. It is characterized by seizures, microphthalmos, coloboma and developmental delays.* |
| sindrome di ambascia respiratoria | **respiratory distress syndrome** *A disease in infants that is caused by a surfactant deficiency.* |
| sindrome di Asperger | **Asperger's syndrome** *A condition characterized by disturbed social interaction; if was named after the Austrian scientist who first described it.* |
| sindrome di Bartter | **Bartter's syndrome** *An autosomal recessive renal disorder with a defect in chloride reabsorption and secondary hyperaldosteronism.* |
| sindrome di Behcet | **Behçet syndrome** *Characterized by recurrent oral and genital ulcers, uveitis, iridocyclitis and frequently arthritis.* |
| sindrome di Boerhaave | **Boerhaave Syndrome** *Rupture of the esophagus from vigorous vomiting, with resultant mediastinitis.* |
| sindrome di Bourneville | **tuberous sclerosis** *An inherited neurocutaneous disorder exhibited by benign hamartomas of the brain, lung, kidney, skin and other organs.* |
| sindrome di Brown-Séquard | **Brown-Séquard syndrome** *Unilateral spinal cord lesions, proprioception loss and weakness occur ipsilateral to the lesion, while pain and temperature loss occur contralateral.* |
| sindrome di Budd-Chiari | **Budd-Chiari syndrome** *Hepatomegaly, severe portal hypertension and ascites related to thrombosis of the hepatic vein.* |
| sindrome di compressione | **crush syndrome** *Rhabdomyolysis occurring as a result of muscle injury from mechanical stress.* |
| sindrome di Down | **Down's syndrome** *A congenital chromosomal defect (trisomy 21) that causes diminished intellectual function, short stature and a broad face.* |
| sindrome di Fanconi | **Fanconi's syndrome** *An idiopathic refractory anemia exhibited by pancytopenia, bone marrow hypoplasia and congenital anomalies.* |
| sindrome di Felty | **Felty syndrome** *Rheumatoid arthritis with leukopenia and splenomegaly.* |

| Italian | English |
|---|---|
| sindrome di Foville | **Foville's syndrome** *Caused by a lesion within the pons, there is ipsilateral facial and abducens nerve paralysis and contralateral hemiplegia.* |
| sindrome di Gerstmann | **Gerstmann syndrome** *Finger agnosia, agraphia and acalculia caused by a lesion between the occipital region and angular gyrus.* |
| sindrome di Goodpasture; pneumopatia interstiziale ed emorragica con nefrite | **Goodpasture' syndrome** *Glomerulonephritis, preceded by hemoptysis. The nephritis can quickly progress to death from renal failure.* |
| sindrome di Guillain-Barré | **Guillain-Barré syndrome** *An acute autoimmune disorder that causes nerve inflammation subsequently muscle weakness.* |
| sindrome di Hamman-Rich | **Hamman-Rich syndrome** *Idiopathic pulmonary fibrosis.* |
| sindrome di Hanhart | **Hanhart's syndrome** *Also referred to as micrognathia with peromelia. There is hypoplasia of the mandible, malformed or missing teeth, birdlike face and severe upper extremity deformities.* |
| sindrome di Henri | **Henri, syndrome of** *Congenital anomaly exhibited by different sized external orifices of the nostrils.* |
| sindrome di Horner | **Horner syndrome** *A lesion of the cervical sympathetic chain causes ipsilateral myosis, ptosis and facial anhidrosis.* |
| sindrome di Job | **Job syndrome** *Also known as hyperimmunoglobulin E syndrome, there are high levels if IgE, a leukocyte chemotactic defect, recurrent staph infections and cold abscess formation in the skin.* |
| sindrome di Libman-Sachs | **Libman-Sachs syndrome** *A verrucous endocarditis associated with disseminated lupus erythematosus; also called nonbacterial verrucous endocarditis.* |
| sindrome di Lyell | **Lyell's syndrome** *Also called toxic epidermal necrolysis, there are large portions of the skin that become erythematous with epidermal necrosis as seen with 2nd degree burns. This reaction can be seen with use of nevirapine or Bactrim.* |
| sindrome di Mallory-Weiss | **Mallory-Weiss syndrome** *Upper GI bleeding related to a laceration at the gastroesophageal junction caused by vigorous vomiting.* |
| sindrome di Marfan | **Marfan syndrome** *A connective tissue disease exhibited by long limbs, joint laxity and cardiovascular defects.* |
| sindrome di Marie-Sainton; disostosi cranioclavicolare | **cleidocranial dysostosis** *A congenital condition exhibited by abnormal ossification of the cranial bones and absence of clavicles.* |
| sindrome di Milkman | **Milkman syndrome** *Osteomalacia with multiple pseudofractures.* |
| sindrome di Morgagni | **Morgagni's syndrome** *Also called metabolic craniopathy and Stewart-Morel syndrome, it is exhibited by hyperostosis frontalis interna, obesity and neuropsychiatric disorders.* |
| sindrome di morte infantile improvvisa | **sudden infant death syndrome** *A leading cause of death of infants from one month to one year; the etiology is unknown.* |
| sindrome di Mucune-Albright | **Mucune-Albright syndrome** *Polyostotic fibrous dysplasia with cutaneous brown patches, endocrine dysfunction that exhibits in females as precocious puberty.* |
| sindrome di Plummer-Vinson | **Plummer-Vinson syndrome** *Also called sideropenic dysphagia. Exhibited by iron deficiency anemia, dysphagia, esophageal stenosis and atrophic glossitis. The cause is not known.* |
| sindrome di Potter | **Potter's syndrome** *A group of findings associated with oligohydramnios. Renal failure is the primary problem but the infant has abnormal limbs, broad nasal bridge, low set ears and receding chin. Death usually ensues due to renal and respiratory failure.* |
| sindrome di Sézary | **Sézary syndrome** *Symptoms are exfoliative dermatitis with intense itching caused by cutaneous infiltration by mononuclear cells,* |
| sindrome femoro-rotulea da stress | **patellofemoral stress syndrome** *Overuse syndrome causing anterior knee pain from excessive lateral motion.* |

| Italian | English |
|---|---|
| sindrome intorpidita del mento | **numb chin syndrome.** *Generally associated with metastatic breast or prostate cancer, it is characterized by unilateral sensory loss of the chin and lower lip.* |
| sindrome mucocutanea linfonodale | **Kawasaki syndrome** *Begins with fever for 5 days, skin rashes, strawberry tongue, lymphadenopathy and swollen hands and feet. It is known to cause coronary artery aneurysms. Also called mucocutaneous lymph node syndrome.* |
| sindrome neurolettica maligna | **neuroleptic malignant syndrome** *A severe reaction to neuroleptic medications characterized by hyperthermia with autonomic and extrapyramidal symptoms.* |
| sindrome premenstruale | **premenstrual syndrome** *A cluster of emotional, behavioral, and physical symptoms that occur in the premenstrual phase of the menstrual cycle and resolve with the onset of menstruation.* |
| sindrome talamico | **thalamic syndrome** *Caused by an infarct of the posteroinferior thalamus, there is transient hemiparesis, severe sensory loss with preserved crude pain in the hypalgic limbs.* |
| sinechia | **synechia** *The adhesion of two body parts, such as synechia vulvae in which the labia minora are congenitally adherent.* |
| singhiozzare | **sob, to** *To cry uncontrollably.* |
| singhiozzo | **hiccup** *Involuntary spasm of the diaphragm with sudden closure of the glottis; this causes a characteristic cough.* |
| single | **single** *Not married.* |
| sinistro | **left** |
| sinistrocardia | **sinistrocardia** *Location of the heart toward the left (more than normally seen).* |
| sinistrotorsione | **sinistrotorsion** *Distortion toward the left; in reference to the eye generally.* |
| sinoviectomia | **synovectomy** *Surgical resection of a synovial membrane.* |
| sinovite | **synovitis** *Inflammation of the synovium.* |
| sinovite cronica ipertrofica | **Brodie's knee** *Also referred to as chronic hypertrophic synovitis of the knee.* |
| sintesi operatorio | **operative note** *A detailed description of a surgical procedure performed on a specific patient.* |
| sintomi lamenti dal al momento della visita | **presenting symptom** *The initial subjective complaint that initiated a visit.* |
| sintomo | **symptom** *A physical feature that is characteristic of disease.* |
| sinusite | **sinusitis** *Inflammation of the sinuses.* |
| sinusoide | **sinusoid** *An irregular vessel having almost no adventitia that is found in the liver, heart, parathyroid, spleen and pancreas.* |
| siringa | **syringe** *A device used for administering medication through various routes.* |
| siringa sonda gastrica | **gavage syringe** *A syringe used for irrigation.* |
| siringomielia | **syringomelia** *A condition exhibited by fluid-filled cavities in the spinal cord.* |
| sistema ABO | **ABO system** *The system using human blood antigens to determine blood type.* |
| sistema metrico | **metric system** |
| sistema motorio extrapiramidale | **extrapyramidal tract** *Motor nerves that are not part of the pyramidal tract.* |
| sistema nervoso autonomo | **autonomic nervous system** *Responsible for regulation of cardiac muscle, smooth muscle and glandular activity.* |
| sistema nervoso centrale | **central nervous system (CNS)** *The brain and spinal cord.* |
| sistema nervoso simpatico | **sympathetic nervous system** *The nerves responsible for the flight or fight response.* |
| sistole | **systole** *The phase of the cardiac cycle in which the ventricles contract.* |

| Italian | English |
|---|---|
| sistolico | **systolic** *Referring to systole or that which occurs during systole.* |
| sito | **site** *Location.* |
| Sjogren, sindrome di | **Sjogren's syndrome.** *Characterized by dryness of the mouth and eyes, it is sometimes linked to rheumatoid arthritis.* |
| smegma | **smegma** *A thick curdled secretion found around the clitoris and the prepuce.* |
| sodio cloruro | **sodium chloride** *A colorless, crystalline compound; also table salt.* |
| soffice, dolce | **soft** *Easy to mold or compress.* |
| soffio | **murmur** *An abnormal heart sound heard with a stethoscope.* |
| soffio cardiaco | **heart murmur** *An abnormal heart sound usually related to valvular disease.* |
| soffio carotide | **carotid bruit** *An abnormal noise heard over the carotid artery that may be a sign of stenosis or aortic valvular disease.* |
| soffocamento | **suffocation** *To die from a lack of air or inability to breathe.* |
| soffrire | **suffer, to** *To be affected by an illness or sickness.* |
| sogno | **dream** *The thoughts or images occurring during sleep.* |
| solco | **sulcus** *A groove, like in the brain.* |
| soleo | **soleus muscle** *Assists with ankle plantar flexion.* |
| solfonamidi | **sulfonamide** *A class of drugs derived from sulfanilamide that are antibacterial.* |
| solidificazione | **consolidation** *An area of fixed secretions in the lung.* |
| sollevare | **lift, to** *Raise to a higher level.* |
| sollevare | **raise, to** *To lift or bring up.* |
| sollevatore | **levator** *A muscle that raises part of the body; the levator labii superioris raised the upper lip.* |
| solo | **single** *Only one.* |
| soluzione fisiologica | **physiological saline** *0.9% normal saline.* |
| solvente | **solvent** *Able to dissolve with other chemicals.* |
| somatico | **somatic** *Referring to the body.* |
| sonda gastrico introdotta del naso | **nasogastric tube placement** *Insertion of a tube that is placed in the stomach via the nostril; it is used for administration of fluid or to suction gastric contents.* |
| sonda nasogastrico | **nasogastric tube** *A tube that is inserted into the nose with the distal tip in the stomach; it is used for irrigation or drainage of gastric contents.* |
| sonnambulisomo | **somnambulism** *Sleepwalking.* |
| sonno | **sleep** *A nap or a snooze.* |
| sonnolenza | **drowsiness** *Sleepiness.* |
| sonnolenza | **somnolence** *Drowsiness.* |
| soporifero | **soporific** *Promoting drowsiness or sleep.* |
| sopracciglio | **eyebrow** *Supercilium.* |
| soprarenale | **adrenal** *Referring to being near the kidney.* |
| sordità | **deafness** *Having impaired hearing.* |
| sordo | **deaf** *Absence of the sense of hearing.* |
| sordomuto | **deaf-mute** *Inability to hear or speak.* |
| sorseggiare | **sip, to** *To slowly take small drinks of a fluid.* |
| sorveglianza | **guarding** *A symptom used to describe a patient resisting an examination because of severe pain; often seen in patients with peritonitis.* |
| sorveglianza prenatale | **prenatal care** *Medical care received while one is pregnant.* |
| sospiro | **sigh** *A long deep exhalation that expresses an emotion, as in relief.* |
| sostanza bianca | **white matter** *The brain tissue consisting of myelin sheaths and nerve fibers.* |

| Italian | English |
|---|---|
| sostanza lipotropo | **lipotrophic substance** *A compound which causes an increase in body fat.* |
| sostegno caviglia | **ankle support** *A mechanical device or banding to support the ankle.* |
| sostegno per ammalati allettati | **bed rest** *A medical order requiring one to stay in bed.* |
| sostenere | **argue, to** *To debate or reason. (quarrel)* |
| sostenere | **sustain, to** *To keep or maintain.* |
| sostituzione dell'anca | **hip replacement** *Both joint surfaces are replaced by high density material such as plastic or metal.* |
| sostonaza grigia che circonda l'acquedotto | **periaqueductal gray matter** *Refers to the brain gray matter adjacent to the periaqueductal.* |
| sottile chiodo metallico | **pin** *Hardware used in surgery.* |
| sotto | **below** *Under.* |
| sotto | **under; infra** *Sometimes used when indicating a patient is "under treatment" for a condition (active treatment).* |
| sottoclaveare | **subclavian** *Refers to the area under the clavicle; the subclavian vein runs below the clavicle.* |
| sottosviluppato | **dwarf** *Abnormally small person.* |
| sovraorbitario | **supraorbital** *Situated above the orbit.* |
| sovrappeso | **overweight** *Defined as BMI over 25 kilograms per meters squared.* |
| sovrapubico | **suprapubic** *Situated above the pubis.* |
| spalla | **shoulder** *The joint were the scapula joins the clavicle and humerus. (right shoulder, left shoulder)* |
| spanna | **span** *A distance between two objects.* |
| spasmo | **spasm** *An involuntary contraction of muscles.* |
| spasmo carpopedale | **carpopedal spasm** *A spasm of the carpus and the foot.* |
| spasmolitico | **spasmolytic** *A substance that diminishes spasms.* |
| spasticità | **spasticity** *Refers to continuous spastic movement.* |
| spastico | **spastic** *Stiff, awkward movement of the muscles.* |
| spazio morto | **dead space** *The area in the respiratory tract where air is not exchanged.* |
| spazio morto anatomico | **anatomical dead space** *The area between the mouth and pulmonary alveoli.* |
| spazio morto fisiologico | **physiologic dead space** *The combination of anatomic and alveolar dead space.* |
| spazzola | **brush** *Implement used for cleaning or for taking a tissue sample.* |
| specchio | **mirror** *A device used for reflecting an image.* |
| specifico | **specific** *Clearly defined.* |
| specillo | **probe** *A device used for exploration.* |
| speculo | **speculum** *A device used to open a canal for inspection. (vaginal speculum)* |
| sperma | **sperm** *Short term for spermatozoon.* |
| spermatocele | **spermatocele** *A cyst in the epididymis containing spermatozoa.* |
| spermatogenesi | **spermatogenesis** *The production of spermatozoa.* |
| spermatozoo | **spermatozoon** *A mature male germ cell that is capable of fertilizing an ovum.* |
| spermicida | **spermicide** *A substance capable of killing sperm.* |
| sperone calcaneare | **calcaneal spur** *A bony protrusion on the calcaneus.* |
| spettrometria | **spectrometry** *The use of a device to measure spectra.* |
| spettroscopio | **spectroscope** *A device for producing and recording spectra.* |
| spicola | **spicule** *A sharp, slender part.* |
| spifferare | **blurt out, to** *To speak without considering the repercussions.* |
| spina dorsale | **spine** *The spinal column or a thorny protrusion.* |

| Italian | English |
|---|---|
| spinale | **spinal** *Referring to the spine.* |
| spirale | **intrauterine contraceptive device (IUD)** *A device used to physically prevent the implantation of a fertilized ovum.* |
| spirografo | **spirograph** *A device used to record respiratory movements.* |
| spirometro | **spirometer** *A device used to measure pulmonary capacity.* |
| splenectomia | **splenectomy** *Surgical excision of the spleen.* |
| splenico | **splenic** *Referring to the spleen.* |
| splenomegalia | **splenomegaly** *An abnormally enlarged spleen.* |
| spogilare | **disrobe, to** *To remove clothing.* |
| spondilite | **spondylitis** *Inflammation of the vertebrae.* |
| spondilite anchilosante | **ankylosing spondylitis** *A type of arthritis found in the spine that is exhibited by bony fusion.* |
| spondilolisi | **spondylolysis** *Dissolution of the vertebra.* |
| spondilolistesi | **spondylolisthesis** *The overlapping of one vertebra over another.* |
| spongiosi | **spongiosis** *Edema of the spongy layer of the skin.* |
| spontaneo | **spontaneous** *Occurring without provocation.* |
| sporco | **dirty** *Unclean.* |
| sporotricosi | **sporotrichosis** *A Sporotrichum schenckii infection manifested by formation of lymphatic and subcutaneous nodules.* |
| spostamento dall abituale posizione | **displacement** *Movement from normal position.* |
| spremere | **squirt, to** *To eject a liquid from a small opening.* |
| spruzzo | **spray** *Liquid blown through the air in the form of fine droplets.* |
| spugna | **sponge** *Sterile fabric used to soak up fluid during surgery.* |
| squalificare | **rule out, to** *To perform a test or exam to exclude an illness or disease.* |
| squama | **squama** *A scale or platelike body.* |
| squamoso | **squamous** *Scaly.* |
| squilibrio fisico | **disequilibrium** *The absence of stability.* |
| stadiazione | **staging** *Refers to a stratification of cancer for example.* |
| stadio tardo | **advanced stage** *A late period of a disease.* |
| staffa (utilizzata durante l'esame pelvico) | **stirrup** *An attachment to an exam table where a woman puts her legs to assist examination of the genitalia.* |
| stafilite | **uvulitis** *Inflammation of the uvula.* |
| stafiloma | **staphyloma** *Protrusion of the cornea due to inflammation.* |
| stafilorrafia | **staphylorrhaphy** *Surgical repair of a defect between the soft palate and uvula.* |
| stampella avambraccio | **forearm crutch** *A long stick with a place for a hand-grip to aid in ambulation when there is lower extremity weakness.* |
| stapediectomia | **stapedectomy** *Surgical excision of the stapes.* |
| stapedio | **stapes** *This auditory ossicle is the innermost of three ossicles and is shaped like a stirrup.* |
| starnutire | **sneeze, to** *To suddenly expel air from the nose and mouth because of nasal irritation.* |
| stasi | **stasis** *Lack of movement.* |
| statico | **static** *Not changing.* |
| stato | **standing** *Position or status.* |
| stato coniugale | **marital status** *Single versus married status.* |
| stato nutrizionale | **nutritional status** *The relative state of one's nutrition.* |
| stato precedente | **prior status** *Referring to a person's previous state of health.* |
| stato, condizione | **status** *Position or condition* |
| stato; condizione | **state** *Status.* |
| steatoma | **steatoma** *A sebaceous cyst or lipoma.* |

| Italian | English |
|---|---|
| steatorrea | **steatorrhea** *Excrement with an abnormally high fat content.* |
| steatosi | **steatosis** *Fatty degeneration; when referring to the liver it involves invasion of fat into hepatocytes.* |
| stecca di immobilizzazione | **splint** *A rigid support used to immobilize and extremity.* |
| stecca di polso dorsiflessione | **cock-up splint** *A splint used to maintain the wrist in dorsiflexion; used for carpal tunnel syndrome.* |
| stenosi | **stenosis** *Narrowing of an orifice.* |
| stenosi mitrale | **mitral stenosis** *Narrowing of the left atrioventricular orifice.* |
| stenosi polmonare | **pulmonary stenosis** *A stricture between the pulmonary artery and the right ventricle.* |
| stenosi valvolare aortica | **aortic stenosis** *Narrowing of the aortic orifice.* |
| stercobilina | **stercobilin** *A substance created by the reduction of bilirubin and gives excrement the brown hue.* |
| sterilizzazione | **sterilization** *A procedure done to prevent production of offspring.* |
| sternale | **sternal** *Referring to the sternum.* |
| sterno | **sternum** *Commonly called the breast bone, it consists of the corpus, manubrium and xiphoid process.* |
| sternocleidomastoideo | **sternocleidomastoid** *The pair of muscles that connect the sternum, clavicle and mastoid process.* |
| sterognosia | **stereognosis** *The ability to identify an object by touch.* |
| sterolo | **sterol** *Unsaturated steroid alcohols such as cholesterol.* |
| stetoscopio | **stethoscope** *Device used to auscultate the heart, lungs and over arteries to assess for abnormalities.* |
| stiletto | **stylet** *A thin wire within a catheter that is removed after the catheter is in place.* |
| stimolo liminale | **liminal stimulus** *Referring to a stimulus of threshold strength.* |
| stimulazione cardiaca | **cardiac pacing** *Electromechanical stimulation of the heart.* |
| stitichezza | **constipation** *A condition exhibited by difficulty in having a bowel movement due to hard stools.* |
| stomaco | **stomach** *Organ of digestion between the esophagus and small bowel.* |
| stomatite aftosa | **aphthous stomatitis** *Grouped small lesions that occur on the tongue or in the mouth.* |
| stomatite di Vincent | **trench mouth** *Inflammation and ulceration of the gingivae.* |
| stomatite gangrenosa | **cancrum oris** *Gangrenous stomatitis.* |
| stoppino | **wick** *A drain using a thin piece of cloth or tubing.* |
| storcersi inguinale | **groin pull** *A muscle strain in the inguinal region.* |
| stordito | **groggy** *Drowsy.* |
| storia di famiglia | **family history** *A review of past medical history of related persons.* |
| storia medica passata | **past history** *Prior medical problems experienced by a patient.* |
| strabismo | **strabismus** *An anomaly of ocular movement.* |
| strabismo interno o convergente | **esotropia** *Medial deviation of the eyes at primary gaze.* |
| strano | **strange** *Unusual in an unsettling way.* |
| strapparsi vaginale | **tear, vaginal** *Referring to a vaginal tear after childbirth.* |
| strascicato | **slurring** *Indistinct yet comprehensible speech.* |
| stratigrafia computerizzata | **CT scan** *Computerized axial tomography.* |
| strato | **layer** *A stratum or thickness.* |
| strato granulare | **granular layer** *A deep layer of the cerebellum.* |
| stravaso | **extravasation** *Referring to a situation in which blood or fluid goes out of a vessel it is normally flowing into.* |

| Italian | English |
|---|---|
| stretto inferiore della pelvi | **inferior pelvis strait** *The pelvic outlet.* |
| stria | **stria** *A narrow bandlike body.* |
| stria | **wheal** *A circumscribed urticarial lesion.* |
| stridore | **stridor** *An abnormal, high-pitched, musical sound caused by an obstruction in the larynx or stenosis of the vocal cords.* |
| stroma | **stroma** *A term used to describe the framework of an organ.* |
| strumento da taglio | **burr or bur** *A rotary cutting instrument.* |
| struttura reticolare spongiosa | **cancellous** *A bony mesh-like structure with many pores.* |
| studio controllato verso il placebo | **placebo controlled study** *When a study is placebo controlled it means part of the group received an inactive treatment while the other group received active therapy.* |
| stupore | **stupor** *A reduced level of consciousness.* |
| subacqueo | **diver** *A person who swims in deep water.* |
| subacuto | **subacute** *A stage between acute and chronic.* |
| subaracnoideo | **subarachnoid** *The layer of the brain covering between the arachnoid and pia mater.* |
| subdurale | **subdural** *The area between the dura mater and the arachnoid membrane.* |
| suberosi | **suberosis** *A type of hypersensitivity pneumonitis related to inhalation of moldy cork dust.* |
| subfrenico | **subphrenic** *Referring to below the diaphragm.* |
| sublinguale | **sublingual** *Situated under the tongue.* |
| submaxillare | **submaxillary** *Situated below the maxilla.* |
| succhiare | **suck, to** *As in, to suction fluid.* |
| succussione | **succussion** *The presence of a splashing sound when a body cavity is moved indicating presence of both air and fluid.* |
| sudamen | **sudamina** *White vesicles noted because of retained sweat in the layers of the epidermis.* |
| sudare 2) accadere | **transpire, to** *To release vapor from the skin or respiratory mucosa. 2) to come about* |
| sudare; traspirare | **sweat, to** *The action of releasing moisture through pores of the skin.* |
| sudorazione | **hidrosis** *The production and secretion of sweat.* |
| sudorazione | **sweat** *Moisture exuded through the pores of the skin.* |
| sudorazioni notturne | **night sweats** *Profuse sweating at night occurring with tuberculosis among other conditions.* |
| sufficiente | **adequate** *Sufficient.* |
| suicidio | **suicide** *To kill oneself intentionally.* |
| suoni e rumori respiratori | **breath sounds** *The noise heard upon auscultation with a stethoscope.* |
| suono breve | **click** *A sound heard by the sudden closure of a heart valve.* |
| superfecondazione | **superfecundation** *The fertilization of two different ova by spermatozoa of two different males.* |
| superficie corporea | **body surface area** *Dubois formula is: (weight in kilograms)to the 0.425th power x (height in centimeters) to the 0.725th power x 0.007184.* |
| superiore | **superior** *In a position above something else.* |
| supinazione | **supination** *Turning the sole of the foot or the palm of the hand upward..* |
| supino | **recumbent** *Lying down.* |
| supino | **supine** *Flat on one's back.* |
| supportare | **bear, to** *To endure or resist.* |
| suppositorio | **suppository** *A delivery system for medication placed in an orifice.* |
| suppurare in superficie | **fester, to** *To become infected.* |

| Italian | English |
|---|---|
| suppurazione | **suppuration** *Formation of purulent material.* |
| surale | **sural** *Referring to the calf of the leg.* |
| surfattante | **surfactant** *A substance that reduces surface tension in the lungs.* |
| surrene | **adrenal gland** *A gland located on the superior aspect of both kidneys.* |
| surrenectomia | **adrenalectomy** *Excision of the adrenal gland.* |
| sussurro | **whisper** *Speech in a volume that is barely discernible.* |
| sutura | **suture** *Thread used for sewing together a wound.* |
| sutura continua | **running suture** *A method of sewing a wound in which there is a knot at each end and continuous otherwise.* |
| sutura coronario | **coronal suture** *The line of intersection of the frontal bone and the two parietal bones.* |
| sutura da materassaio | **mattress suture** *A double stitch that forms a loop and there is eversion of the edges when tied.* |
| sutura nailon | **non-resorbable suture (nylon)** *Suture used to be permanent as it is not removed by normal body processes.* |
| sutura riassorbibile (cromico) | **resorbable suture (chromic)** *Suture that is not intended to be permanent as it is dissolved by normal body processes.* |
| sutura sagittale del cranico | **sagittal suture** *The line where the two parietal bones meet.* |
| sutura sovrapporsi | **overriding suture** *The overlapping of cranial sutures noted on vaginal exam when the head is descended.* |
| sventramento | **eventration** *Protrusion of the intestines from the abdomen.* |
| svolgimento del parto | **parturition** *The process of giving birth.* |
| svuotamento | **voiding** *The act of urinating.* |
| tabacchiera anatomico | **anatomical snuff-box** *The area on the back of the hand near the base of the thumb that is between the extensor pollicus longus and extensor pollicus brevis.* |
| tachicardia | **tachycardia** *Heart rate higher than physiologic normal.* |
| tachicardia ventricolare multiforme | **torsade de pointe** *Ventricular cardiac rhythm disturbance.* |
| tachipnea | **tachypnea** *Breathing faster than normal.* |
| tagliente | **sharp (pain)** *When describing pain, a piercing sensation.* |
| taglietto | **nick** *A small groove or notch.* |
| taglio cesareo | **cesarean section** *Incision of the abdominal and uterine walls in order to deliver a fetus when natural delivery is not possible.* |
| talamo | **thalamus** *A paired structure located adjacent to the third ventricle.* |
| talassemia | **thalassemia** *A hereditary hemolytic anemia first observed in people from the Mediterranean area.* |
| talidomide | **thalidomide** *A drug used originally as a sedative, after it was found to cause congenital anomalies, its use was restricted. Now it is used for a few conditions such as multiple myeloma.* |
| talipo calcaneare | **talipes calcaneus** *A foot deformity exhibited by abnormal dorsiflexion.* |
| talipo equino | **talipes equinus** *A foot deformity exhibited by abnormal plantar flexion.* |
| talipo equinovaro | **talipes equinovaro** *Medical term for what is commonly known as club foot.* |
| talo; astragalo | **talus** *The most superior tarsal bone that articulates with the tibia.* |
| tamponamento 2) tamponamento cardiaco | **tamponade** *1. Stopping bleeding during surgery with a cotton pledget. 2. When referring to cardiac tamponade, it is the limitation of cardiac contraction because of blood or fluid accumulation in the pericardial sac.* |
| tampone | **feminine pad** *Gauze specially designed to absorb menstrual flow.* |
| tampone | **swab** *An absorbent material used for cleaning wounds or applying ointment.* |

| Italian | English |
|---|---|
| tapis roulant | **treadmill** *An exercise machine on a continuous belt used for walking.* |
| tarantola | **tarantula** *A large hairy spider found mainly in the tropics.* |
| tardivo | **late** *A time later than expected.* |
| targa | **target** *An objective towards which efforts are directed.* |
| tarsale | **tarsal** *Referring to any bone in the tarsus.* |
| tarsalgia | **tarsalgia** *Pain in any of the tarsal bones.* |
| tarsectomia | **tarsectomy** *Surgical excision of all or part of the tarsus.* |
| tarso | **tarsus** *The group of seven bones of the ankle or foot (three cuneiform bones, talus, calcaneus, navicular, cuboid bones).* |
| tarsorrafia | **tarsorrhaphy** *Suturing the eyelids in order to tighten the palpebral fissure.* |
| tartaro dentario | **dental calculus** *Calcium phosphate and carbonate adhered to the teeth.* |
| tasca di Douglas | **Douglas' pouch** *A recess in the peritoneum between the rectum and the uterus. Also called the rectouterine pouch.* |
| tasso di natalità | **birth rate** *The number of live births per 1000 of a given population per year.* |
| tattile | **tactile** *Able to be felt.* |
| tatuaggio | **tattoo** *A design made by inserting indelible ink into the skin.* |
| tavoletta, compressa | **tablet** *A small disk of a compressed solid substance.* |
| teca | **theca** *A tendon or ovarian follicle sheath.* |
| tecoma | **thecoma** *A tumor composed of theca cells.* |
| tegumento | **integument** *Outer protective layer.* |
| telangettasia | **telangiectasis** *A condition exhibited by red, dilated capillaries on the skin.* |
| telangiectasia | **angiectasia** *Dilation of a blood or lymph vessel.* |
| telemetria | **telemetry** *Use of radio signals to transmit patient data. The most common form is for electrocardiography in a patient who is ambulatory.* |
| temperatura | **temperature** *The degree of internal heat in a person's body.* |
| tempo di emorragia | **bleeding time** *The time of bleeding after a controlled standardized puncture of the earlobe.* |
| tenaglie | **tongs** *A medical device used for holding or grasping.* |
| tenda a ossigeno | **oxygen tent** *A manner of giving supplement oxygen to a neonate.* |
| tendine | **tendon** *Fibrous tissue that connects muscle to bone.* |
| tendine delimitante la fossa poplitea | **hamstrings** *Tendons of the posterior thigh.* |
| tenesmo | **tenesmus** *The attempt to defecate but attempts elicit pain and are ineffective.* |
| tenoplastica | **tenoplasty** *Surgical repair of a tendon.* |
| tenorrafia | **tenorrhaphy** *The surgical repair with suture of a separated tendon.* |
| tenosinovite | **tenosynovitis** *Inflammation and swelling of an articulation.* |
| tenosinovite scapolo-omerale cronica | **adhesive capsulitis** *Also known as frozen shoulder.* |
| tenosinovite scapolo-omerale cronica; spalla congelata | **frozen shoulder** *Common term for adhesive capsulitis.* |
| tenotomia | **tenotomy** *Incision of a tendon as is done for strabismus.* |
| tensione arteriale | **blood pressure** *Written as the measurement in mmHg at the time of systole of the left ventricle over the time of diastole.* |
| tensione o distensione eccessiva | **strain** *As in a muscle strain.* |
| terapia di mantenimento | **maintenance therapy** *Continuing a form of treatment long-term.* |

| Italian | English |
|---|---|
| terapia elettroconvulsivante | **electroconvulsive therapy (ECT)** *The electrical stimulation of the brain to treat mental disorders.* |
| terapia fisica | **physical therapy** *Treatment of disease by heat, massage and exercise as opposed to medications.* |
| terapia occupazionale | **occupational therapy** *Rehabilitation focusing on activities of daily living.* |
| terapia ossigeno | **oxygen therapy** *Utilization of supplemental oxygen.* |
| teratogene | **teratogen** *A substance that induces fetal anomalies.* |
| teratoma | **teratoma** *A tumor made up of tissue not usually at the location (a mass of hair, teeth and gingival tissue in a leg tumor for instance).* |
| terebrante | **terebrant** *Having a piercing quality.* |
| termometro | **thermometer** *A device used to measure temperature.* |
| terreno di coltura | **culture broth** *A medium used to grow bacteria.* |
| terziario | **tertiary** *Third in order or designating medical care at a specialized hospital.* |
| tessuto | **tissue** *Any of the distinct materials people are made of.* |
| tessuto granulazione | **granulation tissue** *Vascular connective tissue forming granular protrusions on the surface of a healing wound.* |
| test di Coomb | **antiglobulin test (Coombs' test)** *Test used to detect erythroblastosis fetalis.* |
| test di tolleranza al glucosio | **glucose tolerance test** *The oral administration of a carbohydrate load and then evaluation of the blood sugar at timed intervals.* |
| testa | **head** |
| testicolo | **testicle** *One of a pair of organs in the male scrotum that produces sperm.* |
| testosterone | **testosterone** *This steroid hormone produces secondary male sexual characteristics.* |
| tetania | **tetany** *A condition caused by the hypocalcemic effect of hypoparathyroidism, exhibited by periodic muscle spasms, convulsions, and peri-oral numbness.* |
| tetano | **tetanus** *A condition caused by Clostridium tetani which produces spasm and rigidity of voluntary muscles.* |
| tetraciclina | **tetracycline** *An antibiotic used for gram positive and gram negative infections.* |
| tetradattilo | **tetradactylous** *Referring to a condition of having only four digits on a hand or foot.* |
| tetralogia di Fallot | **Fallot, tetrology of** *Congenital cardiac defects including ventricular septal defect, pulmonic valve stenosis or infundibular stenosis, and dextroposition of the aorta.* |
| tetto | **tectum** *A roof-like body.* |
| thrombosi del seno cavernoso | **cavernous sinus thrombosis** *A blood clot in the base of the brain.* |
| tiamina | **thiamine** *Also called vitamin B1; a deficiency causes beriberi.* |
| tibia | **tibia** *The larger of two long bones in the lower leg.* |
| tic | **tic** *Periodic spasmodic facial muscle contractions.* |
| tiepido | **tepid** *Lukewarm.* |
| tifo | **typhoid fever** *A condition caused by ingestion of food or water containing salmonella typhi that is exhibited by fever and abdominal signs and symptoms.* |
| tigna | **tinea** *Medical term for ringworm.* |
| tigna del capo | **tinea capitis** *Ringworm of the scalp, a fungal infection.* |
| tigna del corpo | **tinea corporis** *Ringworm of the body, a fungal infection.* |
| tigna della barba | **tinea barbae** *Ringworm on the face in the region a man shaves.* |
| tigna favosa | **favus** *Tinea capitis caused by Trichopyton schoenleini.* |

| Italian | English |
|---|---|
| tigna piede | **tinea pedis** *Ringworm of the feet, a fungal infection.* |
| timectomia | **thymectomy** *Surgical excision of the thymus.* |
| timina | **thymine** *A chemical with a pyrimidine base found in DNA.* |
| timo | **thymus** *A body organ located in the neck and it produces T cells to improve immune function.* |
| timocito | **thymocyte** *A lymphocyte located in the thymus.* |
| timoma | **thymoma** *A tumor composed of thymic tissue and is sometimes associated with myasthenia gravis.* |
| timpanico | **tympanic** *Referring to the tympanic membrane or having a resonant quality to percussion.* |
| timpanoeustachiano | **tympanic cavity** *The air chamber medial to the tympanic membrane in the temporal bone, between the external acoustic meatus and the inner ear.* |
| timpanoplastica | **tympanoplasty** *Restoration of the tympanic membrane's continuity.* |
| tinea barbae | **barber's itch** *Ringworm that is transmitted by contaminated shaving equipment.* |
| tinea cruris | **jock itch** *Pruritus caused by tinea cruris.* |
| tinea cruris | **tinea cruris** *Ringworm in the inguinal region, a fungal infection.* |
| tinnito | **tinnitus** *Medical term for ringing in the ears. It is associated with Meniere's syndrome among other conditions.* |
| tintura | **tincture** *1. A very small amount of something. 2. A medicine dissolved in alcohol.* |
| tirare | **pull, to** *To exert force on something.* |
| tireotossicosi | **thyrotoxicosis** *Abnormal increase in thyroid activity exhibited by thinning hair, hypertension, tachycardia and at times atrial fibrillation.* |
| tiroidectomia | **thyroidectomy** *Surgical resection of all or part of the thyroid.* |
| tiroideo | **thyroid** *A gland in the neck that secretes hormones regulating metabolism.* |
| tirosina | **tyrosine** *An amino acid important in the synthesis of hormones.* |
| tiroxina | **thyroxine** *An iodine containing hormone, referred to T4.* |
| toccare | **feel, to** *To perceive or discern.* |
| tocoferolo | **tocopherol** *Vitamin E.* |
| togliere il respiro | **choke, to** *To retch, cough or fight for breath.* |
| tomografo a emissione di positroni | **PET scan Positron emission tomography.** *Production of tomographic images revealing biochemical tissue properties by analyzing positrons emitted when radioactively tagged substances are taken in tissues.* |
| tonometro | **tonometer** *A device used to measure ocular pressure in glaucoma.* |
| tonsilla | **tonsil** *A rounded mass of lymphoid tissue, most commonly referring to the pharyngeal tonsil.* |
| tonsillectomia | **tonsillectomy** *Excision of the tonsils.* |
| tonsillite | **tonsillitis** *Inflammation of the tonsils.* |
| torace | **chest** *Thorax.* |
| torace | **thorax** *The part of the body between the neck and abdomen.* |
| torace a imbuto | **funnel chest** *Anterior thorax funnel shaped depression, also called pectus excavatum.* |
| toracentesi | **thoracentesis** *Insertion of a needle into the pleural space to drain and or obtain a specimen for analysis.* |
| toracico | **thoracic** *Referring to the thorax.* |
| toracoplastica | **thoracoplasty** *Surgical removal of ribs.* |
| toracoscopia | **thoracoscopy** *Visualization of the thoracic cavity with a scope.* |
| toracotomia | **thoracotomy** *Surgical incision of the thorax.* |
| torbido | **hazy** *Cloudy.* |

| Italian | English |
|---|---|
| tornasole | **litmus** *A dye that turns red with low pH and blue with high pH.* |
| torpore | **torpor** *Unresponsiveness to normal stimuli.* |
| torsione | **torsion** *Refers to twisting. Testicular torsion is the twisting of the spermatic cord that can lead to ischemia and gangrene of the testicle.* |
| torsione testicolare | **testicular torsion** *Rotation of the spermatic cord resulting in testicular ischemia.* |
| tosse | **cough** *Forceful expulsion of air from the lungs.* |
| tosse secca | **dry cough** *A cough without sputum production.* |
| tosse secca, debole e frequente | **cough, hacking** *A dry, episodic cough.* |
| tossico | **toxic** *Relating to or caused by poison.* |
| tossicodipendenza | **addiction** *An abnormal dependency.* |
| tossicologia | **toxicology** *The study of the nature, effects and detection of poisons.* |
| tossiemia | **toxemia** *The release of toxic substances into the blood stream from a local infection. Toxemia of pregnancy is a synonym for preeclampsia.* |
| tossina | **toxin** *A poison of plant or animal origin.* |
| tossoide | **toxoid** *A chemically modified toxin that can be used as a vaccine.* |
| totale | **absolute** |
| tourniquet | **tourniquet** *A device tied tightly around an extremity to diminish blood flow or blood loss.* |
| toxoplasmosi | **toxoplasmosis** *A disease caused by an organism from the genus Toxoplasma. One can have simple malaise to central nervous system involvement.* |
| trabecola | **trabecule** *A connective tissue strand that goes from a capsule to the enclosed organ.* |
| trabecolotomia | **trabeculotomy** *A surgery for open angle glaucoma.* |
| trachea | **trachea** *The ringed canal between the pharynx and bronchi.* |
| tracheite | **tracheitis** *Inflammation of the trachea.* |
| trachelorrafia | **trachelorrhaphy** *Surgical repair of a lacerated cervix.* |
| tracheobronchite | **tracheobronchitis** *Inflammation of the trachea and bronchi.* |
| tracheostomia | **tracheostomy** *Creation of a surgical opening in the trachea so a tube could be placed in the trachea.* |
| tracheotomia | **tracheotomy** *Surgical incision of the trachea.* |
| tracoma | **trachoma** *An infection of the cornea and conjunctiva caused by Chlamydia.* |
| trago | **tragus** *The fleshy prominence anterior to the opening of the ear.* |
| tranquillante | **tranquilizer** *A medication used to diminish anxiety.* |
| transaddominale | **transabdominal** *Through the abdominal wall.* |
| transaminasi | **transaminase** *An enzyme that facilitates the transfer of an amino group to an amino acid.* |
| transdermico | **transdermal** *Through the skin.* |
| transfusione | **transfusion** *Administration of blood products intravenously.* |
| transfusione sostitutiva | **exchange transfusion** *Treatment of hyperbilirubinemia in neonates.* |
| trapanazione | **trephination** *Cutting away a circular disc of bone or the cornea.* |
| trapano | **drill** *Cylindrical metal tool uses for creating a hole in bone in surgery.* |
| trapiantare | **transplant,to** *To move a body part from one location to another.* |
| trapianto | **graft** *A piece of tissue surgically transplanted.* |
| trapianto | **transplantation** *The grafting of tissues.* |
| trapianto corneale | **corneal transplant** *Surgical replacement of a cornea with a donor cornea.* |
| trapianto osseo | **bone graft** *The transfer of bone to aid in the healing of a complex fracture.* |
| trasparente | **clear** *Transparent.* |

| Italian | English |
|---|---|
| traspirazione | **perspiration** *The process of sweating.* |
| trastornos del equilibrio | **dizziness** *Sensation of losing one's balance.* |
| trasudare | **ooze, to** *To slowly leak.* |
| trasudazione | **transudation** *The movement of body tissue through a membrane that is usually the result of inflammation.* |
| trattamento | **management** *The process of dealing with things or people.* |
| trattamento mediante nebulizzazione | **nebulizer treatment** *Administration of medication such as albuterol via a fine mist using a nebulizer.* |
| trattamento per ascariasi | **ascaricide** *Agent that destroys ascaris.* |
| trattenere | **withhold, to** *To refuse to give something.* |
| tratto | **tract** *A large bundle of fibers or a major passage in the body.* |
| tratto gastrointestinale | **gastrointestinal tract** *The alimentary canal from the distal esophagus to the cecum.* |
| tratto respiratorio superiore | **upper respiratory tract** *Generally considered the part of the respiratory tract superior to the vocal cords.* |
| tratto urinario | **urinary tract** *The organs and canals associated with urine secretion including the kidneys, ureters, bladder and urethra.* |
| travaglio | **labor pains** *The intermittent pain associated with uterine contractions.* |
| traversa | **sheet (bed)** *A rectangular fabric covering a bed.* |
| trazione | **traction** *Sustained pull on a muscle or bone to correct alignment.* |
| trazione scheletrica | **skeletal traction** *Use of a pulley system to reduce a fracture.* |
| tre gemelli | **triplets** *Three infants born during one birth.* |
| Trematoda | **trematoda** *A parasitic fluke such as Schistosoma.* |
| tremore | **tremor** *Involuntary contraction and relaxation of small muscle groups.* |
| tremore intenzionale | **intention tremor** *The tremulous movement noted when a person is beginning to perform a task but not seen at rest.* |
| treonina | **threonine** *An amino acid needed for the growth in infants.* |
| trequarti | **trocar** *A device enclosed in a catheter that is used to withdraw fluid from a body cavity.* |
| triangolo femorale | **femoral triangle** *An area that is bordered by the sartorius muscle, the adductor longus muscle and the inguinal ligament.* |
| trichiasi | **trichiasis** *Inversion of the eyelashes.* |
| Trichinella spiralis | **whipworm** *A parasitic, intestinal nematode worm of the genus Trichuris.* |
| trichinosi | **trichinosis** *A disease caused by meat infected by Trichinella spiralis causing fever and gastrointestinal effects.* |
| Trichomonas vaginite | **trichomoniasis vaginitis** *Infection related to a species of Trichomonas.* |
| tricofitosi | **trichophytosis** *A skin or nail fungal infection caused by Trichophyton.* |
| trigeminale | **trigeminal** *Generally refers to the fifth cranial nerve.* |
| trigono vescicale | **trigone of bladder** *Refers to the area at the base of the bladder between the openings of the ureters and the urethra.* |
| tripanosomiasi | **trypanosomiasis** *A disease caused by a protozoa of the genus Trypanosoma that can cause sleeping sickness and Chagas' disease.* |
| triplegia | **triplegia** *Paralysis of three extremities.* |
| triploide | **triploid** *Referring to a cell with three homologous sets of chromosomes.* |
| tripsina | **trypsin** *An enzyme whose precursor is secreted by the pancreas that breaks down proteins in the intestine.* |
| tripsinogeno | **trypsinogen** *The precursor to trypsin that is secreted by the pancreas.* |
| triptofano | **tryptophan** *An amino acid that is a precursor of serotonin. If present in the body in appropriate levels it can prevent pellagra even if niacin levels are low.* |

| Italian | English |
|---|---|
| trisma | **trismus** *Commonly called lockjaw, it is a spasm of the muscles supplied by the trigeminal nerve and is an early symptom of tetanus.* |
| trisomia | **trisomy** *A general category of congenital anomalies in which there is an extra set of chromosomes in the cell nucleus.* |
| tristezza | **sadness** *The state of being sad.* |
| trocantere | **trochanter** *Refers to the greater or lesser trochanter; the prominences on the femoral neck.* |
| trocicollo | **torticollis** *A condition exhibited by the head being turned to one side continuously.* |
| troclea | **trochlea** *A pulley-shaped structure such as the groove at the distal humerus.* |
| trocleare | **trochlear** *Referring to a trochlea.* |
| trofoblasto | **trophoblast** *A layer of endodermal tissue that helps attach an ovum to the uterine wall.* |
| tromba faringoimpanico | **pharyngotympanic tube** *Synonym for eustachian tube.* |
| trombectomia | **thrombectomy** *Excision of a thrombus from a vein or artery.* |
| trombina | **thrombin** *An enzyme that is a catalyst for the conversion of fibrinogen to fibrin in the formation of a clot.* |
| trombo murale | **mural thrombus** *A thrombus attached to a diseased portion of endocardium.* |
| tromboangioite | **thromboangiitis** *Inflammation and thrombosis in a blood vessel.* |
| tromboarterite | **thromboarteritis** *Thrombosis of an inflamed artery.* |
| trombocitopenia | **thrombocytopenia** *Abnormal decrease in the number of blood platelets.* |
| tromboflebite | **thrombophlebitis** *Inflammation of a venous wall associated with a thrombus.* |
| tromboflebite iliaco-femorale in puerperio | **phlegmasia alba dolens** *Phlebitis of the femoral vein that can occur after pregnancy or typhoid fever.* |
| trombosi | **thrombosis** *Formation of a clot in a vein or artery.* |
| trombosi venoso profonda | **deep vein thrombosis (DVT)** *A blood clot that forms within a vein, typically in the lower extremities.* |
| tronco | **torso** *The trunk of the body.* |
| tronco | **truncal** *Referring to the trunk of a body or a nerve.* |
| tronco cerebrale | **brain stem** *An organ that consists of the medulla oblongata, pons and midbrain.* |
| tubale | **tubal** *Referring to a tube, as in fallopian tube.* |
| tube di falloppio | **fallopian tubes** *Either of a pair of long narrow ducts located in a female's abdominal cavity that transport the male sperm cells to the egg.* |
| tubercolina | **tuberculin** *A solution containing M. tuberculosis or M. bovis that is used to test for tuberculosis by injecting the solution intradermally and looking for a reaction.* |
| tubercolo | **tubercle** *1. A granulomatous nodule produced by Mycobacterium tuberculosis. 2. A small prominence on a bone.* |
| tubercolosi | **tuberculosis** *Any infectious disease caused by Mycobacterium.* |
| tubercoloso | **tuberculous** *Referring to tuberculosis.* |
| tuberosità | **tuberosity** *A protuberance. For instance the iliac tuberosity is a prominence on the surface of the ilium.* |
| tuberuloma | **tuberculoma** *1. A tuberculous growth in the brain. 2. A mass that is produced from enlargement of a caseous tubercle.* |
| tubo drenaggio | **drainage tube** *A cannula used to allow outflow of fluids.* |
| tubo endotracheale con palloncino | **cuffed endotracheal tube** *A cannula that has an balloon on the tip that can be inflated with air and placed into the trachea.* |
| tubo intravenoso | **intravenous tubing** *The tubing used to administer fluids.* |

| Italian | English |
|---|---|
| tubo per trasfusione di sangue | **blood tubing** *(used for infusion of blood)* |
| tubo sonda gastrica | **gavage tube** *A tube used for instillation of liquids into the stomach.* |
| tubo-ovarico | **tubo-ovarian** *Referring to the fallopian tube or ovary.* |
| tubulare | **tubular** *Referring to a hollow, round-shaped organ.* |
| tubuli seminifero | **seminiferous tubules** *Used for transport of semen.* |
| tularemia | **tularemia** *An infectious disease caused by Francisella tularensis. The symptoms range from mild constitutional complaints to septic shock.* |
| tumefazione | **tumefaction** *An area of swelling.* |
| tumefazione; rigonfiamento | **swelling** *An abnormal enlarged from fluid collection.* |
| tumidità | **puffiness** *Having a soft, swollen area.* |
| tumore | **tumor** *A benign or malignant overgrowth of tissue.* |
| tumore di glomus | **glomus tumor** *A reddish-blue painful papule that occurs on the distal aspects of the digits.* |
| tumore, massa | **mass** *Tumor.* |
| tunica | **tunica** *Generally a covering of a body part or organ. The tunica mucosa nasi is the mucous membrane lining the nasal cavity.* |
| turbinectomia | **turbinectomy** *Surgical excision of a turbinate bone.* |
| turgido | **turgid** *Congested and swollen.* |
| turgore | **turgor** *Referring to the elasticity of skin. If one pinches skin and it remains in place the patient is dehydrated.* |
| turno di notte | **night shift** *The late shift, typically beginning at 19:00 or 23:00 hours.* |
| ubriaco | **drunk** *Inebriated.* |
| udito | **hearing** *Auditory perception.* |
| ulcera | **ulcer** *A concave wound caused by a break in the integrity of skin or mucous membrane. (duodenal ulcer)* |
| ulcera duodenale | **duodenal ulcer** *A defect in the lining of the first portion of the small bowel, typically caused by H. pylori.* |
| ulcera gastroduodenale | **gastroduodenal ulcer** *A lesion in the mucosal lining of the stomach or duodenum.* |
| ulcera molle o venerea | **chancroid** *A sexually transmitted disease caused by Haemophilus ducreyi that is exhibited by ulcers without indurated margins.* |
| ulcerativo | **ulcerative** *Referring to ulceration.* |
| ulcerazione della bocca; stomatite aftosa | **canker sore** *An ulceration, usually of the mouth or lips.* |
| ultimo stadio | **end stage** *Terminal stage. End stage cancer means there is no cure possible and death is imminent.* |
| ultrasonografia | **ultrasonography** *Visualization of body structures with the echoes of ultrasound pulses.* |
| ultrasuono | **ultrasound** *A sound or vibration of ultrasonic frequency.* |
| ultrasuono transrettale | **transrectal ultrasound** *Insertion of an ultrasound probe into the rectum to view adjacent structures.* |
| umano | **human** *Homo sapien.* |
| umor acqueo | **humor, aqueous** *The gelatinous fluid circulating between the cornea and lens.* |
| umor vitreo | **humor, vitreous** *The fluid circulating between the lens and retina.* |
| umore | **mood** *A temporary state of mind or feeling.* |
| umore acqueo | **aqueous humor** *The fluid between the cornea and lens, anterior to the globe.* |
| unciforme | **unciform** *Another term for hamate bone in the wrist.* |
| uncinariasi | **uncinariasis** *Hookworm infestation of genus Uncinaria.* |
| unghia | **nail** *The hard surface on the dorsal surface of the toes or fingers.* |

| Italian | English |
|---|---|
| unghia a cucchiaio | **spoon nail** *Also referred to as koilonychia, the nail is concave and is generally associated with anemia.* |
| unghia delle dita dei piedi | **toenail** *The nail at the tip/dorsal aspect of each toe.* |
| unghia di becco di pappagallo | **parrot-beak nail** *A curved fingernail.* |
| unghia di un dito | **fingernail** *Thin horny plate over the dorsal aspect of the end of finger.* |
| unghia incarnita | **ingrown nail** *Also referred to as onychocryptosis.* |
| unguento | **ointment** *A petroleum jelly based topical medication.* |
| unicellulare | **unicellular** *A term describing organisms like protozoans that only have cell.* |
| unità di cura intensiva | **intensive care unit** *The unit where vigorous treatment of the acutely ill takes place.* |
| unità motore | **motor unit** *The complex of one motor cell and its attached muscle fibers.* |
| unzione | **inunction** *The application of lotion with friction.* |
| uomo | **man** *Male human.* |
| uovo | **egg** |
| uraco | **urachus** *A connection between the bladder and the allantois in the fetus.* |
| urato | **urate** *The salt of uric acid.* |
| urea | **urea** *A nitrogenous product of protein metabolism; excreted in urine.* |
| uremia | **uremia** *An excess of urea and creatinine in the blood.* |
| ureterale | **ureteral** *Referring to one of two tubes from the kidneys to the bladder that carry urine.* |
| uretere | **ureter** *The conduit between each kidney and the urinary bladder.* |
| ureterectomia | **ureterectomy** *Surgical resection of one or both ureters.* |
| ureterite | **ureteritis** *Inflammation of the ureter.* |
| ureterocele | **ureterocele** *Protrusion of the distal portion of the ureter into the bladder.* |
| ureterolito | **ureterolith** *Presence of a stone in the ureter.* |
| ureterolitotomia | **ureterolithotomy** *Removal of a ureteral stone.* |
| ureterovaginale | **ureterovaginal** *Referring to the ureter and vagina.* |
| ureterovescicale | **ureterovesical** *Referring to the ureter and urinary bladder.* |
| uretra | **urethra** *The canal connecting the urinary bladder with the outside of the body.* |
| uretrale | **urethral** *Referring to the urethra.* |
| uretrite | **urethritis** *Inflammation of the urethra.* |
| uretrocele | **urethrocele** *A prolapse of the urethra through the meatus.* |
| uretrografia | **urethrography** *Imaging of the urethra after instillation of contrast media.* |
| uretroplasica | **urethroplasty** *Surgical repair of the urethra.* |
| uretroscopio | **urethroscope** *A scope used to visualize the inside of the urethra.* |
| uretrotomia | **urethrotomy** *A surgical opening of the urethra.* |
| urgenza | **urgency** *Emergency or priority.* |
| urina | **urine** *The fluid concentrated by the kidneys and expelled via the urethra.* |
| urina centro della corrente | **midstream urine** *A specimen of urine that is collected after the initial stream of urine is initiated and before one finishes urinating.* |
| urina residuo | **residual urine** *The amount of urine remaining in the bladder after a person voids.* |
| urinario | **urinary** *Referring to the urine.* |

| Italian | English |
|---|---|
| urobiline | **urobilin** *A brownish pigment that is an oxidized form of urobilinogen.* |
| urobilinogeno | **urobilinogen** *A colorless substance produced in the intestines when bilirubin is reduced.* |
| urocromo | **urochrome** *A yellow pigment in the urine that gives urine its color.* |
| urogenitale | **urogenital** *Referring to the urinary and genital systems.* |
| urografia | **urography** *Roentgenography of the urinary tract after administration of contrast media.* |
| urolito | **urolith** *Urinary calculi.* |
| urologia | **urology** *Surgical specialty involving medical and surgical treatment of the urogenital system.* |
| urometro | **urinometer** *A device for measuring urine specific gravity.* |
| ustione | **burn** *An injury caused by exposure to heat.* |
| usuale | **usual** *Typical or normal.* |
| uterino | **uterine** *Referring to the uterus.* |
| utero | **uterus** *The hollow organ in the female pelvis where a fertilized ovum embeds and grows.* |
| utero retroflesso | **retroflexed uterus** *Bending back of the uterus so that the top portion pushes against the rectum.* |
| uterovescicale | **uterovesical** *Referring to the uterus and urinary bladder.* |
| utilizzo dell'ossigeno | **oxygen consumption** *The body's utilization of oxygen per unit of time.* |
| utricolo | **utricle** *A small sac. It can refer to a division of the membranous labyrinth.* |
| uveite | **uveitis** *Inflammation of the uvea.* |
| uvula | **uvula** *A fleshy pendent at the back of the soft palate.* |
| uvulectomia | **uvulectomy** *Excision of the uvula.* |
| vaccinazione | **vaccination** *The act of receiving a vaccine.* |
| vaccino | **vaccine** *A solution of attenuated microorganisms given to prevent or treat a disease.* |
| vacillare | **stagger, to** *To walk in an unsteady fashion.* |
| vacuolo | **vacuole** *A cavity that develops in a cell.* |
| vagale | **vagal** *Referring to the vagus nerve.* |
| vagina | **vagina** *The canal in a female that extends from the vulva to the cervix.* |
| vaginale | **vaginal** *Referring to the vagina.* |
| vaginismo | **vaginismus** *Involuntary contraction of the vagina muscles that causes a painful spasm.* |
| vaginite | **colpitis**; *vaginitis Inflammation of the vagina.* |
| vaginite | **vulvovaginitis** *Inflammation of the vulva and vagina.* |
| vagito | **vagitus** *An infant cry that can be further defined as vagitus vaginalis in which the infant cries while its head is in the vaginal canal.* |
| vagotomia | **vagotomy** *Incision of the vagus nerve.* |
| vaiolo | **smallpox** *Variola.* |
| vaiolo bovino | **cowpox; vaccinia** *A viral disease of cows that was used for an original smallpox vaccine.* |
| vaiolo delle scimmie | **monkeypox** *A viral disease that is similar to smallpox which occurs primarily in monkeys and rarely in humans.* |
| valgo | **valgus** *Refers to a joint being abnormally angulated away from the midline of the body.* |
| valina | **valine** *An essential amino acid that assists with nitrogen equilibrium.* |
| valutazione | **evaluation** *Assessment or evaluation.* |
| valutazione medica | **assessment** *An medical evaluation.* |
| valvola aortica | **aortic valve** *The valve situated between the left ventricle and the aorta.* |

| Italian | English |
|---|---|
| valvola ileocecale | **ileocecal valve** *The membranous folds between the ileum and cecum.* |
| valvola mitrale | **mitral valve** *The valve with two cusps between the left atrium and ventricle.* |
| valvola tricuspide del cuore | **tricuspid valve** *The cardiac valve located between the right atrium and right ventricle.* |
| valvulotomia | **valvulotomy** *Surgical incision of a valve.* |
| vampate di calore | **hot flash** *A symptom of menopause manifested as a sudden sensation of fever.* |
| varice | **varix** *A twisted, distended vein, artery or lymph vessel.* |
| varicelle | **chicken pox, varicella** *A viral disease characterized by extremely pruritus blisters over the entire body.* |
| varicelle | **varicella** *A virus that causes chickenpox and shingles. Also called herpes zoster.* |
| varicocele | **varicocele** *A cluster of varicose veins in the scrotum.* |
| varicose | **varicose** *Referring to an abnormally distended, irregular vein.* |
| varicoso | **cirsoid** *Similar to a tortuous vein, artery or lymph vessel.* |
| vascolare | **vascular** *Referring to a blood vessel.* |
| vasculite | **vasculitis** *Inflammation of a blood vessel.* |
| vasectomia; deferentectomia | **vasectomy** *The surgical separation of each vas deferens with the intent of producing a sterile person.* |
| vasocostrizione | **vasoconstriction** *The process of making the blood vessels smaller which increases blood pressure.* |
| vasodilatazione | **vasodilatation** *The process of making the blood vessels larger which decreases blood pressure.* |
| vasomotore | **vasomotor** *Referring to the constriction or dilation of vessels.* |
| vasopressina | **vasopressin** *A hormone secreted by the pituitary that facilitates the retention of sodium and water and also increases blood pressure.* |
| vasospasmo | **vasospasm** *The abrupt constriction of a blood vessel.* |
| vasovagale | **vasovagal** *Referring to overstimulation of the vagus nerve, exhibited by hypotension, pallor, nausea and diaphoresis.* |
| vecchiaia | **old age** *A relative term for the period of advanced years.* |
| vecchio | **older** *Being around more than compared with another.* |
| vegetazione | **vegetation** *Abnormal growth, such as cardiac valve vegetations as found in endocarditis.* |
| veleno | **poison** *A substance that causes illness or death.* |
| veleno di serpente | **venom** *A term used to describe the toxin injected via a bite or sting.* |
| velo | **velum** *A veil-like part or covering of the palate; soft palate; Velum palatinum.* |
| velocità di eritrosedimentazione | **blood sedimentation rate (ESR)** *The settling time of erythrocytes in a prepared sample. This is a measure of the abnormal concentration of substances that are associated with pathological states.* |
| vena | **vein** *A vessel carrying blood back toward the heart.* |
| vena basilica | **basilic vein** *A vein in the hand that joins the brachial veins to form the axillary vein.* |
| vena cava | **vena cava** *The large vein that carries deoxygenated blood to the right atrium.* |
| vena giugulare | **jugular vein (s)** *Includes the internal, external and anterior jugular veins.* |
| venografia | **venography** *Roentgenography of a vein after administration of contrast media.* |
| venoso | **venous** *Referring to the veins.* |
| ventilatore | **respirator** *A device used to artificially ventilate a patient.* |
| ventilazione | **air flow** *The rate of air movement.* |

| Italian | English |
|---|---|
| ventilazione | **ventilation** *The movement of air into the lungs; generally meant to suggest by an artificial process.* |
| ventilazione meccanica assistita | **assisted ventilation** *The act of helping one breathe through artificial means.* |
| ventrale | **ventral** *Referring to the underside but in humans, a ventral hernia, for example, refers to an abdominal hernia.* |
| ventricolo | **ventricle** *1. One of two chambers of the heart. 2. The four interconnected cavities in the center of the brain.* |
| ventricolografia | **ventriculography** *Roentgenography of the ventricles after administration of contrast media.* |
| ventricolostomia | **ventriculostomy** *A tube placed into the third ventricle to relieve increased intracranial pressure.* |
| venula | **venula** *The vessels that connect the capillary plexuses to veins.* |
| verme | **worm** *Any of long, slender, legless, soft-bodied invertebrates.* |
| verme della Guinea | **guinea worm** *A parasitic nematode worm that, in cases of infection, lives under the skin, formally called Dracunculus medinensis.* |
| verme piatto | **flatworm** *A class of worms that includes parasitic flukes and tapeworms.* |
| verme solitario | **tapeworm** *A parasitic, intestinal flatworm.* |
| verme sottilissimo | **pinworm** *Common term for Enterobius vermincularis; a nematode worm that is a parasite.* |
| verme trematode | **fluke** *Parasitic nematode worm; an example is Schistosoma.* |
| verruca | **verruca** *A hyperplastic epidermal lesion, sometimes referred to as plantar wart.* |
| verruca | **wart** *A flesh colored growth that is also called verruca.* |
| verruca genitale | **genital wart** *The common term for Condylomata acuminata.* |
| verruca plantare | **plantar wart** *A viral epidermal growth on the bottom of the foot.* |
| verruca venereo | **venereal wart** *Common term for condyloma acuminatum.* |
| vertebra | **vertebra** *A term for each bone surrounding the spine.* |
| vertice | **vertex** *The crown of the head.* |
| vertigine paralizzante | **kubisagari** *Vestibular neuronitis.* |
| vertigini | **vertigo** *A sensation of imbalance with many possible causes.* |
| vescica urinaria | **bladder, urinary** *Vestibule for urine prior to being expelled via the urethra.* |
| vescica urinaria | **urinary bladder** *The organ collecting urine from the ureters prior to discharge via the urethra.* |
| vescica urinaria esteso | **distended bladder** *Urinary bladder filled beyond the normal capacity.* |
| vescicale | **vesical** *Referring to the urinary bladder.* |
| vescicola; bolla | **blister** *Common term for bulla.* |
| vescicolite | **vesiculitis** *Inflammation of the urinary bladder.* |
| vescicovaginale | **vesicovaginal** *Referring to the urinary bladder and vagina.* |
| vespa | **wasp** *Any one of a winged hymenopterous insects.* |
| vestibolare | **vestibular** *Referring to a vestibule.* |
| vestigiale | **vestigial** *Rudimentary.* |
| vetrino portaoggetti per microscopio | **slide** *A thin, rectangular piece of glass used for viewing specimen under a microscope.* |
| vettore | **vector** *An organism that transmits disease.* |
| vezzeggiare | **pamper, to** *Indulge with comfort and kindness.* |
| vibrazione | **vibration** *An instance of oscillation of parts.* |
| vicino | **near** *In close proximity.* |
| vigile | **alert** *Being in a watchful, ready state.* |
| villi corionico | **chorionic villi** *Cord-like projections of a fertilized ovum.* |
| villo | **villus** *A small vascular prominence from a membrane surface.* |

| Italian | English |
|---|---|
| villoso | **villous** *Covered with many villi.* |
| violenza carnale | **rape** *Forced sexual relations.* |
| violetto di genziana | **gentian violet** *An antiseptic derived from rosaniline.* |
| virilizzazione | **virilization** *The result of androgen; a process of development of masculine characteristics.* |
| virologia | **virology** *The study of viruses.* |
| virulenza | **virulence** *The potential severity of a disease or poison.* |
| virus del papilloma umano | **HPV human papillomavirus** *The virus that causes genital warts.* |
| viscerale | **visceral** *Referring to the organs in the abdominal or thoracic cavity.* |
| viscosimetro | **viscometer** *A device used to measure viscosity.* |
| viscoso | **viscous** *Having a thick, sticky consistency.* |
| visione | **vision** *State of being able to see.* |
| visione a galleria | **tunnel vision** *Constriction in the visual field as though looking through a tube or hollow cylinder. Also called tubular vision.* |
| visione offuscata | **vision, blurred** *Haziness of the visual field.* |
| vista | **eyesight** *A person's ability to see.* |
| vista offuscata | **blurred vision** *Low visual acuity.* |
| vitale | **viable** *Referring to a fetus that can survive childbirth.* |
| vitellino | **vitelline** *Referring to the yolk of an egg or ovum.* |
| vitiligine | **vitiligo** *The appearance of non-pigmented white patches on otherwise normal skin; hair is usually white in the affected areas.* |
| vitreo | **vitreous** *Glass appearance; used to describe the vitreous body of the eye.* |
| vivace | **brisk** *Rapid or fast.* |
| vivisezione | **vivisection** *Animal surgery done for purposes of research.* |
| vocale | **vocal** *Referring to that which emanates from the vocal cords.* |
| voce | **voice** *The sound produced through the larynx and out the mouth.* |
| volontario | **volunteer** *A person who performs work without expecting compensation.* |
| volume corrente | **tidal volume** *The amount of air inspired with each breath. One can set a ventilator to deliver a preset number of milliliters of oxygenated air with each breath.* |
| volume di riserva espiratoria | **expiratory reserve volume** *Amount of air left in the lung after a maximal exhalation, in liters.* |
| volume di riserva inspiratoria | **inspiratory reserve volume** *The amount of air that can be inhaled after a normal inhalation.* |
| volume ematico | **blood volume** *The amount of blood cells/plasma in the circulatory system.* |
| volume espiratorio massimo in 1 secondo | **forced expiratory volume per second (FEV1)** *The amount of air exhaled with maximal effort, measured in liters, over one second.* |
| volume residuo | **residual volume (RV)** *The amount of air left in the lung after a maximal exhalation.* |
| volvolo | **volvulus** *Twisting of the bowel leading to obstruction and sometimes perforation.* |
| vomitare | **vomit, to** *To expel gastric contents out the mouth.* |
| vomito | **emesis** *Vomiting.* |
| vomito | **vomit** *The gastric contents that are expelled through the mouth.* |
| vulvectomia | **vulvectomy** *Surgical resection of the vulva.* |
| vulvite | **vulvitis** *Inflammation of the vulva.* |
| vuote | **empty** *Containing nothing.* |
| xantina | **xanthine** *A purine derivative that is found in the blood and urine after the metabolism of nucleic acids to uric acid.* |

| Italian | English |
|---|---|
| xantocromia | **xanthochromia** *A yellow tone to the skin or spinal fluid.* |
| xantoma | **xanthoma** *A lipid deposition on the skin exhibited by an irregular yellow patch.* |
| xeroderma | **xerodermia** *A mild form of ichthyosis.* |
| xerooftalmia | **xerophthalmia** *A manifestation of Vitamin A deficiency exhibited by dryness of the cornea and conjunctiva.* |
| xeroradiografia | **xeroradiography** *A form of radiography using photoelectric cells.* |
| xerosi | **xerosis** *Pathological dryness of the skin or mucous membranes.* |
| xerostomia | **xerostomia** *A dry mouth from salivary gland hypofunction.* |
| zaffo di cerume | **cerumen impaction** *External ear canal full of wax resulting in hearing loss until the impaction is removed.* |
| zanzariera | **mosquito net** *A fine mesh fabric hung over a bed as a mosquito repellent.* |
| zecca cervo | **deer tick** *Ixodes scapularis.* |
| zero; nulla | **zero** *No quantity.* |
| zigomatico | **gnathic** *Referring to the jaws.* |
| zigote | **zygote** *A fertilized ovum.* |
| zimogeno | **zymogen** *An inactive compound that is metabolized to an active state.* |
| zinco | **zinc** *A chemical with atomic number 30.* |
| zolfo | **sulfur** *A chemical element with atomic number of 16.* |
| zona | **herpes zoster; shingles** *A unilateral vesicular rash along one dermatome and caused by inflammation of a posterior nerve root by "the chicken pox virus".* |
| zona | **shingles** *A reactivation of herpes zoster.* |
| zonula | **zonula** *A small zone or junction.* |
| zoologia | **zoology** *The study of animals.* |
| zoonosi | **zoonosis** *An animal-born disease that can be transmitted to humans, such as rabies.* |
| zucchero | **sugar** *A sweet crystalline substance made from a plant such as sugar cane.* |

**Other books by A.H. Zemback**
English-Kinyarwanda-French Dictionary
English-Kinyarwanda Dictionary
English-Kirundi-French Dictionary
English-Kirundi Dictionary
English-Swahili-French Dictionary
English-Swahili Dictionary

English-French Medical Dictionary and Phrasebook
English-Spanish Medical Dictionary and Phrasebook
English-German Medical Dictionary and Phrasebook
English-Portuguese Medical Dictionary and Phrasebook

www.ingramcontent.com/pod-product-compliance
Lightning Source LLC
Chambersburg PA
CBHW051627170526
45167CB00001B/85